Stan

Health

Contending Ideas and Opinions

Stand!

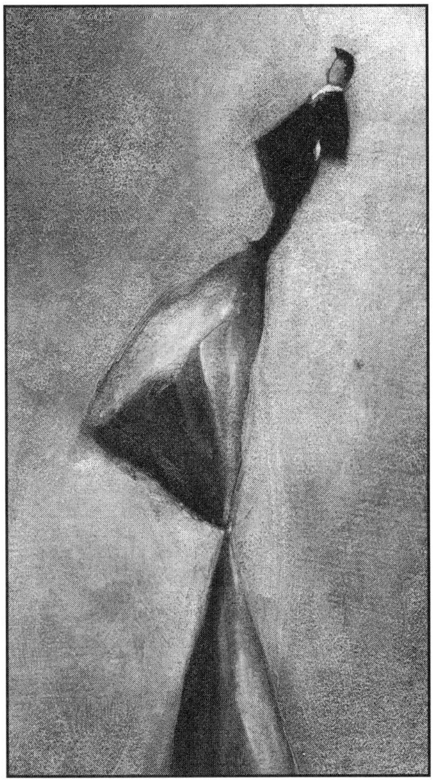

Health

Contending Ideas and Opinions

Academic Editor
Andrew P. Jenkins
Central Washington University

Coursewise Publishing Inc.
Bellevue • Boulder • Dubuque • Madison • St. Paul

Our mission at **Coursewise** is to help students make connections—linking theory to practice and the classroom to the outside world. Learners are motivated to synthesize ideas when course materials are placed in a context they recognize. By providing gateways to contemporary and enduring issues, **Coursewise** publications will expand students' awareness of and context for the course subject.

For more information on **Coursewise,** visit us at our web site: http://www.coursewise.com

To order an examination copy, contact Houghton Mifflin Sixth Floor Media: 800–565–6247 (voice); 800–565–6236 (fax).

Coursewise Publishing Editorial Staff

Thomas Doran, ceo/publisher: Environmental Science/Geography/Journalism/Marketing/Speech
Edgar Laube, publisher: Geography/Political Science/Psychology/Sociology
Linda Meehan Avenarius, publisher: **Courselinks**™
Sue Pulvermacher-Alt, publisher: Education/Health/Gender Studies
Victoria Putman, publisher: Anthropology/Philosophy/Religion
Tom Romaniak, publisher: Business/Criminal Justice/Economics
Kathleen Schmitt, publishing assistant
Gail Hodge, executive producer

Coursewise Production Staff

Lori A. Blosch, permissions coordinator
Mary Monner, production coordinator
Victoria Putman, production manager

Note: Readings in this book appear exactly as they were published. Thus, inconsistencies in style and usage among the different readings are likely.

Cover photo: Ian Lawrence/1998/nonstock

Interior design and cover design by Jeff Storm

Library of Congress Catalog Card Number: 99-067984

ISBN 0-395-97387-2

Printed in the United States of America by Coursewise Publishing, Inc.
7 North Pinckney Street, Suite 346, Madison, WI 53703

10 9 8 7 6 5 4 3 2 1

from the **Publisher**

Sue Pulvermacher-Alt
Coursewise Publishing

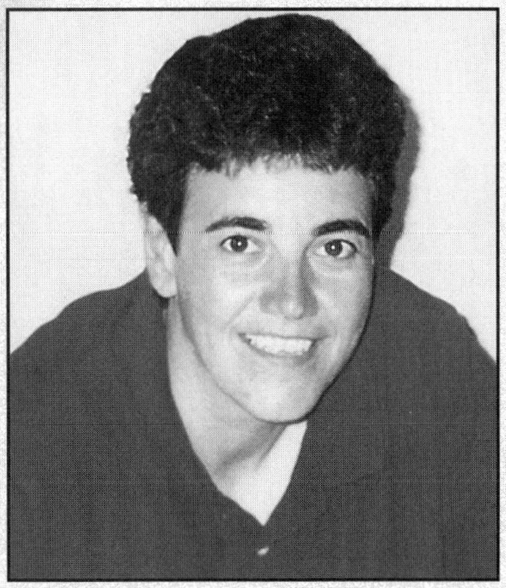

I've always found comfort in basketball. When my dog died, I worked through my eight-year-old grief by shooting hoops. As a thirteen-year-old, I fumed at my too-strict parents by saying nothing but instead loudly chest passing against a target on the basement wall. I learned to hold my own against my big brother playing one-on-one on our gravel driveway court. I gained street smarts playing "21" in college. Now, as a middle-ager, I find so much comfort in basketball that I refuse to miss my weekly WOW (Women on Wednesday) open gym basketball night. I've learned much about myself through the game of basketball.

When I play basketball, I'm deep in my comfort zone. There I'm able to think about and evaluate important matters. In the game I've found the quiet—actual or imagined—that allows me to come away with a clearer understanding.

What gives you comfort? Where do you go or what do you do when you need to reflect? Better take this book to that space. If we've done this volume right, you'll need that comfort zone to get the most out of it. The issues here are complex: How safe are herbal drugs? Is Viagra a benefit or a bane to human sexuality in America? Are addicted pregnant women victims or criminals? Who benefits from managed care? You'll need your best thinking to evaluate these controversial issues.

In addition to the readings in this volume, you'll find resources at the **Courselinks**™ web site for Health that we hope will expand your understanding of the issues. It's your comfort zone and your understanding though. Read our annotations and decide if a site is worth visiting. Do the www.orksheets so you can get to know the site better. Search the **Courselinks** site by key topic and find the information you need to be better informed.

As publisher for this volume, I had the good fortune to work with Andy Jenkins as the Academic Editor. I first knew of Andy through the Friday inspirations he sent to a listserv I joined. He didn't know of me until I responded to his **Coursewise** web site query. He and I agreed this was a good project for him. He's passionate about health education. Add to that his affable attitude and personal sense of responsibility, and I found a great Academic Editor.

We were helped by a top-notch Editorial Board. Take a look on pp. viii and ix at the breadth of experience this board brought to the project. At **Coursewise,** we work hard to publish "connected learning" tools—connecting theory to practice and the college classroom to the outside world. Readings and web sites are selected with this goal in mind. My thanks to Andy and the entire Editorial Board.

As you use our print and online resources and continue to build your understanding of these and other issues surrounding health, I invite you to share your reactions to our materials. How'd we do in representing these complex issues? What worked and what didn't work in this *Stand! Health* volume and the accompanying **Courselinks** site? Let me know what you think. I'll meet you on the court, and we can talk about it over a game of HORSE.*

Sue Pulvermacher-Alt, Publisher
suepa@coursewise.com

*O.K., an email would be fine, too!

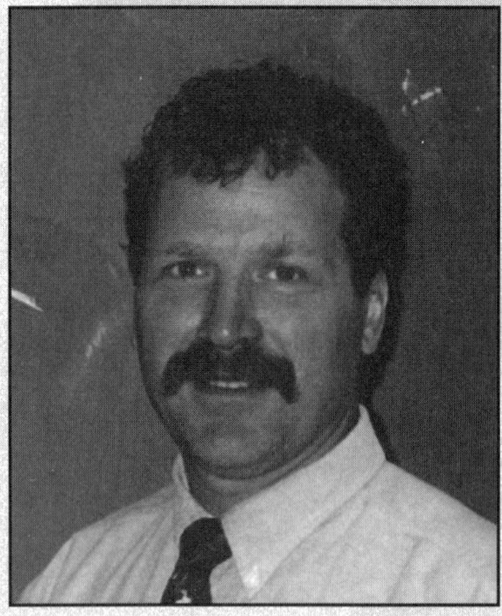

Andrew Jenkins is an associate professor in the Department of Health Education at Central Washington University, where he teaches courses in drug abuse and exercise science. He is an American Red Cross HIV/AIDs instructor, and he also serves as a volunteer firefighter/EMT and Mountain Rescue member. Jenkins received his Ph.D. in community health education from The Pennsylvania State University.

from the **Academic Editor**

Andrew P. Jenkins
Central Washington University

I took on the task of editing this *Stand! Health* reader as a result of an "awakening" I had in my professional career as a university health education professor. I had prepared a lecture on the six stages of program planning. As a joke to lighten things up, I added a seventh stage to my overhead: "Praise for the uninvolved administrators." No one laughed—not because my joke wasn't funny—but because they weren't really listening to me. They weren't even thinking about what they were copying down!

I had always held that the most important job we have as university faculty is to teach our students to *think*. It may seem self-evident that the very nature of being a student is to be a thinker, but it dawned on me that day in class that my students weren't thinking at all. They weren't analyzing what I was presenting them, weren't honing their critical thinking skills—they were merely acting as human Xerox™ machines!

I pledged that day to do all I could to provide my students with the educational experience they really needed—opportunities to develop informed opinions based on factual information and intellectual debates and discussions. I created and developed a new seminar class called "Controversial Issues in Health Education" as a forum for free and critical thinking.

Health education is surrounded by controversial issues, problems, and approaches. The mark of a competent professional is the ability to discuss and debate these issues from an informed standpoint based on a thorough knowledge of all sides of an issue. The goal of *Stand! Health* is to increase your awareness, knowledge, and appreciation of the significant issues facing health educators and other health professionals. This reader will give you a chance to explore issues and to develop and defend your personal informed viewpoints.

When I took on the responsibility of being the Academic Editor of *Stand! Health,* I set out to stir the emotions, challenge the intellect, and initiate contemplation, discussion, and debate. The readings in this collection reflect varied and contrasting points of view on each topic. Each reading was selected for its ability to present a variety of opinions, facts, and methods of persuasion. Sometimes, the issues in this book are presented with just two opposing opinions, but more often, the readings present not oppositional but *contrasting* points of view. Some of the readings are solely informative. They provide a factual basis for discussion and allow for exploration of more subjective matters, such as the ethics and values related to the issues.

In 1948, the World Health Organization developed a constitution that, in its preamble, stated that: "Health is a state of complete physical, mental and social well-being and not merely the absence of disease. . . ." *Stand! Health* is organized into seven sections derived from this multidimensional concept of wellness and comprehensive health education. Within each of the seven topic areas are one to four issues posed as questions for consideration. The issues reflect a whole-person approach to health and wellness, and encourage you to consider the psychosocial and cultural aspects of health, in addition to the physical aspects.

Take a moment to read the biographies of the members of the Editorial Board of *Stand! Health*. You'll find a wide variety of talents and backgrounds. I wanted the book to reflect more than the opinions of college faculty and Ph.D.s, so I assembled an Editorial Board of individuals from a variety of backgrounds. The Editorial Board is comprised of four college professors, an RN and EMS instructor, a nurse anesthesiologist in private practice, a public health administrator, an independent health education consultant, and a retired advertising and public relations expert. All of the board members have practiced for at least 15 years in their respective fields. This diverse panel ensured that the book would include a variety of opinions and perspectives.

In the aforementioned preamble of its constitution, the World Health Organization also stated: "Informed opinion and active cooperation on the part of the public are of the utmost importance in the improvement of the health of the people." Glance outside your classroom and into the hallway, and you'll see a variety of students passing by. Each of them probably has an opinion on any given health topic. Some might even have very strong opinions and might voice them firmly and with conviction—but how many would be equipped to argue from an *informed standpoint*? How many could state well-documented facts supporting their position?

The fact is, almost everyone has feelings and opinions surrounding the various controversial health topics that confront our field every day, but few people are well informed on the actual facts surrounding the issues. Informed opinion is the hallmark of a well-educated professional. We in the health fields have a duty to provide accurate, well-supported factual information, which, in turn, enables our clients and students to make positive health behavioral choices. By exploring the various contrasting viewpoints presented in *Stand! Health,* you will be better equipped to enhance your personal critical thinking skills, as well as those of your future clients or students.

Reading *Stand! Health* will produce one of three results: (1) you will change your point of view, (2) you will alter your point of view, or (3) your knowledge base will allow you to become more concrete and resolved in your point of view. To this end, I offer only one caveat: Remember that the mind is like a parachute—it works best when opened.

STAND!

Editorial Board

We wish to thank the following instructors for their assistance. Their many suggestions not only contributed to the construction of this volume, but also to the ongoing development of our Health web site.

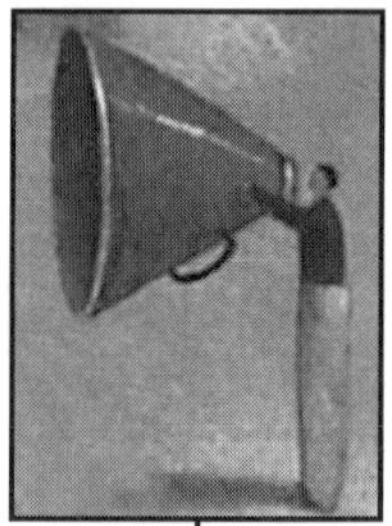

Carolyn Booth, RN

Central Washington University

Carolyn Booth is an assistant professor in the Department of Physical Education, Health, and Leisure Services at Central Washington University, where she teaches first aid and courses for paramedics and community health majors. Before assuming a full-time teaching position, she held several positions at Kittitas Valley Community Hospital over a 22-year period: assistant administrator/director of patient care services, acting hospital administrator, critical care and emergency department nurse manager, and nurse manager for the medical-surgical department. She serves as an alternate on the Kittitas County Board of Health and is an ACLS affiliate faculty member of the American Heart Association, Washington Affiliate.

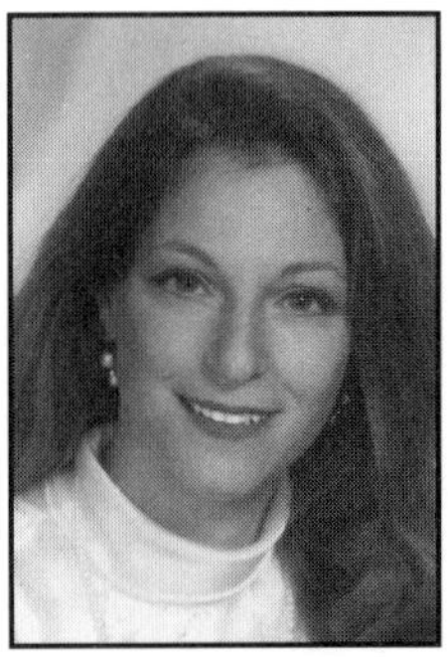

Isabel Burk, M.A., CHES,

The Health Network

Isabel Burk, director of The Health Network, is a nationally known expert on health, prevention, and education issues. Formerly the safe and drug-free schools coordinator for 117 school districts in southern New York State, she now provides technical assistance, program consultation, and training to schools and organizations in many states, and has made presentations to more than 25,000 people in twenty-three states. Burk's professional achievements have been honored with awards from the U.S. Department of Health and Human Services, the Northeast Regional Training Center for Safe and Drug-Free Schools, the Commission for a Healthy New York, and the New York State Department of Health. She is vice-chair of the American School Health Association Council on Alcohol, Tobacco and Other Drugs and training director of the National Inhalant Prevention Coalition.

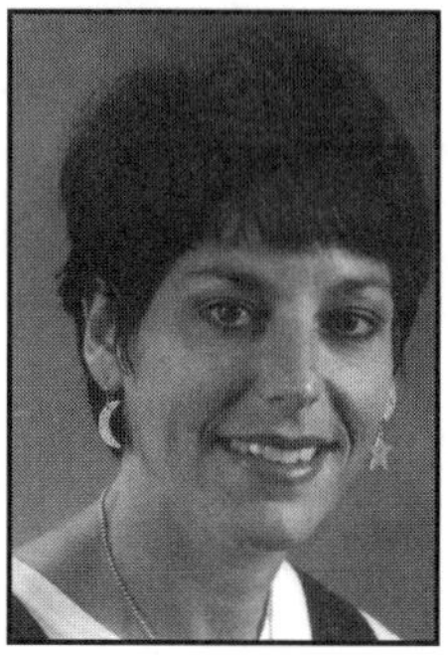

Joanne Chopak

Georgia Southern University

Joanne Chopak is an assistant professor in the Department of Health and Kinesiology at Georgia Southern University. Her research interests focus on adolescent and women's health issues, including eating disorders, adolescent pregnancy and sexual health, curriculum development in health education, and health issues facing rural communities.

Brenda J. Dunn, CRNA, RN

Brenda J. Dunn is enrolled in the Central Washington University graduate program in health education, and she is currently employed as a certified registered nurse anesthetist. She received her B.A. from the University of South Carolina, a diploma from the Durham County General Hospital School of Anesthesia for Nurses, and an A.A.S. in nursing from Alfred State University of New York.

Stephen C. Goodwin, Ph.D.

University of Delaware

Stephen C. Goodwin is an assistant professor in the College of Physical Education, Athletics, and Recreation at the University of Delaware. He has made presentations throughout the nation, and his articles have appeared in professional journals, such as *Journal of Health Education, Journal of School Health, The Physical Educator,* and *Journal of Physical Education, Recreation, and Dance.* Goodwin received his Ph.D. from The Pennsylvania State University.

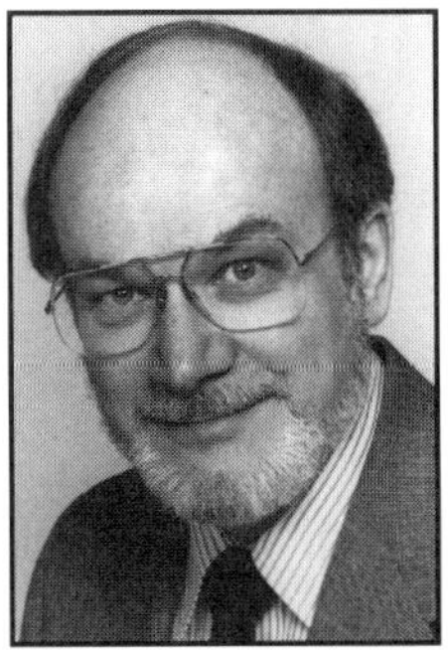

D. Joseph Jenkins

Joe Jenkins is a specialist in marketing communications, advertising, and public relations, with a wide background of diversified experiences. He has counseled hundreds of organizations in manufacturing, industrial, retail, services, and consumer products. During his long career, he created and produced advertising and public relations for many clients, such as Weyerhaeuser, Seafirst, Nalley Foods, Fisher's, and Aplets & Cotlets. He is a past president of the Pacific Northwest Speaker's Association and is a member of the National Speakers Association. Jenkins also volunteers for many nonprofit organizations, such as the American Cancer Society, Community Services for the Blind, and the American Association of Retired Persons.

Holly Hanson Lenz, Ph.D., CHES

California State Department of Health

Holly Hanson Lenz is the community health manager at the Shasta County Public Health Department in Redding, California, where she is responsible for organizing, developing, administering, and evaluating the countywide public health education programs for the Public Health Department. Her professional interests include public health promotion and education, community health promotion and education, social marketing, and risk communication strategies and implementation. Other areas of interest include applying health communication and marketing techniques to public health and health policy development. Lenz received her Ph.D. from Oregon State University.

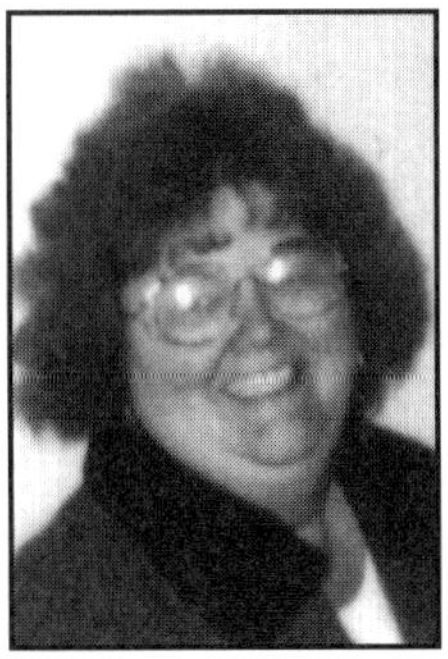

Shelley Wilkerson Smith, M.S.Ed., CHES

Southern Illinois Healthcare—St. Joseph Memorial Hospital

Shelley Wilkerson Smith is currently employed by Southern Illinois Healthcare as the community health coordinator, based at St. Joseph Memorial Hospital in Murphysboro, Illinois. She previously taught for over 10 years at John A. Logan College. Wilkerson Smith received both her B.S. and M.S. in health education from Southern Illinois University at Carbondale.

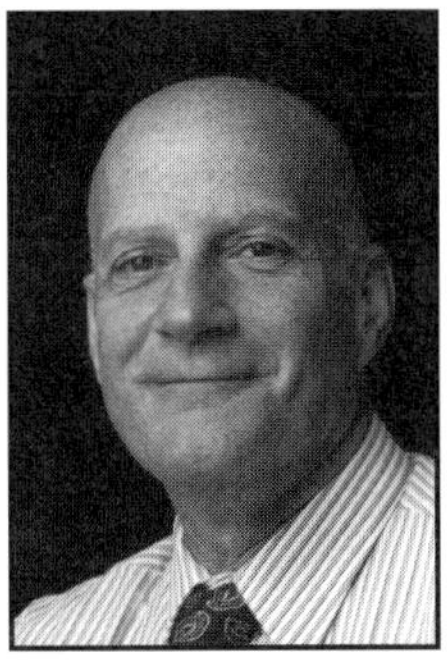

Martin S. Turnauer

Radford University

Martin S. Turnauer is a professor in the Department of Physical and Health Education at Radford University, where he has taught since 1973. His teaching expertise centers on personal health and wellness, drug education, human sexuality, stress management, sexual harassment, and consumer health. He has served as chair of the health section for the Virginia Health, Physical Education and Recreation Association, and he has been a member of the board of directors of the Virginia Alcohol Safety Action Program since 1986. Turnauer received his Ph.D. from Southern Illinois University.

WiseGuide Introduction

Critical Thinking and Bumper Stickers

Question Authority

The bumper sticker said: Question Authority. This is a simple directive that goes straight to the heart of critical thinking. The issue is not whether the authority is right or wrong; it's the questioning process that's important. Questioning helps you develop awareness and a clearer sense of what you think. That's critical thinking.

Critical thinking is a new label for an old approach to learning—that of challenging all ideas, hypotheses, and assumptions. In the physical and life sciences, systematic questioning and testing methods (known as the scientific method) help verify information, and objectivity is the benchmark on which all knowledge is pursued. In the social sciences, however, where the goal is to study people and their behavior, things get fuzzy. It's one thing for the chemistry experiment to work out as predicted, or for the petri dish to yield a certain result. It's quite another matter, however, in the social sciences, where the subject is ourselves. Objectivity is harder to achieve.

Although you'll hear critical thinking defined in many different ways, it really boils down to analyzing the ideas and messages that you receive. What are you being asked to think or believe? Does it make sense, objectively? Using the same facts and considerations, could you reasonably come up with a different conclusion? And, why does this matter in the first place? As the bumper sticker urged, question authority. Authority can be a textbook, a politician, a boss, a big sister, or an ad on television. Whatever the message, learning to question it appropriately is a habit that will serve you well for a lifetime. And in the meantime, thinking critically will certainly help you be course wise.

Getting Connected

This reader is a tool for connected learning. This means that the readings and other learning aids explained here will help you to link classroom theory to real-world issues. They will help you to think critically and to make long-lasting learning connections. Feedback from both instructors and students has helped us to develop some suggestions on how you can wisely use this connected learning tool.

WiseGuide Pedagogy

A wise reader is better able to be a critical reader. Therefore, we want to help you get wise about the articles in this reader. Each section of a *Stand!* reader has three tools to help you: the WiseGuide Intro, the WiseGuide Wrap-Up, and the Frame the Debate review form.

WiseGuide Intro

WiseGuide Intro

In the "Introduction" to each section, the Academic Editor gives you an overview of the issues covered in that section. In the "WiseGuide Intro" for each issue, the Academic Editor explains why particular articles were selected and what's important about them. You'll also find questions designed to stimulate critical thinking.

Wise students will keep these questions in mind as they read the articles for each issue. When you finish reading the articles for an issue, check your understanding. Can you answer the questions? If not, go back and reread the articles. The Academic Editor has written sample responses for many of the questions, and you'll find these online at the **Courselinks**™ site for this book. More about **Courselinks** in a minute. . . .

WiseGuide Wrap-Up

Be course wise and develop a thorough understanding of the topics covered in this course. The WiseGuide Wrap-Up at the end of each issue will help you do just that with concluding comments or summary points that repeat what's most important to understand from the articles you just read.

In addition, we try to get you wired up by providing a list of select Internet resources—what we call R.E.A.L. web sites because they're **R**elevant, **E**nhanced, **A**pproved, and **L**inked. The information at R.E.A.L. sites will enhance your understanding of a topic. (Remember to start at http://www.courselinks.com so that if any of these sites have changed, you'll have the latest link.)

Frame the Debate Review Form

At the end of the book is the Frame the Debate review form. Your instructor may ask you to complete this form as an assignment or for extra credit. If nothing else, consider doing it on your own to help you critically think about the readings for each issue.

Prompts at the end of each article encourage you to complete this review form. Feel free to copy the form and use it as needed.

The Courselinks™ Site

The **Courselinks** site for your course area is a wonderful world of integrated web resources designed to help you with your course work. This is where the readings in this book and the key topics of your course are linked to an exciting array of online learning tools. Here you will find carefully selected readings, web links, quizzes, worksheets, and more, tailored to your course and approved as connected learning tools. The ever-changing, always interesting **Courselinks** site features a number of carefully integrated resources designed to help you be course wise. These include:

http://www.courselinks.com

- **R.E.A.L. Sites** At the core of a **Courselinks** site is the list of R.E.A.L. sites. This is a select group of web sites for studying, not surfing. Like the readings in this book, these sites have been selected, reviewed, and approved by the Academic Editor and the Editorial Board. The R.E.A.L. sites are arranged by topic and are annotated with short descriptions and key words to make them easier for you to use for reference or research. With R.E.A.L. sites, you're studying approved resources within seconds—and not wasting precious time surfing unproven sites.
- **Editor's Choice** Here you'll find updates on news related to your course, with links to the actual online sources. This is also where we'll tell you about changes to the site and about online events.

- **Course Overview** This is a general description of the typical course in this area of study. While your instructor will provide specific course objectives, this overview helps you place the course in a generic context and offers you an additional reference point.
- **Take a Stand!** Register your opinion about the issues presented in your *Stand!* reader online. You can see what students and faculty members across the country are thinking about the controversial issues presented in your text. Then add your own vote.
- **www.orksheet** Focus your trip to a R.E.A.L. site with the www.orksheet. Each of the 10 to 15 questions will prompt you to take in the best that site has to offer. Use this tool for self-study, or if required, email it to your instructor.
- **Course Quiz** The questions on this self-scoring quiz are related to articles in the reader, information at R.E.A.L. sites, and other course topics, and will help you pinpoint areas you need to study. Only you will know your score—it's an easy, risk-free way to keep pace!
- **Topic Key** The online Topic Key is a listing of the main topics in your course, and it correlates with the Topic Key that appears in this reader. This handy reference tool also links directly to those R.E.A.L. sites that are especially appropriate to each topic, bringing you integrated online resources within seconds!
- **Message Center** Share your ideas with fellow students and instructors, in your class or in classes around the world, by using the Message Center. There are links to both a real-time chat room and a message forum, which are accessible all day, every day. Watch for scheduled CourseChat events throughout the semester.
- **Student Lounge** Drop by the Student Lounge, a virtual "hangout" with links to professional associations in your course area, online article review forms, and site feedback forms. Take a look around and give us your feedback. We're open to remodeling the Lounge per your suggestions.

Building Better Stand! Readers

Please tell us what you think of this *Stand!* volume so we can improve the next one. Here's how you can help:

1. Visit our **Coursewise** site at: http://www.coursewise.com
2. Click on *Stand!* Then select the Building Better *Stand!* Readers Form for your book.
3. Forms and instructions for submission are available online.

Tell us what you think—did the readings and online materials help you make some learning connections? Were some materials more helpful than others? Thanks in advance for helping us build better *Stand!* readers.

Student Internships

If you enjoy evaluating these articles or would like to help us evaluate the **Courselinks** site for this course, check out the **Coursewise** Student Internship Program. For more information, visit: http://www.coursewise.com/intern.html

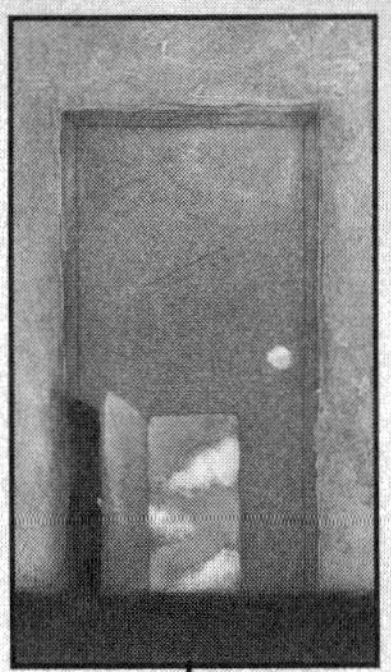

Brief Contents

Contents

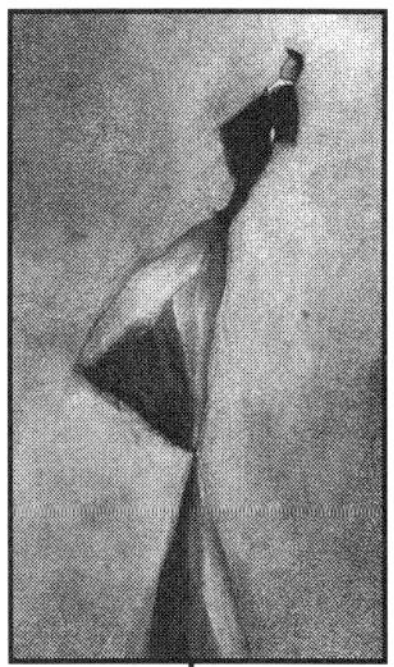

At **Coursewise,** we're publishing connected learning tools. That means that the book you are holding is only a part of this publication. You'll also want to harness the integrated resources that **Coursewise** has developed at the fun and highly useful **Courselinks**™ web site for *Stand! Health.* Visit http://www.coursewise.com.

section 1

Consumer Health

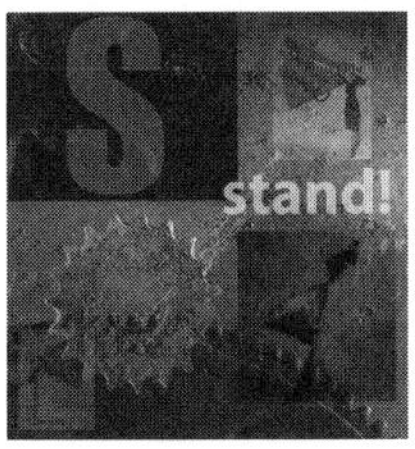

section 5

Drugs and Alcohol

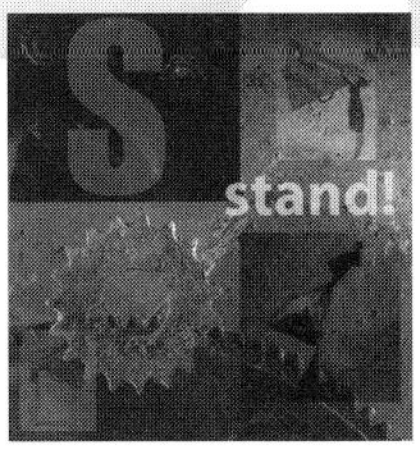

Issue 11: Should the Legal Limit for Blood Alcohol Concentration for Drunk Driving Be Lowered?

Issue 12: Is It Time to Reexamine Our Approach to Addictions?

section 6

Health Care in America

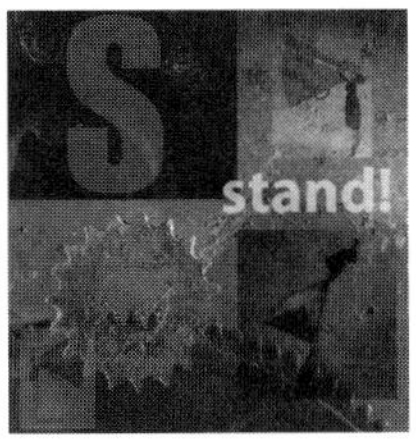

section 7
Spiritual Health

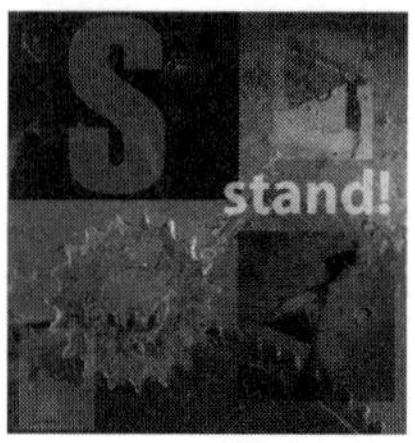

Topic Key

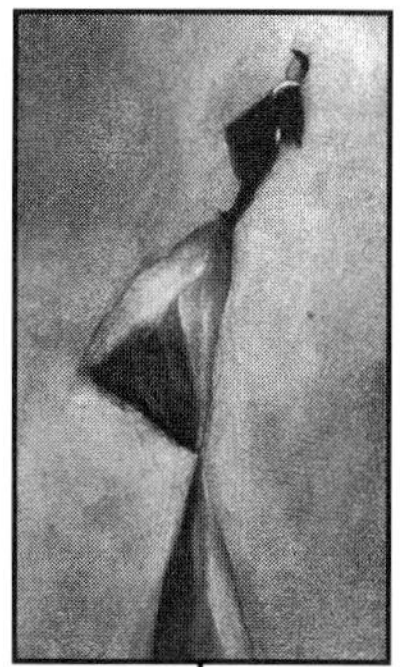

This Topic Key is an important tool for learning. It will help you integrate this reader into your course studies. Listed below, in alphabetical order, are important topics covered in this volume. Below each topic you'll find the reading numbers and titles, and R.E.A.L. web site addresses, relating to that topic. Note that the Topic Key might not include every topic your instructor chooses to emphasize. If you don't find the topic you're looking for in the Topic Key, check the index or the online topic key at the **Courselinks**™ site.

Abstinence

20 The Failure of Sex Education
21 What's Wrong with Abstinence-Only Sexuality Education Programs?

A Case for Abstinence Education
http://www.family.org/cforum/hotissues/A0000990.html

SIECUS Believes
http://www.siecus.org/about/abou0002.html

The Sinclair Intimacy Institute's Online Encyclopedia of Sex
http://www.sexualitydata.com/

Alcoholism

31 The End to Addictions: A Startling New Treatment for Reversing All Addictions
32 Half Steps vs. 12 Steps
33 Alcohol Abuse and Dependence

Alcohol—an Interactive Assessment
http://www.mayohealth.org/mayo/9707/htm/alcohol.htm

Alcoholism Runs in Families
http://www.health.org/pubs/alcruns/index.htm

Alternative Medicine

36 Why Unconventional Medicine?
37 An Interview with Dr. Andrew Weil: Natural Medicine, Natural Health
38 Be Wary of "Alternative" Health Methods
42 Faith and Healing: Making a Place for Spirituality
43 Can Spirituality Uplift Your Health?
44 Health and Spirituality: Medicine Ponders How the Two May Interact
45 Can Prayer Heal?

Alternative Health News Online
http://www.altmedicine.com/

Quackwatch
http://www.quackwatch.com/

Alternative Health
http://www.bewell.com/healthy/alternative/index.asp

Ask Dr. Stoll
http://bcn.net/~stoll/index.html

Spirituality and Health: Pathfinders
http://www.spiritualityhealth.com/path/xpat.html

Yahoo! Health—Alternative Therapies
http://health.yahoo.com/health/Alternative_Medicine/Alternative_Therapies/Meditation/

Birth Defects

26 Abuse Laws Cover Fetus, a High Court Rules
27 Why the Supreme Court Should Rule against Mandatory Treatment: Five Good Reasons

Social Drinking during Pregnancy Risks Infant Health
http://www.pslgroup.com/dg/404de.htm

Fetal Alcohol Syndrome—Why Caution Makes Sense
http://www.mayohealth.org/mayo/9810/htm/fetal.htm

Breast Cancer

13 Love's Labor's Lost?
14 Hormone-Replacement Therapy: Weighing the Benefits and Risks
15 Is Progesterone Good For Your Breasts?
16 Hard-Won Consensus on Screening Younger Women
17 The Mammogram Debate
18 Concerns about Recommending Routine Screening Mammograms for Women Ages 40 to 49
19 Deceiving Numbers: Breast Cancer Risk often Overestimated

Breast Cancer
http://www3.cancer.org/cancerinfo/main_cont.asp?st=wi&ct=5

Decisions, Decisions: The Fortysomething Mammography Mess
http://www.acsh.org/publications/priorities/0903/decisions.html

Health by Web MD, Menopause
http://content.health.msn.com/topic_summary/1370

Caffeine/Coffee

22 Caffeine: Not So Bad for Your Bones after All
23 What Caffeine Can Do for You—and to You
24 Caffeine: The Inside Scoop
25 Study Finds Coffee May Help Battle Colon Cancer

Coffee Science Source: The Online Source for Coffee, Caffeine, and Health Information
http://www.coffeescience.org/

Naturopathic Medicine: Caffeine, Sugar and Bone Loss
http://www.healthy.net/library/articles/naturopathic/art.CaffeineBone.np.htm

International Food Information Council: Caffeine Myths and Facts
http://ificinfo.health.org/insight/fi1112b.htm

Cancer

1 Sunscreens, Suntans, and Skin Cancer
2 Too Little Sun?
3 New Sunscreens
13 Love's Labor's Lost?
14 Hormone-Replacement Therapy: Weighing the Benefits and Risks
15 Is Progesterone Good For Your Breasts?
16 Hard-Won Consensus on Screening Younger Women
17 The Mammogram Debate
18 Concerns about Recommending Routine Screening Mammograms for Women Ages 40 to 49
19 Deceiving Numbers: Breast Cancer Risk Often Overestimated
25 Study Finds Coffee May Help Battle Colon Cancer

The Darker Side of Tanning
http://www.aad.org/aadpamphrework/darker.html

Breast Cancer
http://www3.cancer.org/cancerinfo/main_cont.asp?st=wi&ct=5

Decisions, Decisions: The Fortysomething Mammography Mess
http://www.acsh.org/publications/priorities/0903/decisions.html

Sunscreens
http://www.ftc.gov/bcp/conline/pubs/health/sun.htm

Health by Web MD, Menopause
http://content.health.msn.com/topic_summary/1370

Menopause
http://bewell.com/hic/menopause/index3.asp

STAND!

section 1 Consumer Health

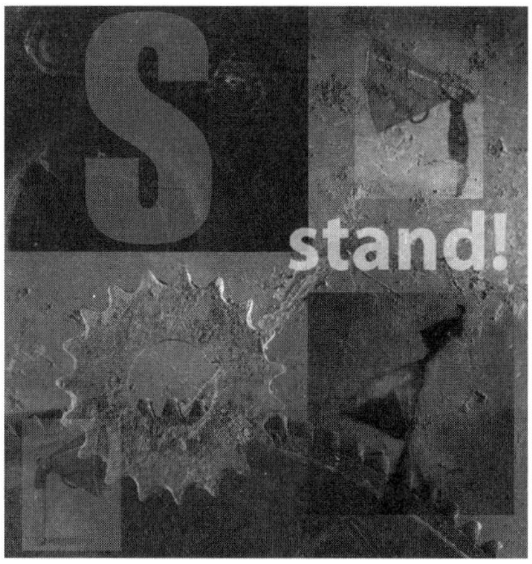

Learning Objectives

- Examine the contrasting opinions regarding the use of sunscreens and food supplements.
- Learn the health benefits and detriments of vegetarianism.
- Recognize the use of persuasive techniques, such as pseudo-science, superlatives, and vague terms, in the health marketplace.
- Separate proven fact from unsubstantiated claims about health products or practices.

Introduction

One only needs to flip through the Sunday paper or turn on the television to see that Americans are currently bombarded with a barrage of health advice—much of it conflicting and confusing. What was recommended last year is considered out-of-date this year. We receive health advice from physicians and scientists, movie stars and fashion models, athletes and alternative health-care providers. We buy vitamins, food supplements, ultrasonic toothbrushes, and exercise equipment—all guaranteed to make us healthier and happier.

Nearly every American college student has heard the Latin term *caveat emptor,* which means, "Let the buyer beware." Consumer health strives to do just that! Consumer health is the process by which we, the consumers of health-related goods and services, become better informed and thus better prepared to make positive decisions regarding our involvement in the health marketplace. Consumer health is perhaps the single best area for sharpening your health-related *critical thinking* skills. This section provides insight into three contemporary consumer health issues of special interest to college students.

Are Sunscreens Really Safe and Effective for Preventing Skin Cancer?

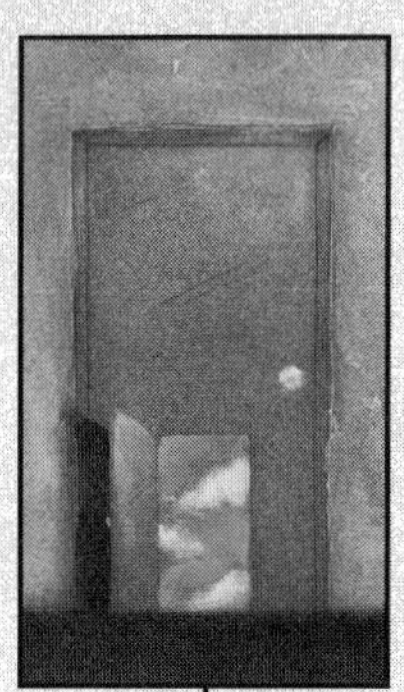

ISSUE 1

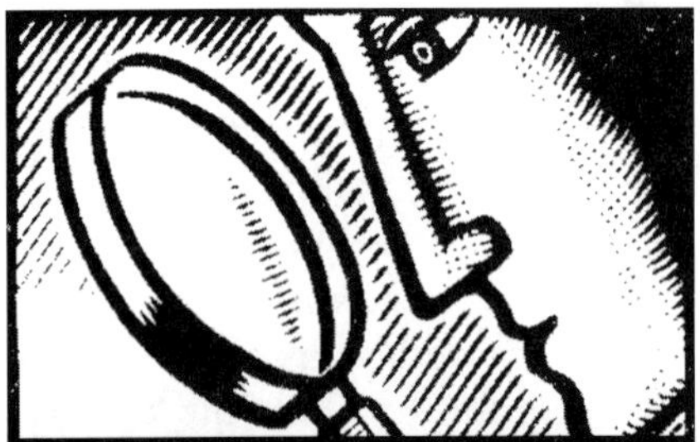

Take a Closer Look

1. What type of sun rays is most responsible for sunburn?
2. According to McGregor and Young in Reading 1, what is the major shortcoming of most popular sunscreens?
3. Do light-skinned people have a greater risk of skin cancer than darker-skinned people?
4. What do the words "Slip, Slop, Slap" stand for in terms of sun protection?

WiseGuide Intro

Skin cancer afflicts over a million Americans each year and claimed about 9,200 lives in 1998. Although many Anglo-Americans still perceive sun-tanned skin as "healthy" and "fit looking," overexposure to the sun's ultraviolet rays is the major risk factor in the development of basal and squamous cell carcinomas, as well as melanoma, the most deadly of skin cancers. The rate of new melanomas diagnosed per year has doubled since the 1970s—from 6 per 100,000 to 12 per 100,000—and melanomas killed approximately 7,300 Americans in 1998, according to the American Cancer Society.

In hopes of lowering their skin cancer risks while still enjoying the outdoors, many well-intentioned consumers use various types of lotions containing sunscreens such as PABA and Parsol 1789. The American Cancer Society and National Cancer Institute promote sunscreen use for skin cancer prevention. Currently, however, the relative effectiveness of these lotion-based sunscreens is under debate. Some of this debate stems from the role of ultraviolet A rays in causing skin cancer and the hypothesis that sunscreens may actually be causative factors in some types of skin cancer. Still further debate centers around the health benefits of sun exposure. Too much sun avoidance may place some people at risk of disorders stemming from a lack of vitamin D synthesis, which is in part dependent on exposure to the sun.

In Reading 1, "Sunscreens, Suntans, and Skin Cancer," J. M. McGregor and A. R. Young review the possible link between skin cancers and sunburn and the need for protection from both ultraviolet A and ultraviolet B rays. Their most salient point is that sunscreen users may actually be at greater risk for developing certain types of skin cancer.

Reading 2, "Too Little Sun?," suggests that health professionals may have gone too far in recommending that people avoid sun exposure. Lack of sun may be a factor in increased risks of arthritis, osteoporosis, and even cancer. The reading provides some specific consumer recommendations for balancing the positive and negative effects of sun exposure.

In Reading 3, "New Sunscreens," Christine Gorman outlines the current thinking on cancer prevention through sunburn protection and introduces the theory that ultraviolet A rays may be a factor in the development of skin cancer. Parsol 1789, a new ingredient in lotions, is intended to block ultraviolet A rays.

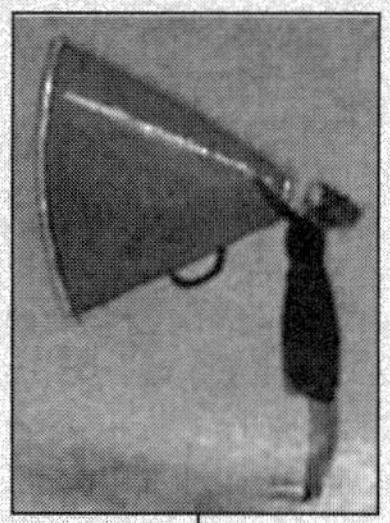

Issue 1: Are sunscreens really safe and effective for preventing skin cancer?

Sunscreens, Suntans, and Skin Cancer

J. M. McGregor and A. R. Young

J. M. McGregor is a senior lecturer in dermatology and A. R. Young is a senior lecturer in photobiology, Department of Photobiology, St. John's Institute of Dermatology, St. Thomas's Hospital, London SE1 7EH

Sunlight causes sunburn, photoaging, and skin cancer,[1] the price many people seem prepared to pay for a tan. Yet recent studies suggest that tanning is a direct consequence of damage to DNA caused by ultraviolet radiation.[2] Even seemingly trivial sun exposure, enough just to turn the skin red, causes considerable damage to both keratinocytes[3] and melanocytes and is sufficient for many cells in the skin to sustain lethal doses of ultraviolet radiation. Patients with xeroderma pigmentosum, who are unable to repair this damage, develop skin cancer in the first 5–10 years of life, but the accumulation of genetic alterations sufficient to cause skin cancer normally takes 50–60 years. Despite the efficiency of our DNA repair machinery, the rising incidence of skin cancer in fair skinned populations suggests that DNA repair is not always able to keep pace with 20th century lifestyle.

Sunscreens should not be seen as a safe way to prolong sun exposure.

In recognition of the economic and public health concerns, the government's strategy document, Health of the Nation, has as one of its major targets the reversal of the year on year increase in melanoma and non-melanoma skin cancer by 2005. The key to achieving this target is public health education, to increase awareness of the dangers of sun exposure, even in Britain, and to promote a healthier, less "sun seeking" lifestyle. The slogan of Britain's Health Education Authority, "Shift to the Shade," emphasises that the safest way to reduce sun exposure is by changing behaviour. The use of sunscreens to prevent skin cancer is more controversial, not least because by preventing sunburn they may encourage longer exposure to the sun.

Sunscreens work mainly by blocking solar ultraviolet B wavelengths (295–320 nm), which (despite accounting for less than 5% of solar ultraviolet radiation) are primarily responsible for sunburn. There is increasing evidence that ultraviolet A (320–400 nm) can also damage the skin, and most sunscreens in Britain now contain good ultraviolet A blocking agents. A sunscreen's ability to prevent sunburn is designated by its "sun protection factor" (SPF), which is defined as the ratio of the minimum erythemal dose of simulated sunlight on protected skin compared with unprotected *skin.* In reality, it is widely perceived as how many times longer it takes to obtain a mild sunburn, the *skin's* early warning system, while wearing a sunscreen. But we know little about the precise relation between sunburn and skin cancer.

Studies in hairless albino mice have shown that, as with sunburn, ultraviolet B is the main cause of non-melanoma skin cancer.[4] This suggests that sunscreens used to prevent sunburn might also prevent non-melanoma skin cancer. Mouse experiments[5] as well as preliminary human sunscreen studies,[6] show that the incidence of malignant and premalignant lesions is indeed reduced by the use of sunscreens, although the "cancer protection factor" of sunscreens may be lower than their "sunburn protection factor."

The complex relation between sunscreens and skin cancer is further illustrated by reports of an increased risk of malignant melanoma in sunscreen users.[7,8] One possible explanation is that some sunscreens fail to provide adequate protection from ultraviolet A. Studies on fish models,[9] supported by limited evidence that sunbeds are a risk factor for melanoma,[10] suggest that ultraviolet A wavelengths may be particularly important in the induction of this tumour type. The sunscreens used were almost certainly primarily ultraviolet B blocking agents. Sunscreens containing only ultraviolet B blocks would protect against sunburn and therefore enable greater exposure to ultraviolet A than would otherwise be possible to obtain. Another possibility is that sunscreens may

This article was first published in the STUDENT BRITISH MEDICAL JOURNAL, J. M. McGregor and A. R. Young, Sunscreens, Suntans, and Skin Cancer, August 1996 (Volume 4, Issue 43) and is reproduced by permission of the British Medical Journal.

afford insufficient protection against the immunosuppressant effects of ultraviolet radiation.[11] This immunosuppression is thought to have an important role in the promotion of non-melanoma skin cancer and may also be involved in melanoma.

Whatever the potential shortcomings of sunscreens in preventing skin cancer, they do provide an important way of reducing cumulative exposure to solar ultraviolet radiation if they are used in conjunction with other photoprotective measures. However, all photoprotection is lost if sunscreens are used to prolong sun exposure to the maximum achievable by the sun protection factor; so that, for example, sunburn develops over five hours instead of 30 minutes. Thus the marketing of sunscreens as a safe way to stay out in the sun longer may be misleading. Indeed, animal[12] and human studies[7,8] suggest that this approach may actually increase the risk of both melanoma and non-melanoma skin cancer for the same daily exposure dose.

A recent survey by Britain's Health Education Authority showed that 57% of the public had bought or used sunscreens in the past two to three years. Most people claimed an interest in the photoprotective aspects of sunscreens against sunburn (80%) and skin cancer (53%) rather than their use to get a good tan (35%).

Along with the ongoing trend for buying products with higher sun protection factors, this suggests that the public increasingly regards sunscreens as health rather than cosmetic products. Though this is certainly encouraging, the role of sunscreens in preventing skin cancer still needs clarifying.

Notes

1. Green A, William G. Ultraviolet radiation and skin cancer: Epidemiological data from Australia. In: Young AR, Bjorn LO, Moan J, Nultsch W, eds. *Environmental UV Photobiology.* New York: Plenum, 1993:233–54.
2. Eller MS, Yaar M, Gilchrest BA. DNA damage and melanogenesis. *Nature* 1994; 372:413–4.
3. Young AR, Chadwick CA, Harrison GI, Hawk JLM, Nikaido O, Potten CS. The in situ repair kinetics of epidermal thymine dimers and 6–4 photoproducts in human *skin* types I and II. *J Invest Dermatol* 1996; 106:1307–13.
4. De Gruijl FR, Van der Leun JC. Estimate of the wavelength dependency of ultraviolet carcinogenesis in humans and its relevance to the risk assessment of a stratospheric ozone depletion. *Health Phys* 1994: 67:1–8.
5. Forbes PD, Davies RE, Sambuco CP, Urbach F. Inhibition of ultraviolet radiation-induced skin tumours in hairless mice by topical application of the sunscreen 2-ethyl hexyl-p-methoxycinnamate. *J Toxicol Cut Ocular Toxicol* 1989; 8:209–26.
6. Thompson SC, Jolley D, Marks R. Reduction of solar keratoses by regular sunscreen use. *N Engl J Med* 1993; 329:1147–51.
7. Autier P, Dore JF, Schifflers E, Cesarini J-P, Bollaerts A, Koelmel KF, et al. Melanoma and use of sunscreens: an EORTC case-control study in Germany, Belgium and France. *Int J Cancer* 1995; 61:749–55.
8. Westerdahl J, Olsson H, Masback A, Ingvar C, Jonsson N. Is the use of sunscreens a rick factor for malignant melanoma? *Melanoma Res* 1995; 5:59–65.
9. Setlow RB, Grist E, Thompson K, Woodhead AD. Wavelengths effective in the induction of malignant melanoma. *Proc Natl Acad Sci USA* 1993; 90:6666–70.
10. Westerdahl J, Olsson H, Masback A, Ingvar C, Jonsson N, Brandt L, et al. Use of sunbeds or sunlamps and malignant melanoma in Southern Sweden. *Am J Epidemiol* 1994; 140:691–9.
11. Young AR, Walker SL. Photoprotection from UVR-induced immunosuppression. In: Krutmann J, Elmers CA, eds. *Photoimmunology.* Oxford: Blackwell Science: 1995: 285–97.
12. Kelfkens G, van Weelden H, de Gruijl FR, van der Leun JC. The influence of dose rate on ultraviolet tumorigenesis. *J Photochem Photobiol Biol* 1991; 10:41–50.

FRAME the DEBATE

Form at end of book

Issue 1: Are sunscreens really safe and effective for preventing skin cancer?

Too Little Sun?

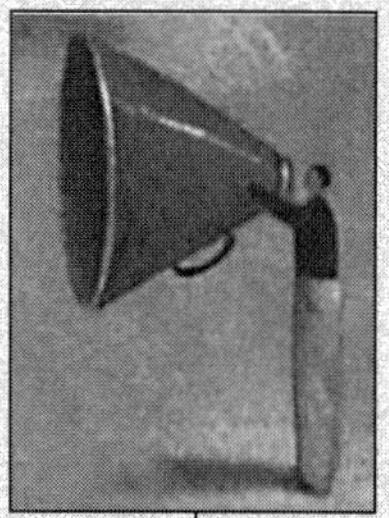

Overexposure can cause wrinkles and skin cancer. But underexposure can dangerously lower vitamin-D levels.

Americans have been warned repeatedly to cover up or use sunscreens to avoid the dangers of too much sun. But they're seldom warned about the consequences of too *little* sun. Sunlight stimulates the skin to synthesize vitamin D. Insufficient exposure to sunlight can lead to insufficient levels of the vitamin, since many people don't get enough from diet alone. Indeed, recent evidence suggests that insufficient vitamin-D levels may be far more prevalent than previously believed, particularly in older people. It may be far more harmful as well, weakening the bones, possibly worsening arthritis, and perhaps even increasing the risk of cancer.

The Dangers of Little D

Here's what research shows about the three most important risks, proven or potential, of getting too little vitamin D.

Weakened Bones

Vitamin D helps the body absorb calcium from food; that, in turn, increases calcium absorption by the bones. Outright deficiency of the vitamin causes a condition known as rickets in children, osteomalacia in adults, in which new bone tissue fails to harden due to lack of calcium. Vitamin-D deficiency also worsens osteoporosis, or porous bones, through direct and indirect effects on existing bone tissue.

But mounting evidence indicates that even moderately low levels of the vitamin, traditionally considered within the normal range, may also weaken the bones. Such "low normal" levels stimulate secretion of a hormone that pulls calcium out of the skeleton; some research suggests that such levels increase the risk of fractures as well. Clinical trials have shown that boosting consumption of vitamin D, with or without extra calcium, can slow bone loss or increase bone density in older women who have low-normal blood levels of the vitamin. And one large clinical trial has proved that boosting consumption of both vitamin D and calcium can actually reduce the risk of fractures in such women.

Arthritis

Osteoarthritis, the most common kind of arthritis, develops when the cartilage lining the joints breaks down, causing painful friction between the bare ends of the bones. As the disease progresses, the bone itself may start to break down or develop spurs, increasing the pain. In theory, vitamin D might slow that progression, by helping the bones maintain their normal shape and possibly helping the remaining cartilage stay healthy. In the first test of that theory, published last September, Boston researchers studied 75 arthritic knees for up to 10 years. They found that the risk of the disease worsening was three times greater in people with average or lower blood levels of vitamin D than in those with higher levels. Both bone and cartilage deteriorated faster in those with less of the vitamin.

Getting enough vitamin D may be harder for older people.

Cancer

Vitamin D has inhibited the development and growth of many different cancers in both test-tube and animal studies. In humans, the risk of various cancers—notably breast, colon, and prostate, the three most common kinds in nonsmokers—is substantially lower in sunny regions than in areas with less sunlight, both around the world and within the U.S. One possible reason: The skin produces more vitamin D in sunnier climes. Studies of vitamin-D consumption tentatively support that explanation. Four of five large observational studies have found at least some evidence linking low intake with an increased risk of colorectal cancer. Studies of blood levels, the most accurate measure of vitamin-D status, have yielded mixed results: One study of colon cancer and another study of prostate cancer linked relatively low levels of the vitamin with increased risk, but two other prostate-cancer studies found no such link.

Who's at Risk?

Younger people almost always get enough vitamin D, either from sunshine or from diet. But getting enough may be harder for older people, for several reasons. First, they need more than younger people do, to fight bone loss. And the rate of vitamin-D synthesis by the skin is two to four times slower in older than in younger individuals. Many older people, fearing skin cancer and other damaging effects of the sun, wear protective clothing and apply strong sunscreens whenever they go outside. Others simply don't like to bare their arms or legs in public, or seldom go outdoors in the first place. Further, older people are more likely to take certain drugs, notably laxatives and the cholesterol-lowering drug cholestyramine (*Questran*), that interfere with the absorption or action of vitamin D.

Despite those obstacles, healthy older residents of sunny regions, including the American South, generally get adequate amounts of vitamin D from sunshine alone, just by going about their daily affairs—even if they wear sunscreen (apparently because it's rarely applied perfectly and at all times). Only those Southerners who never get outdoors need to be concerned about vitamin D. (Note that sitting by a window doesn't help, since glass absorbs virtually all ultraviolet light, the component of sunshine that stimulates vitamin-D synthesis.) But getting enough sunlight is somewhat harder in the North.

Northern Exposure

The best time to expose the skin in the northern U.S. is mid-morning or mid-afternoon during the spring, summer, and fall. That's because the sunlight is too weak to stimulate much vitamin-D production in the early morning or late afternoon—or to stimulate any production during the winter. And the skin is more susceptible to damage or sunburn at midday.

At the optimal hours, a light-skinned older person in Boston or Chicago would need roughly 15 to 20 minutes of exposure—on the face, hands, and lower arms—about three times a week during the warmer months to produce an adequate year-long supply of vitamin D. (The body can store extra vitamin D for the winter.) Briefer, more frequent exposure would work equally well. But a darker-skinned person would need up to 50 percent more exposure. And the requirement is higher in regions north of Boston or Chicago—50 percent higher in Toronto, for example—and lower in regions to the south. In general, you produce enough vitamin D in about one-third the time it takes for your skin to start turning red.

Many older Northerners may not get even that much exposure, and thus may not get enough vitamin D. Studies have found insufficient levels of the vitamin—low enough to increase bone loss—in at least 25 percent of healthy older people in Boston. The numbers are even higher during the dark, winter months. (Indeed, average bone density drops and fracture risk rises in winter, an increase that's only partly due to slips on ice and snow.) And more than half of people who never get outside—due to illness, frailty, or disease—have low levels of vitamin D.

Directions for D

If you're an older person in the North, you may need to change your habits to ensure an adequate supply of the vitamin. One way is to expose your skin to the sun as described above. Such modest exposure is generally safe. If you stay out longer than that, however, be sure to apply sunscreen with a SPF (sun-protection factor) of 15 to 30 after the initial period.

You may be able to get all the vitamin D you need from your diet (see table). People with insufficient sun exposure probably require about 400 IU (International Units) per day during their 50s and 60, 600 to 800 IU during their 70s and 80s. Fortified milk is supposed to contain 100 IU per cup. A few years ago, studies found that milk often contains significantly less than that. While the fortification process has improved since then, studies have not confirmed that milk is now a fully reliable source of the vitamin. Still, it's wise to drink several cups of low-fat or skim milk per day: The milk generally supplies at least a moderate amount of vitamin D and invariably supplies lots of calcium. People who do consume plenty of milk and often eat fatty fish, the other main source of vitamin D, are almost surely meeting the 400 IU daily requirement. However, meeting the higher requirement from dietary sources alone may be difficult.

If the guidelines presented in this report suggest that you're not getting enough vitamin D—either the full amount from sunlight or diet, or a partial contribution from both—consider taking a supplement.

That's particularly appropriate during the winter and for people who are at increased risk for osteoporosis. The risk is much higher for older women than older men, especially if their menopause started early or they consumed little calcium before menopause. Other factors increase risk in both sexes: lack of weight-bearing exercise, heavy alcohol consumption, cigarette-smoking for many years, being thin, and being white or Asian. Individuals

Vitamin D in the Diet[1]

Food	Serving Size	Vitamin D (IU)
Dairy		
Milk[2]	1 cup	100[3]
Egg, whole	1	26
Fish and Shellfish		
Oysters	3 oz	544
Col liver oil	1 tsp	452
Catfish	3 oz	424
Mackerel	3 oz	394
Salmon	3 oz	238
Sardines, canned in oil	3 oz	231
Tuna, bluefin	3 oz	170
Halibut	3 oz	170
Tuna, canned in water	3 oz	136
Shrimp	3 oz	122
Sole/flounder	3 oz	51
Cod	3 oz	48
Bass, freshwater	3 oz	34
Swordfish	3 oz	34
Clams	3 oz	7
Mushrooms (fresh)		
Shiitake	2 oz	57
Chanterelle	2 oz	48
Button (common)	2 oz	0

Source: USDA and ESHA Research, Salem, Ore.

IU = International Units

[1] In addition to milk, other foods that may have added amounts of vitamin D include breads, breakfast cereals, fruit drinks, chocolate beverages, and cocoa powder.

[2] Whole, reduced-fat, low-fat, or nonfat milk.

[3] While each cup of milk is supposed to be fortified with 100 IU of vitamin D, studies have not yet proved the reliability of the fortification process.

Summing Up

Insufficient vitamin-D levels appear to be more common and more hazardous than previously believed. Young people and Southerners generally don't need to worry, unless they never go outside. But older Northerners need to ensure an adequate supply, by taking any of these steps:

- Regularly expose your skin for a short while; the older you are, the darker your skin, and the father north you live, the more exposure you need. (But cover up or apply sunscreen before you start to redden.)
- Consume plenty of milk and fatty fish.
- Consider taking a supplement if you're not meeting at least one of the preceding requirements fully, or both of them partly—particularly if you are an older postmenopausal woman or have other risk factors for osteoporosis. The pill should contain no more than you need to reach the total suggested intake for someone your age.

over age 70 or so who rarely or never gets outdoors generally need a supplement, regardless of where they live or what they eat.

If you do take a vitamin-D pill, be sure it contains no more than the dose that brings you up to roughly the suggested intake (including diet) for your age group. Too much vitamin D can lead to elevated calcium levels in the blood and, in turn, to severe kidney damage and calcium deposits in many parts of the body. However, you can't get a toxic dose of vitamin D from sun exposure, even if you consume lots of the vitamin; that mechanism is self-regulating.

FRAME the DEBATE

Form at end of book

Issue 1: Are sunscreens really safe and effective for preventing skin cancer?

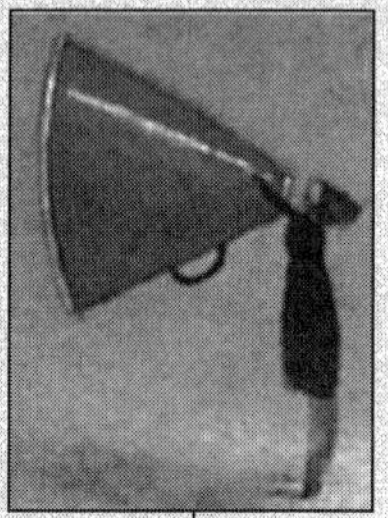

New Sunscreens

They help block both types of harmful rays. But don't rely only on potions for your protection.

Christine Gorman

As a fair-haired descendant of freckled Irishmen, I once got scorched in just 10 minutes on the Texas coast. So, I take the risk of skin cancer pretty seriously. I jog in the morning, when the sun's rays are least intense, wear a hat when I'm out all day and try to keep my arms and legs covered. But if you're like me, you may discover that the hardest part of staying out of the red this summer is picking the right sunscreen. At my local drugstore last week, I counted no fewer than 66 formulas with nearly as many competing claims. How do you choose?

One way is to look for the new products, just out this year, that protect against both types of harmful sun rays. It used to be that the only part of the ultraviolet spectrum you had to worry about was short-intensity, UV-B radiation, which is primarily responsible for sunburns and the most likely cause of skin cancer. But then researchers discovered that UV-A, which has a longer wavelength than UV-B, does more than just promote wrinkles. It can also damage the skin's underlying connective tissue and possibly even dampen the body's immune system. Could UV-A, therefore, play a role in triggering cancer?

That question hasn't been answered yet—and probably won't be for another couple of decades. But already this year some manufacturers are adding to their sunscreens a new anti-UV-A ingredient called Parsol 1789. The new products are about twice as expensive as regular formulas but offer protection against the whole spectrum of ultraviolet radiation.

Or for a little less money, you can get all the UV-A and UV-B protection you need from titantium dioxide, a tried-and-true chemical agent that physically blocks the sun's rays (hence the name sunblock) from reaching the skin, rather than absorbing them, like most sunscreens. You remember titanium dioxide. Like zinc oxide, it's one of those gunky white pastes that lifeguards used to plaster all over themselves. Both chemicals have been reformulated so that they no longer leave a residue. But some people find that these sunblocks clog their pores or feel sticky on their skin, so they may prefer one of the new products with Parsol 1789, like Ombrelle, PreSun, Ultra or Shade UVA Guard.

Slip, Slop, Slap

To lower your risk of sunburn and skin cancer:

- **Slip** on a shirt
- **Slop** on lots of sunscreen with an SPF of 15 or higher. Consider new products that contain Parsol 1789
- **Slap** on a hat

Whether you prefer sunscreen or sunblock, choose one with an SPF rating of at least 15. Light-skinned people should opt for an SPF rating of 30. If it normally takes you 10 minutes to burn at the beach without any protection, an SPF-15 product will let you frolic in the sun for 15 times 10 minutes, or 2 1/2 hours. After that, you've had your radiation dose for the day. Stay out any longer, even if you reapply sunscreen, and you will burn, just as a turkey cooked too long will eventually burn, no matter how much you baste it.

That's why you should never rely on sunscreen as your only protection. Stay out of the midday sun (from 10 to 3), and you will avoid 60% of the UV-B that hits the earth. Slip on a long-sleeve shirt to protect those vulnerable areas on the shoulders and back. When you use sunscreen, slop it on thick and often. And slap on a wide-brimmed hat, and you can keep 70% of the sun's rays off your face and neck. After decades of their "Slip, Slop, Slap" campaign, Australians are starting to see a decrease in their rate of deaths from melanoma, a particularly deadly form of skin cancer. That's an example worth following.

FRAME the DEBATE

Form at end of book

WiseGuide Wrap-Up

While ultraviolet rays clearly cause melanoma and various skin cancers, the role of sunscreens in preventing sun-related skin cancer may be overrated. To be effective, sunscreens must be applied more liberally than most people currently apply them. However, in our zeal to prevent skin cancer, we may be placing ourselves at risk of developing health problems related to vitamin D deficiency, for which sun exposure is an asset and not a liability. Moderation and prudence are the keys for balancing the advantages and disadvantages of sun exposure.

R.E.A.L. Sites

This list provides a print preview of typical **Coursewise** R.E.A.L. sites. (There are over 100 such sites at the **Courselinks**™ site.) The danger in printing URLs is that web sites can change overnight. As we went to press, these sites were functional using the URLs provided. If you come across one that isn't, please let us know via email to: webmaster@coursewise.com. Use your Passport to access the most current list of R.E.A.L. sites at the **Courselinks** site.

Site name: Sunscreens

URL: http://www.ftc.gov/bcp/conline/pubs/health/sun.htm

Why is it R.E.A.L.? This government-sponsored site has specific information on the risks of sun exposure. According to the Federal Trade Commission, "Any tan is a sign of skin damage." The site also has specific recommendations for sunscreen use.

Key topics: suntanning, sunscreens, ultraviolet A rays, ultraviolet B rays

Try this: Take the True or False sunscreen test. How well did you score? Read the article on sunscreens. What exposure times, sunscreens, and sunscreen use are recommended for adults? Are the recommendations for children any different? What three concerns might you, as a critical thinking consumer, have regarding these recommendations?

Site name: The Darker Side of Tanning

URL: http://www.aad.org/aadpamphrework/darker.html

Why is it R.E.A.L.? The American Academy of Dermatology is a professional organization of physicians whose scope of practice is limited to the health of human skin. The site offers advice on avoiding skin cancer and provides a table for determining skin type with regard to melanoma risk.

Key topics: sunscreens, tanning, skin cancer

Try this: Go to the site and read the article "The Darker Side of Tanning." Determine your skin type and your relative risk of developing skin cancers.

ISSUE 2

How Safe Are Herbal Drugs and Food Supplements?

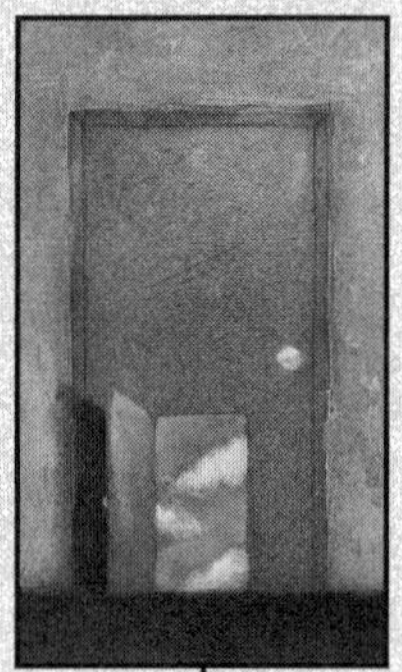

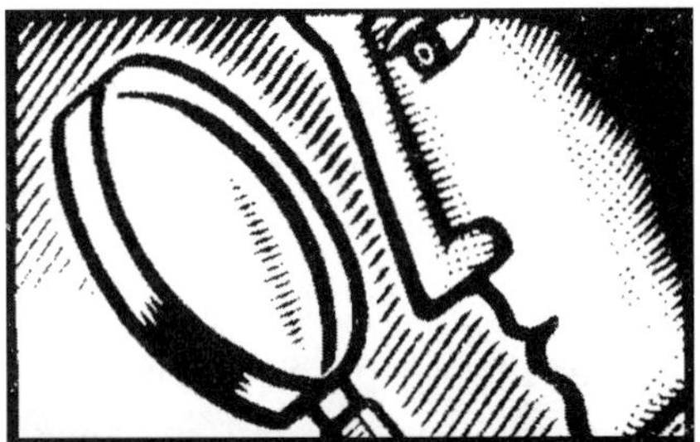

Take a Closer Look

1. According to Long in Reading 4, how many herbs has the Food and Drug Administration found to be safe and effective? List at least two of these.
2. According to Graham Woolf, quoted in Reading 4, what is the critical mistake that most people who become ill from herbals make?
3. In Reading 5, what are Barrett's three criteria for making a rational decision about an herbal product?
4. According to Jenkins in Reading 6, what are sympathomimetic substances?
5. What is Ma Huang, and what does it do in the human body?
6. Name five specific risks to athletes who take herbal supplements, as listed by Jenkins in Reading 6.

WiseGuide Intro

In the 1990s, many Americans have been shying away from mainstream medicine and seeking alternatives to medical doctors and to pharmaceutical medicines. One of the popular treatment options is "herbal medicine." So popular are herbal remedies that in 1995 they represented $1.6 billion in sales. Many consumers are concerned and distrustful of "chemical" or "artificial" drugs. They often seek herbal or Chinese medicines, which they perceive to be more natural and therefore less harmful or toxic than modern manufactured pharmaceuticals.

Consumer advocates and most mainstream health-care professionals are concerned that, although herbal remedies may be natural, they are not necessarily safe. Some herbals have caused severe illnesses and even death. Although some herbs are effective at treating certain symptoms, such as garlic for lowering cholesterol, most have not undergone rigorous scientific and clinical study, and therefore, the applications, prescriptions, and doses are usually based on testimonials, folklore, and hearsay. The positive results, say the critics, are likely placebo effects or spontaneous remission.

In Reading 4, "The Naturals," Patricia Long explores the current interest in herbal remedies and makes several comparisons to pharmaceuticals. She cites experts in herbology who feel that herbs are less harmful than prescription drugs—but not completely safe. Long provides examples of scientific research and compares herbal remedies in several European countries. She also lists several specific herbs and gives their reputed medicinal uses.

In Reading 5, "The Herbal Minefield," consumer advocate Dr. Stephen Barrett argues against jumping on the herbal bandwagon. He raises concerns about untested herbal drugs and unqualified practitioners of herbal medicine. Barrett points out that scientific research in this area is lacking and that most information is based on folklore, tradition, and testimonials. He concedes that some herbal medicines may help but also warns that others may be toxic and that many are wastes of the consumer's time and money.

The first half of Reading 6, "Herbal Energizers: Speed by Any Other Name," is aimed at educating the reader on the nature, use, and side effects of over-the-counter stimulants. Andrew Jenkins classifies the drugs and reviews the main effects and potentially harmful side effects of sympathomimetic amines.

He also presents the Food and Drug Administration dosage regulations and discusses the side effects of overdoses. The second half of the reading is directed at specific over-the-counter stimulants and "herbal supplements" that are cleverly sold as "safe" sports enhancers. Jenkins exposes several advertising and marketing strategies that purveyors of herbal and chemical stimulants use. He contends that insidious packaging and clever marketing allow many ordinary over-the-counter but potentially dangerous stimulants, antihistamines, and cold medications to be sold as herbal or natural supplements to unwary teens and athletes. He emphasizes the relative risks for athletes in competition and outlines physical and legal ramifications. Jenkins closes with specific advice for teachers, parents, administrators, and coaches to prevent over-the-counter stimulant abuse by teens.

Issue 2: How safe are herbal drugs and food supplements?

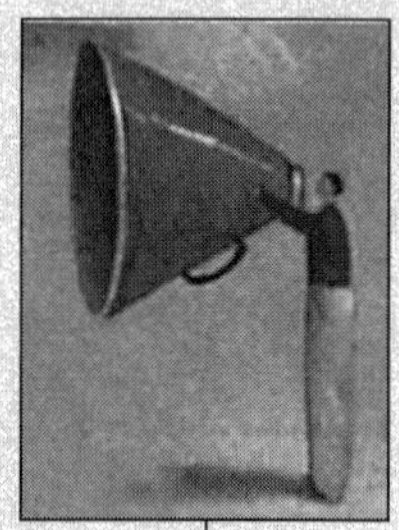

The Naturals

Herbal remedies really can fight off colds, headaches, and other ills—if you know how to use them safely.

Patricia Long

Patricia Long is a staff writer.

Hanging around my friend Patti's kitchen, I sometimes come across the strangest things. Just this past weekend, for example, I noticed a little bottle of brown tablets on her kitchen table.

"Yin Chiao," she explained. "It's a Chinese herb for colds."

"Does it work?"

"I think so. I take it when my throat gets scratchy, and it seems to make it better. Of course, it's hard to tell for sure, because I also take echinacea, which does the same thing."

I scanned the items ranged along her shelves. There was a bottle labeled *Arnica montana* Medicated Pellets ("for bruises and muscular tiredness," explained Patti) and a dusty tin of dried, crushed valerian ("to help me sleep").

Patti, who works at a software development company, isn't exactly a devotee of natural medicine. She heads for her doctor's office at the first sign of a serious illness. It's just that when it comes to staving off mild conditions, like a cold or hay fever, she prefers herbal remedies to over-the-counter drugs.

"Cold pills make me feel drowsy, and they dry up my nose and throat too much," she said. "Herbs don't affect me as strongly, they're more natural."

No doubt about it, Mother Nature's remedies—the leaves, flowers, bark, berries, or roots of plants—are fast becoming the treatment of choice for millions of Americans. Packaged as capsules, tablets, concentrated extracts, teas, tinctures, and salves, these botanicals, as they're also called, are trumpeted as a natural and safer alternative to drugs. What's more, proponents say, herbs can treat a handful of conditions that drugs generally can't help, including viral infections like influenza.

Apparently, a lot of us are buying this message. Herbal products rang up a healthy $1.6 billion in sales last year, making botanicals the fastest-growing category in drugstores.

"Fifteen years ago, when I told people I worked for an herb company, they'd make some joke about pot," says Michael McGuffin, president of McZand Herbal, in Santa Monica, California. "Now they say, 'Really? What company?' "

In the view of many believers, all this excitement about herbs is merely a case of Americans finally catching up with the rest of the world. Andrew Weil, a physician at the University of Arizona College of Medicine in Tucson and the author of several books on natural medicine, points out that in Europe botanicals have long been considered an important complement to conventional drugs. In Germany, for instance, doctors routinely prescribe herbal preparations for insomnia, colds, heart problems, constipation, and depression. In fact, half the prescriptions German doctors write for antidepressants are for Saint-John's-wort, an herb whose active ingredient hypericin is under study in this country as an AIDS drug.

Weil himself frequently recommends botanicals in his private practice, mostly to patients who have common complaints such as headaches or allergies or who simply want to stay well. "People come to me because they don't want to take pharmaceutical drugs," says Weil. "Almost all say they've been hurt by medicines prescribed by standard practitioners. In fact, I see a surprising number of doctors' wives."

Even some mainstream doctors, although still wary about exaggerated claims, acknowledge that there just might be something to all this herbal hoopla. It was Patti's family doctor, after all, who suggested she try echinacea for her sniffles—along with rest, fluids, and vitamin C.

"The proper use of herbs can add another dimension to health care," says Varro Tyler, a pharmacognocist at Purdue University and one of the country's leading experts on herbal medicine. He points out, for instance, that it's better to take echinacea—a mild immune stimulant—

to lessen flu symptoms than antibiotics, which are worthless against viral illnesses.

Botanicals are also cheaper than drugs. Saw palmetto, a proven treatment in Europe for an enlarged prostate, costs only 40 cents a day, compared to the drug finasteride, at about $1.75 a day. Similarly, cholesteramine, a cholesterol-lowering drug, costs nearly $4 a day more than simple garlic tablets, which have been shown to lower cholesterol and other blood lipids. At least two big insurance companies have taken notice. American Western Life Insurance Company and Blue Cross of Washington and Alaska recently announced new health plans that will cover the cost of herbal medicines prescribed by health practitioners.

Even the notoriously conservative federal government seems intrigued by the promise of botanicals. This past December, the Office of Alternative Medicine sponsored the first-ever conference to bring together two historical antagonists—representatives of the herbal industry and officials of the U.S. Food and Drug Administration—to work out better ways to regulate and sell botanicals in this country. To the astonishment of many attendees, the FDA officials said they'd welcome any botanical that could treat conditions for which there are currently no effective drugs. Specifically, they pointed to a need for sleep-inducing agents that aren't addictive, safeguards against migraine, and aids to improve memory, especially in the elderly.

Of course, there was one catch: Before you can make a therapeutic claim for a product, they told the herbal manufacturers, you must prove that it's safe—and that it's *effective.*

Do Herbs Work?

If you put an ear to the herbal grapevine, you'll discover seemingly endless uses for botanicals: Andrew Weil's favorite remedy for hay fever symptoms is freeze-dried stinging nettles. James Duke, a Department of Agriculture botanist and recognized authority on medicinal plants, recommends, among other things, feverfew for migraine headaches and ginkgo for tinnitus (ringing in the ears). My own mother swears by garlic pills, which she swallows each morning with her juice. If it weren't for them, she says, she'd still be plagued with sinus trouble.

Do these natural remedies really work? There's every reason to think they might. For one thing, plants already give us about a quarter of all drugs. Painkillers such as morphine or codeine, for example, are derived from the opium poppy. Atropine, a muscle relaxant, comes from belladonna; and the cancer drugs vincristine and vinblastine from periwinkle. Even aspirin is derived from the salicin in willow bark. What's more, at least 16 herbs have been judged by the FDA to be both safe and effective, allowing them to carry health claims and be sold as over-the-counter drugs. Among them are slippery elm bark (sold as Throat Coat Tea) and two laxatives, senna (Senokot) and psyllium seeds (Metamucil).

Drugs that have undergone extensive testing are one thing, of course; herbal remedies that rely on testimonials and tradition are quite another. For most herbs, scientific proof is hard to come by. Indeed, of the roughly 600 botanicals sold here, fewer than a dozen have been tested in costly controlled clinical trials, which determine whether an herb is safe and works better than a placebo. Researchers say there's sketchy clinical trial evidence on another 50 or so botanicals.

Scientists worldwide are striving to fill the gaps. The Office of Alternative Medicine recently funded several studies on traditional Chinese herbal remedies to determine whether they are effective treatments for premenstrual syndrome, hot flashes, warts, and chronic congestion in people with the AIDS virus. Meanwhile the German Commission E—composed of pharmacists, physicians, and toxicologists, among others—has been busy piecing together information from field studies, clinical trials, and doctors themselves on known medicinal herbs. So far, they've written more than 400 monographs, each a page or two long, containing information on the action of the herb, side effects, dosage, and cautions.

Does my mother's sinus remedy have any scientific backing? Not exactly. There's plenty of evidence that garlic lowers cholesterol, but it has yet to prove its ability to unstuff sinuses. The news on freeze-dried stinging nettles is also mixed: Only half the volunteers in a 1990 study gave it a thumbs-up as a hay fever remedy. However, feverfew does seem to fend off migraines. And studies showing ginkgo's ability to improve conditions associated with impaired blood circulation in the brain—such as headaches, memory loss, and tinnitus—fill an entire book. But that still leaves nearly 600 herbs available in this country whose effectiveness remains in doubt.

"I'm open to the possibility that some herbal remedies don't work at all," says Ted Kaptchuk, a doctor of Oriental medicine at Boston's Beth Israel Hospital and the author of *The Web That Has No Weaver,* a popular primer on Chinese medicine. "Let's find out what really works and get rid of what doesn't."

Are Herbs Safe?

Many people who have qualms about swallowing a single aspirin don't think twice about popping herbal capsules like candy—a practice that worries both mainstream doctors and herbal supporters. Indeed, if there's one thing everyone agrees on, it's this: An herb that has the ability to heal also has the ability, if misused, to harm.

Picking an Herbal Remedy

Feel an itching in your throat? Queasiness in your stomach? Before you reach for a natural remedy, make sure you know what to expect. Here's the latest information on 13 of the best-selling herbs in the country.

	Uses	Safety/Remarks
Chamomile *Matricaria recutia* (teas, ointments, lotions, inhalations)	Used as a mild sedative and to treat digestive disorders, menstrual cramps, various skin conditions, and minor infections. Used in bathwater for skin care and to treat yeast infections. Clinical trials show chamomile to be effective against inflammations and spasms in the digestive tract.	In rare cases can cause allergic reactions; otherwise, considered safe.
Echinacea *E. angustifolia, E. purpurea, or E. pallida* (tinctures, powders)	Used at first sign of cold or flu to ward off full-blown illness. Clinical studies show that echinacea has a mild stimulatory effect on the immune system.	Best used intermittently; the body is less responsive after eight weeks of continual use. Tinctures appear more effective than powdered capsules, which often contain the herb prairie dock instead of the real thing.
Feverfew *Tanacetum parthenium* (tablets, powders, extracts)	Used to prevent migraine and for arthritis, menstrual irregularities, stomachache, and fever. Clinical trials suggest it can relieve migraine pain.	Don't take for a long period of time without consulting a physician, because there are no long-term studies on toxicity. Products vary in the concentrations of parthenolide, one of the active ingredients.
Garlic *Allium sativum* (tablets, capsules)	Evidence suggests garlic can fight bacteria, lower high blood pressure, prevent blood clots, and protect against certain cancers (in animal and population studies). Clinical studies mainly support its ability to lower cholesterol.	Moderate doses pose little risk. Large amounts can reduce blood clotting time, a problem for anyone taking anticoagulants. Some experts recommend "enteric-coated" capsules, which allow the active ingredients to pass into the intestines intact. Garlic supplements vary in potency.
Ginger *Zingiber officinale* (capsules, teas, candied ginger)	Used to prevent nausea and to aid digestion. Some clinical studies have found it effective against motion sickness, morning sickness, and postoperative nausea. Lab findings suggest it can help stave off and fight colds.	There have been no reports of toxicity.
Ginkgo *Ginkgo biloba* (tablets, capsules, extracts)	Used in Europe as a conventional drug for treating short-term memory loss, headache, tinnitus, and depression. Also used as an antioxidant. Claims are backed by numerous clinical trials.	Recommended doses of standardized extracts (in tablet form) are safe. Large doses may cause restlessness, stomach upset, diarrhea, nausea, and vomiting.

Generally speaking, herbs *are* safer than drugs—most of which have potentially serious side effects. Illnesses associated with herbal use are relatively uncommon, and deaths rare. Still, even the safest of herbs carry risks. "Herbal medicine is like any other medicine," says Duke. "It should be used with discretion."

One way to look at the relative safety of herbs, he says, is to compare them to coffee, America's favorite herbal beverage. Drinking two cups of coffee a day is generally safe; five cups can cause headaches and nervousness; 15 can cause dizziness, ringing ears, even temporary hearing loss.

The question is, how much is too much? That depends on the herb. Each has its own safe dose, Duke says. He rates particular herbal teas, for instance, according to whether he believes they're more or less safe than coffee, which he would limit to two cups a day. A score of zero, for example, means he wouldn't touch the stuff. Water hemlock and belladonna, both long known to be deadly, rate zeros. A tea that scores one—goldenseal, for example—he would take only with great caution. A score of two—which he give lemon verbena—indicates he's no more leery of the herb than he is of coffee. And a rating of three—bestowed on herbs like feverfew and chamomile—means he would not be afraid to drink three cups. There's little problem with the herbal teas sold in grocery stores, he says, because they contain small amounts of herbs blended for flavor only, not for medicinal effects.

Picking an Herbal Remedy *(continued)*

	Uses	Safety/Remarks
Ginseng *Panax ginseng* (teas, powders, capsules, tablets, extracts)	Promoted for building up the body's resistance to stress and disease and for enhancing sexual potency. There's no strong clinical documentation for such claims.	The ginseng market is so rife with abuses—with cornstarch mixed into capsules of powdered ginseng, for example—that reputable companies fed up with the situation are helping to fund a major evaluation.
Goldenseal *Hydrastis canadensis* (teas)	Beneficial as a mouthwash to relieve canker sores. Tea is also widely used for eye inflammations and for respiratory conditions, like sinusitis. Active ingredients exert minor effects on circulation and on the central nervous system, but only in almost toxic doses. In animal studies, the herb has been shown to be effective against certain yeasts, bacteria, and protozoa, such as giardia.	No clinical studies on its safety when ingested rather than used as a rinse. Goldenseal should be taken only for acute conditions, not for long periods of time. Do not take during pregnancy.
Milk Thistle *Silybum marianum* (capsules)	Approved in Germany for treating liver conditions such as cirrhosis. In lab studies, active ingredient appears to prevent toxins from entering the liver and to help liver cells regenerate. Clinical trials show its effectiveness in treating jaundice and cirrhosis.	There are no known toxic effects.
Peppermint *Mentha x piperita* (teas)	Widely used for improving digestion and treating menstrual cramps. Some evidence backs claims for its digestive properties, especially for gas pains, and for giving relief to cold sufferers.	Safe to drink, but unless greatly diluted should not be given to infants or very young children, because the menthol may cause choking.
Saw Palmetto *Serenoa repens* (extracts)	Used in Europe to treat enlarged prostate or benign prostate hyperplasia, a condition that can cause blocked urinary flow, kidney damage, and infection. Controlled clinical trials on 2,000 German patients have confirmed its effectiveness.	Use standardized gel capsules. Whole fruit (in capsules or bulk powders) may be as effective but not backed by clinical studies. Because the active ingredients are fat-soluble, saw palmetto is less effective as a water extract, tea, or tincture.
Valerian *Valeriana officinalis* (teas, tinctures, extracts)	Approved in Germany as a minor tranquilizer for restlessness and for sleep disturbances. Not related to the drug Valium.	No significant side effects have been reported. Unlike other sedatives, it doesn't interact with alcohol to intensify drowsiness.
Willow Bark *Salix alba, S. purpurea, S. fragilis* (coarse or powdered bark)	Traditionally steeped as a tea for headache, fever, muscle pain, and arthritis. The concentration of active ingredients may be too low for it to be an effective medication.	Willow bark and aspirin belong to a class of compounds called salicylates and so may share similar side effects, including stomach irritation, bleeding during pregnancy, stroke, and Reye syndrome.

—*P.L.*

Most of the handful of people who get seriously ill or injured from herbs each year make the mistake of believing that if something is natural, it's safe at any dose, says Graham Woolf, a specialist in liver diseases at Cedars-Sinai Medical Center, in Los Angeles. The liver, he points out, can detoxify small amounts of a substance but gets overwhelmed with large doses—whether it's a drug or an herb. "Just about everyone takes acetaminophen, and they're not walking around with liver failure," says Woolf. "But if you down, say, sixteen 500-milligram tablets, you can develop acute liver failure within four days."

Toxicities that build up over months or years are another worry, though harder to predict. Centuries of use can rule out herbs that are acute poisons, but they can't always identify those that cause cancer or other chronic ills. Only in the last 30 years, for instance, have researchers learned that comfrey, coltsfoot, and borage, herbs used for hundreds of years for a variety of ills, contain toxins called pyrrolizidine alkaloids that, over time, damage the liver. Similarly, six cases of liver failure reported in the past few years have been linked to the long-term use of chaparral, an herb widely used for everything from arthritis to cancer.

One case, reported this past February, involved a 60-year-old Chicago woman who took just one or two daily capsules of chaparral for ten months, then upped the dose to six capsules when she developed flulike symptoms. She eventually required both liver and kidney transplants.

Some experts worry that chronic liver toxicity, though still rare, may be more common than generally acknowledged—a concern supported by observations from a Swedish medical laboratory. Five years ago, doctors in Gotene noticed that blood tests were turning up a lot of liver abnormalities in patients who used herbal preparations. So they asked 53 patients with early signs of liver damage to stop using all herbs. When the 12 who'd agreed returned to the lab six weeks later, all but one had normal liver tests.

"Nature *is* potentially dangerous," says Subhuti Dharmananda, director of the Institute for Traditional Medicine, in Portland, Oregon. "But just as it's unfair to expect herbs to be totally safe, it's unfair not to offer reasonable precautions."

Can You Trust What's on the Market?

Not always. At least not to the degree that the FDA, doctors, and many herbal enthusiasts would like. The trouble is, botanicals don't have to be proved safe before they're put on store shelves. It's only after a problem occurs that a product is withdrawn. What's more, only since last October has the herbal industry had FDA approval to list on their labels dosage, side effects, and contraindications. But many companies have been slow in making the switch—and the lack of warnings can lead consumers to believe that a product is perfectly safe no matter how it's used.

A 37-year-old San Francisco woman, for instance, died after drinking an herbal "dieter's tea" over a period of several months. The tea, it turns out, contained senna (a laxative) and ura ursi (a diuretic), both of which can deplete potassium, an electrolyte needed to regulate heartbeat. Yet none of the standard warnings against taking laxatives and diuretics for more than a week without medical supervision appeared on the label; nor did the directions mention any upper limit. One lab estimated that the woman got three times the maximum dose advised for senna in over-the-counter laxatives.

Products also can contain harmful or undesirable substances, whether added by mistake or design. Ayurvedic herbs, imported from India, are boiled down in clay or metal pots, often leaving residues of lead, mercury, arsenic, gold, or cadmium. Chinese herbal remedies—typically blends of many different herbs brewed into teas—are sometimes laced with prescription drugs. Misidentified plants can also be a problem. From 1991 to 1993, 48 Belgian women suffered severe kidney damage after taking a Chinese herbal preparation for weight loss that mistakenly contained a toxic plant instead of the herb stephania.

Even at its best, the botanicals industry faces questions about the quality and consistency of its products. One reason modern medicine moved away from herbal preparations in the first place was that drugs were easier to purify and standardize. When you take a 325-milligram aspirin tablet, you get 325 milligrams—no more, no less. Herbs, on the other hand, can vary widely in their concentrations of active ingredients, depending on where the plant was grown, the time of harvest, how it was handled and stored, and what part of the plant was used. "I've seen anywhere from a ten- to a 10,000-fold variation in active ingredients in herbs," says James Duke.

A case in point: Canadian researchers studying feverfew, a remedy for migraine widely used in Canada and Europe, established that the herb is effective when the concentration of parthenolide, one of its active ingredients, is 0.2 to 0.4 percent. But many feverfew preparations sold in this country contain little parthenolide.

In Germany, manufacturers have gotten around the problem by selling tinctures and extracts with standardized amounts of certain active ingredients. But this practice raises the hackles of some U.S. manufacturers, who argue that herbs contain a potent cocktail of hundreds of active ingredients. Standardizing for just one or two, they say, reduces an herb to a drug, possibly limiting its effectiveness.

Duke and other experts disagree. "It's true that a standardized product won't be as natural," he says, "but it's *more* likely to be effective."

Not to mention more predictable. Just as some botanicals are short on active ingredients, others may have too much. Graham Woolf recalls a woman who sipped Chinese tea for a cold. "After she took it," says Woolf, "she thought she was going to die. Her heart began racing, and she started hyperventilating." The tea was loaded with ephedrine, a potent stimulant in the Chinese herb ma huang and a chemical cousin of pseudoephedrine, used in over-the-counter decongestants. "If I had a choice whether to take ma huang or Sudafed," says Woolf, "I'd take Sudafed. At least I'd know how much of it to take."

Even popular herbs, when sold in a variety of forms, can leave consumers bewildered. For example, studies show that echinacea boosts the immune system, but nobody knows which ingredients are responsible or which

The Safe Use of Herbs

Most experts say it's best to take herbal remedies on your own only for minor, short-term discomforts such as colds. For everything else, see a doctor—if only to make sure you're not simply alleviating the symptoms of a potentially serious illness. Here are some other things to keep in mind:

Don't take herbs if you're pregnant, trying to become pregnant, or nursing. And don't give herbs to your baby. Fetuses and babies lack some of the liver enzymes needed to detoxify harmful chemicals in herbs. When adults drink a cup of coffee, for example, caffeine is cleared from the body in less than five hours. But a baby takes 80 hours to clear a comparable dose.

Don't overdo it. Damage to the liver, kidneys, and other organs occurs more often when botanicals are consumed in large amounts or over a long period of time. Generally, early symptoms of liver damage resemble the standard flu or cold symptoms; jaundice may show up a little later.

Don't regularly use a large variety of herbs. No botanicals have been checked for safety when combined with other herbs or drugs, whether prescription or over-the-counter. Get advice from knowledgeable people. Good sources include physicians or pharmacists who've taken courses on herbal remedies, and licensed naturopaths, who take extensive coursework in botanical medicine. (For a referral, call the American Association of Naturopathic Physicians, 206/323-7610.) If you're looking for Chinese herbs, get them prescribed by a licensed acupuncturist trained in Chinese medicine. (For more information, call the National Commission for the Certification of Acupuncturists, at 202/232-1404).

Learn as much as you can about the herbs you're taking. Two helpful sources are *Peterson Field Guides Eastern/Central Medicinal Plants* by Steven Foster and James Duke (Houghton/Mifflin) and *The Honest Herbal* by Varro Tyler (Haworth Press).

If you do have an adverse reaction, such as fever, nausea, or a headache, report it. Call the Food and Drug Administration, at 800/332-1088, and the American Herbal Products Association, at 512/469-6355.—*P.L.*

form is most potent. Alcohol tinctures, for instance, may contain little of what I'll call agent X ("high-molecular-weight polysaccharides" is too unwieldy), an ingredient known to stimulate the immune system but not soluble in alcohol. But they do contain an immune stimulant I'll call agent Z (or "isobutylamides"), although no one knows how its effectiveness compares to agent X's. So are capsules better? Not necessarily. They're often adulterated with cheaper herbs, in which case you're not getting any active ingredients.

Recognizing that such problems could scare consumers away just as they're discovering the promise of botanicals, both retailers and manufacturers are scrambling to solve these thorny issues. Fresh Fields, the country's second largest chain of health food supermarkets, no longer sells supplements that carry unproven claims or that it considers unsafe. That includes any product containing pennyroyal, comfrey, yohimbe, kola nut, and ma huang.

For its part, the American Herbal Products Association, a trade group of herbal manufacturers, has asked its members to voluntarily recall comfrey and to temporarily suspend sales of chaparral. By next year, it hopes to complete a consumer reference manual on 600 herbal ingredients, including directions for safe use.

"Industry, science, and government will have to work these problems out, because consumers want these products," says Mark Blumenthal, executive director of the nonprofit American Botanical Council, in Austin, Texas. "The Pandora's box of herbs has been opened, and you're not going to get it closed again."

FRAME the DEBATE

Form at end of book

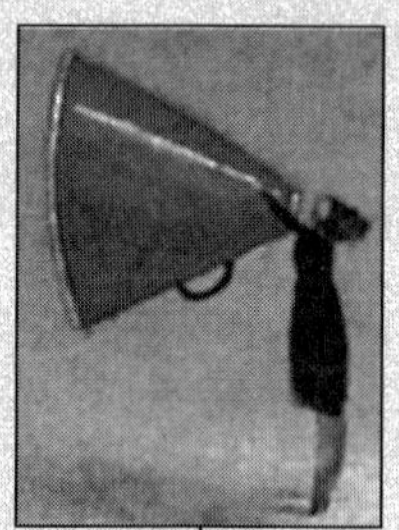

Issue 2: How safe are herbal drugs and food supplements?

The Herbal Minefield

Stephen Barrett, M.D.

In 1997, health-food-store patrons spent over a billion dollars for capsules, tablets, bulk herbs, and herbal teas. Although many of these items are consumed for their flavor, most are probably used for supposed medicinal qualities. Sales by multilevel distributors and pharmacies amount to hundreds of millions more for products that are obviously intended for self-medication. Herbs are also marketed by naturopaths, acupuncturists, iridologists, chiropractors, and unlicensed herbalists, many of whom prescribe them for the entire gamut of health problems. Many such practitioners are not qualified to make appropriate medical diagnoses or to determine how the products they prescribe compare to proven drugs.

Herbal advocates like to point out that about half of today's medicines were derived from plants. (Digitalis, for example, was originally derived from leaves of the foxglove plant.) This statement is true but misleading. Drug products contain specified amounts of active ingredients. Herbs in their natural state can vary greatly from batch to batch and often contain chemicals that cause side effects but provide no benefit.

When potent natural substances are discovered, drug companies try to isolate and synthesize the active chemical in order to provide a reliable supply. They also attempt to make derivatives that are more potent, more predictable, and have fewer side effects. In the case of digitalis, derivatives provide a spectrum of speed and duration of action. Digitalis leaf is almost never used today because its effects are less predictable. Many herbs contain hundreds or even thousands of chemicals that have not been completely catalogued. Some of these chemicals may turn out to be useful as therapeutic agents, but others could well prove toxic.

In the United States, herbs intended for preventive or therapeutic use would be regulated as drugs under federal laws. To evade the law, these products are marketed as "foods" or "dietary supplements" without health claims on their labels. Since herbs are not regulated as drugs, no legal standards exist for their processing, harvesting, or packaging. In many cases, particularly for products with expensive raw ingredients, contents and potency are not accurately disclosed on the label. Many products marked as herbs contain no useful ingredients, and some even lack the principal ingredient for which people buy them. Some manufacturers are trying to develop industrywide quality-assurance standards, but possible solutions are a long way off.

The Dietary Supplement Health and Education Act of 1994 included herbal products in its definition of "dietary supplements," even though herbs have little or no nutritional value. (The bill was spearheaded by the health-food industry in order to weaken FDA regulation of its products.) Herbal or other botanical ingredients include processed or unprocessed plant parts (bark, leaves, flowers, fruits, and stems) as well as extracts and essential oils. They are available as teas, powders, tablets, capsules, and elixirs, and may be marketed as single substances or combined with other herbs, vitamins, minerals, amino acids, or non-nutrient ingredients. The fact that an herb is known to be toxic does not ensure its removal from the marketplace. When the FDA concludes that an herb is dangerous, it usually issues a warning rather than a ban. The FDA Center for Food Safety and Applied Nutrition maintains a searchable database of reports the FDA has received of adverse events associated with the use of dietary supplements and herbal products.

To make a rational decision about an herbal product, it would be necessary to know what it contains, whether it is safe, and whether it has been demonstrated to be as good or better than pharmaceutical products available for the same purpose. For most herbal products this information is incomplete or unavailable. Even worse, most published information about herbs is unreliable. Varro E. Tyler, Ph.D., former dean of the Purdue University School of Pharmacy and a leading authority on pharmacognosy (the science of medicines from natural sources), has observed:

> More misinformation about the safety and efficacy of herbs is reaching the public currently than at any previous time, including the turn-of-the-century heyday of patent medicines. The literature promoting herbs includes pamphlets, magazine articles, and books ranging in quality from cheaply printed flyers

to elaborately produced studies in fine bindings with attractive illustrations. Practically all of these writings recommend large numbers of herbs for treatment based on hearsay, folklore, and tradition. The only criterion that seems to be avoided in these publications is scientific evidence. Some writings are so comprehensive and indiscriminate that they seem to recommend everything for anything. Even deadly poisonous herbs are sometimes touted as remedies, based on some outdated report or a misunderstanding of the facts. Particularly insidious is the myth that there is something almost magical about herbal drugs that prevents them, in their natural state, from harming people.

Two of Tyler's books (*The Honest Herbal* and *Herbs of Choice*) summarize what is known about many commonly used herbs. The recent entry of drug companies into the herbal marketplace is likely to improve standardization of dosage for some products. However, with safe and effective medicines available, treatment with herbs rarely makes sense, and many of the conditions for which herbs are recommended are not suitable for self-treatment.

Books to Avoid

- *The Complete Medicinal Herbal* (Ody)
- *Earl Mindell's Herb Bible* (Mindell)
- *The English Physician* (Nicholas Culpeper)
- *Natural Healing with Herbs* (Santillo)

FRAME the DEBATE

Form at end of book

Issue 2: How safe are herbal drugs and food supplements?

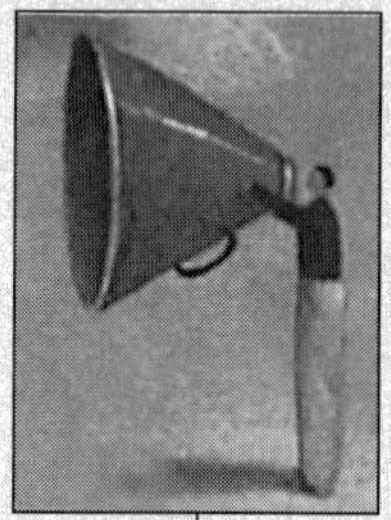

Herbal Energizers: Speed by Any Other Name

Andrew P. Jenkins

Andrew P. Jenkins is an associate professor of health education at Central Washington University, Ellensburg, WA 98926.

Currently, more than one hundred types of over-the-counter (OTC) stimulants are sold in the United States (Consumers Union, 1995). This article focuses on stimulants sold to high-school-age athletes and dieters. These OTC stimulants are sold as "herbal energizers," food supplements, and fatigue reducers. The advertising often makes these products appear healthful and harmless; however, all of these stimulants belong in the class sympathomimetic amines, a potentially dangerous and addictive class of drugs similar in structure and actions to amphetamines.

Main Effects of Sympathomimetic Amines

Sympathomimetic amines are a class of drugs that imitate the actions of the sympathetic nervous system (Crimson & Jermain, 1993, Knoben & Anderson, 1988). The sympathetic nervous system stimulates the "fight or flight" response that readies the human body for extreme muscle activity—such as battling a foe or running for one's life. During a fight or flight response, all nonbattle activities or functions, such as digestion and sexual function, are shut down (see table 1).

The fight or flight response is what teenagers often call an "adrenaline rush." Most of the effects on the sympathetic nervous system are the result of two hormones that are released—epinephrine (adrenaline) and norepinephrine (nor-adrenaline) (Marieb, 1995). Drugs that directly stimulate the sympathetic nerves or receptors, or cause the release of these excitatory hormones, are termed sympathomimetic because they *mimic* the sympathetic nervous system hormones and its subsequent stimulatory actions (Hanson & Venturelli, 1995). Short-term stimulation of the sympathetic nervous system is not harmful because it is usually resolved promptly and control of the body systems is returned to parasympathetic (relaxation) nervous system domination. Most side effects and risks of sympathomimetic amines are tied to abnormally high or chronic stimulation of the sympathetic nervous system.

Table 1 Summary of Sympathetic Nervous System Arousal

Increases	Decreases
Alertness	Saliva production (cotton mouth)
Anxiety	Digestion
Heart rate	Sexual function
Cardiac output	Blood to internal organs
Blood pressure	Sleep and REM cycle
Respiration rate	Appetite
Muscle tension	Fatigue
Perspiration	Concentration
Urination	
Blood supply to skeletal muscles and brain	
Dilation of pupils and bronchioles	
Blood sugar production	

The most common types of stimulants used in OTC stimulants are caffeine, ephedrine, pseudoephedrine, and phenylpropanolamine. These drugs have legitimate use as antihistamines and cold medications, and for asthma relief, and are found in over-the-counter medicines such as Actifed, Allerest, Contac, Nyquil, and Drixol. The desired main effects are bronchial dilation, sinus drying, and drowsiness (Knoben & Anderson, 1988). The FDA requires that over-the-counter medications have clear instructions and warnings. Unfortunately, these side effects often appear even when these drugs are taken within the recommended doses (see table 2). Reactions to all drugs vary from person to person.

This article is reprinted with permission from the JOURNAL OF PHYSICAL EDUCATION, RECREATION & DANCE, volume 68, number 2, pp. 39–45. JOPERD is a publication of the American Alliance for Health, Physical Education, Recreation and Dance, 1900 Association Drive, Reston, VA 20191.

Table 2 Common Over-the-Counter Stimulants (Sympathomimetic Amines)

Drug	Cold Medicine/ Antihistamine	Exercise/ Diet Aid
Chlorprenaline	Asthone (Japanese)	
*Ephedrine (includes Ma Huang Chinese herbal ephedra)	Bonkaid, Bronkotabs, Primatene, Vitronol Nose Drops	High Energy Herbal Energy Formula, High Energy Max. Strength, Diet Now: Sensible Diet & Wt. Management Plan, E'Ola Drops
Phenylephrine	Codimal, Coridicin, Dristan, Neo-Synephrine, Robitussin	
Pseudoephedrine	Actifed, Afrinol, Sudafed, Drixol, Chlortrimeton	
*Phenylpropanolamine	Allerest, ARM, Contac, Dimetapp, 4 Way Formula, Nyquil, Sine-Off, Vicks Nighttime Cold Medicine	Acutrim, Dexatrim, Metabolift Thermogenic Formula, Permathin-16 Maximum Strength
*Caffeine (xanthine with sympathetic actions)	Anacin, Excedrin, No-Doz	Caffedrine

*Most common over-the-counter stimulants.

Note: The sale of the combination of these three has been banned by the FDA.

Adverse Effects of Over-the-Counter Stimulants

The onset and nature of side effects from OTC stimulants are dependent on individual drug reactions, dose, duration of use, and tolerance. All of these drugs can cause an increase in physical tolerance with repeated use; therefore, the individual will need to increase the dosage progressively to attain the desired results. With increased dosages comes an increased risk of side effects. Physical tolerance and prolonged use will also be followed by withdrawal syndrome upon cessation of use. Withdrawal symptoms can include depression, fatigue, irritability, nausea, and headache (Holtzman, 1990).

The most common effect and side effects of OTC stimulant use include, but are not limited to, anxiety to agitation, alertness to disorientation, increased muscle tension and shakes, mildly elevated heart rate to tachycardia or dangerously elevated heart rate levels (Boyd, 1986). Appetite is suppressed although the large intestine and bowel may be stimulated. Urine production is increased as is blood glucose production. Temperature elevation can range from mild to severe hyperthermia (overheating) (Appelt, 1993; Heishman & Henningfield, 1992).

Ephedrine is particularly dangerous. Following twelve reported deaths due to ephedrine overdose, the FDA is currently examining how to tighten the regulations controlling its sale and distribution (*Substance Abuse Funding News,* 1995). Ephedrine can cause heart palpitations, hypertension, nerve damage, muscle injury, psychosis, stroke, and death. Ohio has passed laws restricting all sales of ephedra and ephedrine following the overdose death of a high school athlete (Consumers Union, 1995). There is also strong concern over the use of ephedrine in the manufacture of illegal forms of methamphetamine known as "crank" and "crystal meth" (Kleiner, 1994). Currently, the FDA prohibits the sale of ephedrine in large quantities, but nothing prohibits drug chemists from purchasing multiple quantities of over-the-counter ephedrine from multiple distributors.

Pseudoephedrine is nearly identical in structure and in effects to ephedrine. It is derived from plant sources of the genus, Ephedra. Like ephedrine, it may be sold as a "natural" herbal stimulant and manufacturers may tout its ergogenic or sports-enhancing effects, none of which are supported by research (Clemons & Crosby, 1993; Collins, 1993). The main effects, side effects, and risks are essentially the same for ephedrine and pseudoephedrine. Both drugs are on the banned lists for most athletic unions.

A false sense of security may surround the use of OTC stimulants, but these drugs are only safe when used as recommended and in the doses recommended. The uninformed user of these drugs may accidentally overdose as the result of the combined or synergistic effects of multiple drug use. The deadly triple combination of ephedrine, caffeine, and phenylpropanolamine (PPA) has been banned by the FDA since 1982. The potential still exists, however, for an individual to combine phenylpropanolamine and ephedrine, wash them down with a cup or two of coffee or a double latte and end up in a critical overdose situation!

Phenylpropanolamine (PPA) by itself can cause nervousness, restlessness, insomnia, headache, nausea, elevated blood sugar, and elevated blood pressure. PPA is the active ingredient in Acutrim and Dexatrim, two diet aids often used by teenage girls.

Most research indicates that low doses of caffeine in the 100–300 mgs/day (1 to 3 cups/day) range do not likely cause any serious side effects (Heishman & Henningfield, 1992). However, it should be noted that an individual's reaction to any drug can vary. Hypercaffeinism results from high or prolonged doses of caffeine. Doses in excess of 300 mgs/day may produce elevated heart rate, blood pressure, diarrhea, gastric upset, insomnia, REM-deprived sleep, anxiety, tension, nervousness, and muscle twitches. Extremely high doses in excess of 500 mgs/day (more than 5 cups/day) can result in psychotic disorders, convulsions, muscle spasms, extreme anxiety, paranoia, respiratory collapse, heart palpitations, even death (Consumers Union, 1994; Heishman & Henningfield, 1992; Wisconsin Clearinghouse, 1986).

Caffeine is an addictive substance and tolerance is developed over time. Also, increased tolerance causes a need for progressively larger doses over time. Acute withdrawal will set in within 24 hours of cessation of use resulting in headache, fatigue, lethargy, decreased alertness, nervousness, flu-like symptoms, muscle pain, and nausea. Most withdrawal symptoms pass within 7 days of cessation of caffeine use (Holtzman, 1990).

Caffeine side effects of greatest concern for high school coaches and school medical personnel include: inability to concentrate, anxiety, tachycardia (high heart rate), dehydration from increased urine output, and loss of muscle coordination (Knoben & Anderson, 1988). Although early research on caffeine indicated that caffeine may increase the availability of certain fatty acids under aerobic conditions (Costill, Dalsky, & Fink, 1978; McNaughton, 1987), the possible performance-enhancing effects of caffeine and other OTC stimulants are usually negated by the side effects (Casal & Leon, 1985; Rogers, 1985). Recent research does not indicate any ergogenic effects to caffeine use during prolonged low or moderate intensities (Engels and Haymes, 1991; Szurgot et al., 1991). Further, caffeine may actually cause a decrease in fine motor function (Jacobson, Edwards, & Kulling, 1991).

Regardless of the cause, whether it is drug- or stress-induced, prolonged stimulation of the fight or flight response results in chronic stress syndrome. Chronic fatigue, anxiety, adrenal depletion, and even paranoid delusions and psychosis may result (see table 3).

Table 3 Summary of Risks to OTC Stimulant Abuse

- Acute psychiatric disorders
- Addiction/dependence
- Anxiety disorders
- Cardiac disorders and arrhythmia's
- Chronic fatigue syndrome
- Chronic stress syndrome
- Dehydration
- Depression
- Disqualification from athletic event
- Heart failure
- Hyperthermia (high body temperature)
- Hypertension (high blood pressure)
- Nervousness
- Muscle spasms and injury
- Respiratory collapse
- Stroke
- Shakes and tremors
- Tolerance
- Withdrawal syndrome

Stimulants and Sport Drug Testing Limits

Most drug testing programs for amateur athletics are modeled after the International and U.S. Olympic Committees' (IOC and USOC) drug testing programs. The lists of banned substances such as anabolic steroids, amphetamines, and other stimulants are comparable, if not identical, in most cases.

Most, if not all, of the common stimulants found in over-the-counter medications and herbal energizers are listed as banned substances by the International and U.S. Olympic Committees (USOC) and the National Collegiate Athletic Association (NCAA) (Benson, 1991; NCAA, 1996; USOC, 1996). These stimulants include, but are not limited to, ephedrine in both natural and synthesized form, pseudoephedrine, phenylpropanolamine, and caffeine.

The caffeine limit established by the U.S. Olympic Committee (1996) is any concentration greater than 12 mcg/ml in the urine, which would be equal to 6 to 8 cups of drip brew coffee in a 2-hour period. However, it is entirely possible for an athlete to use several stimulants and to drink a variety of beverages and reach this limit, unknowingly. Two cups of coffee would result in 3 to 6 mcg/ml in the urine. Two colas would produce .59 to .70 mcg/ml in the urine. And, one No-Doz would produce 1.5 mcg/ml in the urine. Only 1 cup of guarana tea, which contains as high as 6 percent caffeine, could cause an unacceptable level of caffeine in an athlete's urine (Merdink & Wooley, 1990).

It is suggested that the athletic union and/or the team physician be contacted before an athlete takes any over-the-counter or prescription antihistamine, asthma medication—including mists, cold medicine, or stimulants. The U.S. Olympic Committee reports that over-the-counter cold medications and antihistamines can be detected up to 72 hours after last use (USOC, 1996).

Advertising Ploys

Advertisers of food supplements, some of which contain stimulants, target young weightlifters, bodybuilders, and athletes by using words and phrases that remind the reader of anabolic steroids such as " . . . has twice the anabolic effect." They use terms like "herbal," "natural," and "nutrition supplement" to give the impression that these are healthful and harmless substances.

The advertisers balance these safe and gentle words and phrases with powerful hyperbole meant to appeal to the sports minded, hard working, young athlete: "T & M Delivers!," "performance-enhancing," "high intensity," "explode," and "break through." "Kickers" are ephedra tablets packaged in a bright orange and silver envelope with a karate champion on the front to emphasize the power of the drug and to make the sports link. These packs sell for a dollar a piece at mini-markets and are one of the most popular OTC stimulants on the market.

Some of the advertising campaigns are fully confrontational and appeal to an athlete's risk-taking tendencies and sense of pride. One advertisement, aimed at young bodybuilders, even states outright, this product is "Not for every Pencil-Necked Ding Dong in your gym" and then challenges the athlete, "If you're sick and tired of taking mamby pamby-feel nothing-do little supplements . . . then [this product] is for you."

Diet aids aimed at women and girls are now being sold out of home businesses. Signs are appearing on lawns and telephone poles which call their product, "Will Power in a Bottle." The signs claim "Lose up to 30 lbs. in 30 days . . . without exercising!," "Great for men's spare tire," and "Lose weight and inches." Most of these products contain ephedrine and caffeine and most of the home dealers of these stimulants have no medical training. The home dealers usually have little or no knowledge of the effects of sympathomimetics.

What's in a Name?

Packaging and advertising of diet products aimed at young women and dieters are no less suggestive than those aimed at athletes. Names like "Dexatrim," "Diet Now," "Mini-Thin," and "Permathin" give the clear impression that the drug is going to contribute to significant weight loss and "thinness." Some of the stimulants advertised in the back of fashion magazines have powerful and dangerous names such as "357 Magnums," ".44's," and "White Crosses." These OTC stimulants are sold mail order at discount prices to women as "diet aids," in large volumes up to 1,000 count. The low, mail-order prices and large volumes may precipitate overdose and abuse of these drugs among young women.

For the student studying late, or the drowsy driver, there are products sold over-the-counter at truck stops and mini-marts, called "Super Ener-Max," "Super Pep Extra Strength," and "Mega-Blast," "Ultra Energy Now," and simply, "UP-Time." The packaging of these drugs as "herbal" or "natural" supplements is often used to soften or hide the drug qualities of these products. The buyer may think of them as vitamins or harmless food supplements. Some manufacturers, however, take a full frontal approach. The OTC stimulants are often shaped to resemble more powerful and dangerous prescription amphetamines. For example, Mini-Thins are white with a fine cross on the top to imitate the prescription stimulant, Benzedrine.

Common "Herbal" Stimulants

Many of the herbs sold in food supplement packages are benign and probably only yield food value; however, many of the vitamin and supplement combinations contain central nervous system stimulants disguised as "herbal" supplements (see table 4). Despite advertising ploys intended to sell herbal stimulants as "safe and natural" products, many of these herbs carry dangerous side effects if used excessively or improperly. The following is a list of the most common herbal stimulants sold in over-the-counter herbal energizers, vitamin packs, and food supplements.

- **Ma Huang (ephedra)** contains the drug, ephedrine, in its natural form. There is no pharmacological difference in the natural or synthesized form of the drug—the effects are the same on the human body.
- **Guarana (paullnia cupana)** is a bean much like the coffee bean; however, it contains much more caffeine. Caffeine content in the guarana bean is between 2 and 6 percent.
- **Green tea (camellia sinensis)** contains between 3 and 4 percent caffeine.
- **Coffee (coffea arabica)** is a bean and contains between 0.8 and 2.4 percent. The average cup of drip coffee contains 110 to 150 mgs of caffeine.
- **Kola nut** contains only a minuscule amount of caffeine. Most of the 33 to 60 mgs of caffeine found in cola soft drinks is added in its synthetic form.
- **Cocoa (theobroma cacao)** contains small amounts of caffeine, which is present in chocolate candy and coca drinks. Chocolate bars contain approximately 22 mgs of caffeine, whereas hot cocoa contains around 5 mgs of caffeine.

Concerns for Teachers, Parents, and Youth Coaches

Over-the-counter stimulants carry health risks for adults as well as teenagers, but when approaching teen stimulant use/abuse, special considerations often need to be made.

Table 4 Common Herbal Stimulants (Often Sold at Mini-Marts and Gas Stations)

Brand Name	Drug	Dose
Kickers Chinese Herbs	Ma Huang (Chinese ephedrine)	Not revealed
Ultra Energy Now	Ma Huang (Chinese ephedrine)	Not revealed
	Guarana extract (caffeine)	Not revealed
	Kola (caffeine)	Not revealed
Mini-Thin	Ephedrine HCL (stimulant, antihistamine)	25 mgs
Gin Zing	Ma Huang (Chinese ephedrine)	1000 mgs
	Guarana (caffeine)	500 mgs
Mega BLAST High Energy formula	Ma Huang (Chinese ephedrine)	450 mgs
	Gota Kola (caffeine)	225 mgs
	Caffeine	150 mgs
Super PEP Extra Strength	Kola nut (caffeine)	Not revealed
	Guarana (caffeine)	Not revealed
	Gota Kola (caffeine)	Not revealed
Super Ener-Max	Ma Huang (Chinese ephedrine)	220 mgs
	Green tea extract (caffeine)	100 mgs
	Kola nut extract (caffeine)	80 mgs
UP Time Food Supplement	Caffeine	Not revealed

The following is a summary of eight important concerns to consider when educating and preventing OTC stimulant abuse among teenagers.

1. Teenage athletes are particularly susceptible to persuasive marketing and claims.
2. Teenage girls are at the highest risk for anorexia and bulimia nervosa and overuse of diet aids.
3. Teenagers are susceptible to overuse attitudes: "If one works, ten will work ten times better."
4. Terms like "herbal," "natural," and "no caffeine" are used by manufacturers and advertisers to give a false sense of security.
5. The distribution, sale, and use of these products by minors is not controlled or regulated.
6. The combination of symptoms and conditions associated with the use of OTC stimulants may become fatal. Example: Athletes or dieters who are dehydrated may suffer cardiac arrest from the combined effects of low blood volume and high heart rate.
7. The combined (synergistic) effects of OTC stimulants and caffeine can be fatal. Example: The deadly combination of ephedrine, caffeine, and phenylpropanolamine has been banned by the FDA since 1982.
8. The purpose of using OTC stimulants to gain an athletic advantage will be of no use when athletes fail drug tests and/or become disqualified from athletic events. Any possible advantage gained will be lost if the athlete is banned, penalized, or relegated.

What Can Be Done?

Parents, coaches, and teachers can take action in two ways: First, they should educate themselves and then educate teens on the marketing ploys, the main effects and side effects, and the risks of OTC stimulants. The American Council for Drug Education and the National Federation of Parents for Drug-Free Youth can be contacted for information and teaching resources. Many states have coalitions such as The Wisconsin Clearinghouse for Drug Information and the Washington State Substance Abuse Coalition that readily provide information, education, and referrals for teachers, parents, and coaches working with and educating youth.

Second, concerned adults can request gyms, stores, and mini-markets to place these dangerous stimulants out of reach of minors and to voluntarily agree to sell them only to adults. While most businesses are acting within the limits of the current laws, many business owners are unaware of the potential dangers of OTC stimulants, although they may be receptive to community concerns.

Organized citizen groups can appeal to city councils who can pass ordinances restricting or prohibiting businesses from selling OTC stimulants to minors. The state pharmaceutical board can also be contacted. The groups can ask vendors for voluntary compliance with restricted sale of OTC stimulants to minors.

Through a coordinated effort between coaches, parents, teachers, and business people, the abuse of OTC stimulants by student athletes and teenagers can be curbed.

Resources

American Council for Drug Education, (301) 294-0600
National Clearinghouse for Alcohol & Drug Information, PO Box 2345, Rockville, MD 20852
National Federation of Parents for Drug-Free Youth, (800) 554-KIDS
National Institute on Drug Abuse, (800) 662-HELP
National Institute on Drug Abuse, U.S. Dept. of Health and Human Services. (800) 638-2045
Parents Resource Institute for Drug Education, (404) 577-4500
PRIDE Drug Information Line, (800) 241-9746
United States Olympic Committee Drug Hotline, (800) 233-0393
Wisconsin Clearinghouse, (608) 263-2797
Washington State Substance Abuse Coalition, (800) 662-9111
Washington State Pharmacists Association, (206) 228-7171
Washington State Board of Pharmacies, (206) 753-6834
Schools Without Drugs: The Challenge, (202) 732-4161
Wisconsin Clearinghouse (1986). *Mood altering chemical series: Caffeine.* Fact sheet available from Wisconsin Clearinghouse, PO Box 1468, Madison, WI 53701

References

Appelt, G. (1993). Weight control products. In Covington, T. (Ed.), *Handbook of nonprescription drugs,* 10th ed. (pp. 339–349), Washington, DC: American Pharmaceutical Association.
Benson, M. (1991). *NCAA drug testing/education programs.* Overland Park, KS: The National Collegiate Athletic Association.
Boyd, J. R. (1986). Nonprescription drug screening. *American Pharmacology, 26,* 22–24.
Casal, D. C., & Leon, A. S. (1985). Failure of caffeine to affect substrate utilization during prolonged running. *Medicine and Science in Sports and Exercise, 17*(1), 174–179.
Clemons, J., & Crosby, S. (1993). Cardiopulmonary and subjective effects of a 60 mg. dose of pseudoephedrine on graded treadmill exercise. *The Journal of Sports Medicine and Physical Fitness, 33*(4), 405–412.
Collins, L. H. (1993, July/August). Doping in sports, *Journal of the American Academy of Physician Assistants,* 465–476.
Consumers Union (1995, November). Herbal roulette. *Consumer Reports,* 698–705.
Consumers Union (1994). *Complete Drug Reference, 1994 Edition.* Yonkers, NY: Author.
Costill, D., Dalsky, G., & Fink, W. (1978). Effects of caffeine ingestion on metabolism and exercise performance. *Medicine and Science in Sports and Exercise, 10,* 155–158.
Crimson, M., & Jermain, D. (1993). *Handbook of Nonprescription Drugs,* 10th ed. (pp. 135–146) Washington, DC: American Pharmaceutical Association.
Hanson, G., & Venturelli, P. (1995). *Drugs and society,* (4th ed.), Boston, MA: Jones and Bartlett Publishers.
Heishman, S., & Henningfield, J. (1992). Stimulus functions of caffeine in humans: Relation to dependence potential. *Neuroscience and Biobehavior Review, 16,* 273–287.
Engels, H., & Haymes, E. (1991). Effects of caffeine on metabolic responses of aerobically trained males during prolonged exercise at low and moderate intensities. Abstracts of research papers of the American Alliance for Health, Physical Education, and Dance Convention 1991 (p. 90). Reston, VA: AAHPERD.
Holtzman, S. (1990). Caffeine as a model of drug abuse. *Trends in Pharmacological Sciences, 11,* 355–356.
Jacobson, B., Edwards, S., & Kulling, F. (1991). Effects of caffeine on delicate motor performance. *Supplement to Medicine and Science in Sports and Exercise, 23*(4), 76.
Kleiner, K. (1994). Drug laws crack down on crank. *New Scientist, 147*(94), 9.
Knoben, J., & Anderson, P. (1988). *Handbook of clinical drug data.* Hamilton, IL: Drug Intelligence Publications.
Marieb, E. (1995). *Human anatomy and physiology,* 3rd ed., Redwood City, CA: The Benjamin/Cummings Publishing Company, Inc.
McNaughton, L. (1987). Two levels of caffeine ingestion on blood lactate and free fatty acid responses during incremental exercise. *Research Quarterly for Exercise and Sport, 58*(3), 255–259.
Merdink, J., & Wooley, B. (1990). Drug testing: history, philosophy, and rationale. In Tricker, R. & D. Cook (Eds.), *Athletes at Risk: Drugs and Sport* (pp. 161–171). Dubuque, IA: W. C. Brown.
National Collegiate Athletic Association (1996). *1996–97 NCAA Manual* (pp. 496–499). Overland Park, KS: The National Collegiate Athletic Association.
Public Citizen Health Research Group (1991). Do not use phenylpropanolamine-containing products. *Public Citizen Health Research Group Newsletter, 7*(1), 3.
Rogers, C. C. (1985). Cyclists try caffeine suppositories. *The Physician and Sports Medicine, 13*(3), 38–39.
Substance Abuse Funding News (1995, October 18). FDA may tighten ephedrine limits. *Substance Abuse Funding News,* 10.
Szurgot, B., Knowton, R., Brown, D., Perkins, R., & Sanjabi, P. (1991). The ergogenic influence of venous infused caffeine on cardiovascular and metabolic dynamics during exercise. *Supplement to Medicine and Science in Sports and Exercise, 23*(4), 76.
U.S. Olympic Committee (1996, March). *USOC guide to prohibited substances and methods.* Colorado Springs, CO: USOC Drug Control Administration.
U.S. Olympic Committee (1996, May). *Drug free: Examples of prohibited and allowable medications.* Colorado Springs, CO: USOC Drug Control Administration.
Wisconsin Clearinghouse (1986). *Mood altering chemical series: Caffeine.* Madison, WI: Author.

FRAME the DEBATE

Form at end of book

WiseGuide Wrap-Up

Herbal drugs and food supplements are flooding the health marketplace. With them comes the hope of natural, nonchemical treatments and cures for common health problems. This is especially true since the 1993 Dietary Supplement Health and Education Act. Consumers often view herbals and food supplements as safe alternatives to potentially hazardous drugs. Several herbals have even received Food and Drug Administration approval for the treatment of minor health problems.

Herbal drugs are not without certain risks and liabilities, however. Many herbals are ineffective, and several carry potential health risks. In some cases, little or no scientific evidence supports their effectiveness or safety, and some herbal proponents lack proper training in the health or botanic sciences. Consumer caution and critical thinking appears to be the middle ground that both sides agree on.

R.E.A.L. Sites

This list provides a print preview of typical **Coursewise** R.E.A.L. sites. (There are over 100 such sites at the **Courselinks**™ site.) The danger in printing URLs is that web sites can change overnight. As we went to press, these sites were functional using the URLs provided. If you come across one that isn't, please let us know via email to: webmaster@coursewise.com. Use your Passport to access the most current list of R.E.A.L. sites at the **Courselinks** site.

Site name: Editor's Choice Herbal Remedies

URL: http://www.courselinks.com/archives/health/ec12.cfm

Why is it R.E.A.L.? At this site is a discussion of the proliferation of herbal remedies on the market today. Various possible hazards regarding the use of herbals are presented, and caution when selecting an herbal remedy is recommended.

Key topics: herbals, alternative medicine

Try this: Read the article on herbal remedies. Go to the UC Davis Health Journal web site (linked) and read about each of the herbs that show medicinal promise. Select one that you might consider using yourself. What questions should you, as an informed consumer, ask before purchasing and using these supplements?

Site name: Ask Dr. Stoll

URL: http://bcn.net/~stoll/index.html

Why is it R.E.A.L.? This site is a collection of brief essays written by a medical doctor who was trained in allopathic (Western) medicine but now espouses the benefits of alternative medical practices. The site includes an interactive bulletin board that promises that "Dr. Stoll personally reads and responds to all posts directed to him within three days (unless he is ill or travelling)."

Key topics: alternative medicine, aromatherapy, American Medical Association conspiracy, health coaching

Try this: Read the articles "How to Be Healthy," "Modern Medical Interpretation of Stress," and "Why My License Was Revoked." Does Dr. Stoll offer sufficient valid evidence to support his contentions? Discuss the relative strengths and weaknesses of his arguments.

Site name: Viagra Alternatives

URL: http://www.mdhealthline.com/cgi/deliver.cgi?viagra_alternatives-mdp1208

Why is it R.E.A.L.? This commercial site offers both conventional pharmaceuticals and herbal remedies for a variety of ailments. It provides health consumers with an opportunity to examine sales and persuasion techniques used to sell two different types of products.

Key topics: alternatives, Viagra, herbals

Try this: Preview a few of the product pages. What persuasive techniques are being used? Are the sales pitches based on provable facts or on emotional appeals? Are different techniques used to advertise the herbal remedies than the prescription medications? What questions might a critical-thinking consumer want to ask before purchasing these products over the Internet?

Site name: Medicine Chest: Herbal Drugs

URL: http://www.dml.georgetown.edu/patientinfo/medchest/mcherbal.htm

Why is it R.E.A.L.? At this site, the article, "Medicine Chest: Herbal Remedies Can Be Drugs, Too" reviews many of the possible side effects associated with common herbal supplements and remedies. The article presents several testimonials on the hazards of herbal supplements by physicians who caution, "As with prescription drugs, herbal remedies are, by and large, safe, if prescribed by a health-care professional trained in herbal medicine and if taken with proper observation and caution."

Key topics: herbal remedies

Try this: How well do the authors support their positions? What persuasive techniques do they use? Are the arguments based on provable facts or emotional appeals?

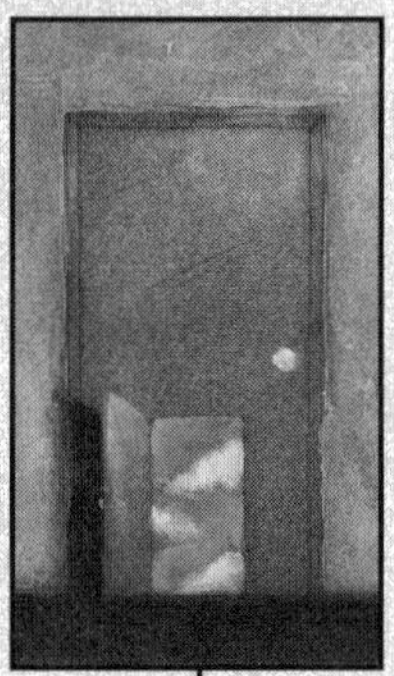

Is Vegetarianism Really Healthful?

ISSUE 3

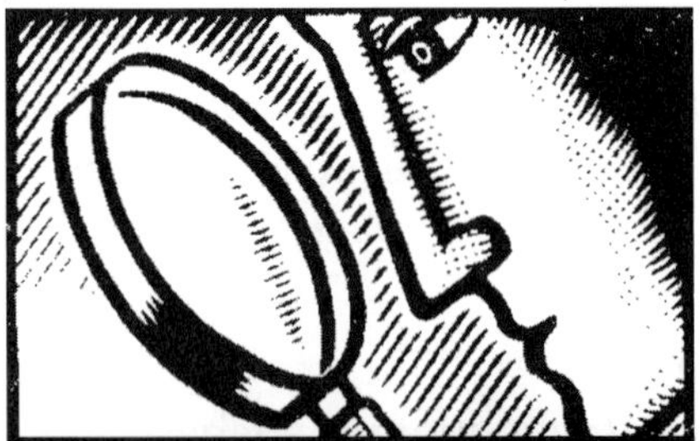

Take a Closer Look

1. What does the American Dietetic Association recommend that vegan breast-feeding mothers give their babies?
2. Into what two behavioral classes does Jarvis (Reading 8) classify vegetarians? Which of these is more likely to make health-related dietary decisions?

WiseGuide Intro

In the past twenty years, hundreds of thousands of Americans have switched to vegetarianism for health, humanitarian, and spiritual reasons. Not all vegetarian regimens are alike. Variations of vegetarianism are based on certain dietary prescriptions and proscriptions. Strict vegetarians— "vegans"—eat only vegetables and no animal products of any type. Lacto-vegetarians, however, eat vegetables and consume dairy products; ovo-vegetarians also eat eggs; lacto-ovo-vegetarians eat a combination of vegetables, dairy products, and eggs; and pesco-vegetarians eat vegetables and fish. Strict vegans make up the smallest number of vegetarians, as most allow for small quantities of animal products other than flesh in their diets.

The reasons for adopting and adhering to vegetarianism are varied. Some people are concerned about the effects of saturated fats and cholesterol from animal flesh on health risks, such as coronary heart disease and cancers. Other people see the consumption of animal products as unnecessary, cruel, and inhumane, and some call it a demonstration of "species-ism," the assumption that one species has the right to prey upon and consume another.

Compelling data show that the risks of heart attack are lower among vegetarians, as is the risk of some types of cancers. While vegetarianism may be healthful in many ways, concerns exist about the nutritional adequacy of many vegetarian diets, particularly with regard to infant and child development. Some have challenged the conclusions made from research on vegetarians, noting that vegetarians may be healthier because they also tend to participate in other healthful behaviors, such as exercising regularly and avoiding smoking. The debate over the true need and moral ramifications of consuming animals for food remains an ethical and ecological debate.

Reading 7 is the position statement of the American Dietetic Association (ADA) on vegetarian diets. The American Dietetic Association supports the concept that vegetarianism may lower risks of heart disease, hypertension, colon and breast cancer, and noninsulin dependent diabetes. The ADA acknowledges that vegetarians tend to be closer to ideal body weight than nonvegetarians and also tend to be less likely to smoke. The organization is cautious, however, regarding the nutritional adequacy of vegetarianism for what they consider to be "groups with special needs," such as infants, children, and pregnant and lactating women. The reading lists specific recommendations in terms of food groups, serving sizes, and daily servings to meet the needs of a nutritionally "adequate" vegetarian diet.

In Reading 8, "Why I Am Not a Vegetarian," William Jarvis, M.D. takes a somewhat humorous approach to discrediting what he identifies as "flawed axioms" and beliefs about vegetarianism. Jarvis uses a point-by-point approach to his rebuttals and cites scientific journal articles that support his points. He identifies two basic types of vegetarians: the "ideological vegetarian," who avoids meat for ethical reasons, and the "pragmatic vegetarian," who avoids meat for health reasons. Jarvis discusses and critiques both types of vegetarianism. He is especially critical of the ideological vegetarian, stating that vegetarianism may act as a religion built around self-denial, guilt, and asceticism. While he acknowledges that vegetarianism is not inherently unhealthy, he also points out that neither is carnivorism. Included in his critique is a discussion of the diets and Biblical philosophies of early vegetarian enthusiasts, such as John Harvey Kellogg, Mary Harmon White, and the Seventh-Day Adventists.

R E A D I N G 7

Issue 3: Is vegetarianism really healthful?

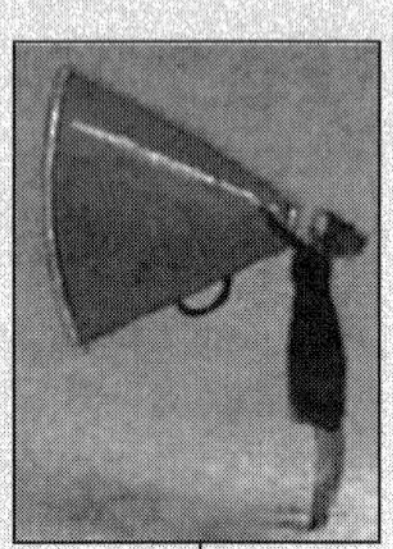

Position of the American Dietetic Association: Vegetarian Diets

Virginia K. Messina, M.P.H., R.D., and Kenneth I. Burke, P.h.D., R.D.

Scientific data suggest positive relationships between a vegetarian diet and reduced risk for several chronic degenerative diseases and conditions, including obesity, coronary artery disease, hypertension, diabetes mellitus, and some types of cancer. Vegetarian diets, like all diets, need to be planned appropriately to be nutritionally adequate.

Position Statement

It is the position of The American Dietetic Association (ADA) that appropriately planned vegetarian diets are healthful, are nutritionally adequate, and provide health benefits in the prevention and treatment of certain diseases.

Vegetarianism in Perspective

The eating patterns of vegetarians vary considerably. The lacto-ovo-vegetarian eating pattern is based on grains, vegetables, fruits, legumes, seeds, nuts, dairy products, and eggs, and excludes meat, fish, and fowl. The vegan, or total vegetarian, eating pattern is similar to the lacto-ovo-vegetarian pattern except for the additional exclusion of eggs, dairy, and other animal products. Even within these patterns, considerable variation may exist in the extent to which animal products are avoided. Therefore, individual assessment is required to accurately evaluate the nutritional quality of a vegetarian's dietary intake.

Studies indicate that vegetarians often have lower morbidity[1] and mortality[2] rates from several chronic degenerative diseases than do nonvegetarians. Although nondietary factors, including physical activity and abstinence from smoking and alcohol, may play a role, diet is clearly a contributing factor.

In addition to the health advantages, other considerations that may lead a person to adopt a vegetarian diet pattern include concern for the environment, ecology, and world hunger issues. Vegetarians also cite economic reasons, ethical considerations, and religious beliefs as their reasons for following this type of diet pattern. Consumer demand for vegetarian options has resulted in increasing numbers of foodservices that offer vegetarian options. Presently, most university foodservices offer vegetarian options.

Health Implications of Vegetarianism

Vegetarian diets low in fat or saturated fat have been used successfully as part of comprehensive health programs to reverse severe coronary artery disease.[3,4] Vegetarian diets offer disease protection benefits because of their lower saturated fat, cholesterol, and animal protein content and often higher concentration of folate (which reduces serum homocysteine levels),[5] antioxidants such as vitamins C and E, carotenoids, and phytochemicals.[6] Not only is mortality from coronary artery disease lower in vegetarians than in nonvegetarians,[7] but vegetarian diets have also been successful in arresting coronary artery disease.[8,9] Total serum cholesterol and low-density lipoprotein cholesterol levels are usually lower in vegetarians, but high-density lipoprotein cholesterol and triglyceride levels vary depending on the type of vegetarian diet followed.[10]

Vegetarians tend to have a lower incidence of hypertension than nonvegetarians.[11] This effect appears to be independent of both body weight and sodium intake. Type 2 diabetes mellitus is much less likely to be a cause of death in vegetarians than nonvegetarians, perhaps because of their higher intake of complex carbohydrates and lower body mass index.[12]

Incidence of lung and colorectal cancer is lower in vegetarians than in nonvegetarians.[2,13] Reduced colorectal cancer risk is associated with increased consumption of fiber, vegetables, and fruit.[14,15] The environment of the colon differs notably in vegetarians compared with non-

Position of the American Dietetic Association: Vegetarian Diets. JOURNAL OF THE AMERICAN DIETETIC ASSOCIATION, 1997; 97: 1317–1321. Reprinted by permission.

vegetarians in ways that could favorably affect colon cancer risk.[16,17] Lower breast cancer rates have not been observed in Western vegetarians, but cross-cultural data indicate that breast cancer rates are lower in populations that consume plant-based diets.[18] The lower estrogen levels in vegetarian women may be protective.[19]

A well-planned vegetarian diet may be useful in the prevention and treatment of renal disease. Studies using human being and animal models suggest that some plant proteins may increase survival rates and decrease proteinuria, glomerular filtration rate, renal blood flow, and histologic renal damage compared with a nonvegetarian diet.[20,21]

Nutrition Considerations for Vegetarians

Plant sources of protein alone can provide adequate amounts of essential amino acids if a variety of plant foods are consumed and energy needs are met. Research suggests that complementary proteins do not need to be consumed at the same time and that consumption of various sources of amino acids over the course of the day should ensure adequate nitrogen retention and use in healthy persons.[22] Although vegetarian diets are lower in total protein and a vegetarian's protein needs may be somewhat elevated because of the lower quality of some plant proteins, protein intake in both lacto-ovo-vegetarians and vegans appears to be adequate.[16]

Plant foods contain only nonheme iron, which is more sensitive than heme iron to both inhibitors and enhancers of iron absorption. Although vegetarian diets are higher in total iron content than nonvegetarian diets, iron stores are lower in vegetarians because the iron from plant foods is more poorly absorbed.[23] The clinical importance of this, if any, is unclear because iron deficiency anemia rates are similar in vegetarians and nonvegetarians.[23] The higher vitamin C content of vegetarian diets may improve iron absorption.

Although plant foods can contain vitamin B-12 on their surface from soil residues, this is not a reliable source of B-12 for vegetarians. Much of the vitamin B-12 present in spirulina, sea vegetables, tempeh, and miso has been shown to be inactive B-12 analog rather than the active vitamin. Although dairy products and eggs contain vitamin B-12, research suggests that lacto-ovo-vegetarians have low blood levels of vitamin B-12. Supplementation or use of fortified foods is advised for vegetarians who avoid or limit animal foods.[24]

Because vitamin B-12 requirements are small, and it is both stored and recycled in the body, symptoms of deficiency may be delayed for years. Absorption of vitamin B-12 becomes less efficient as the body ages, so supplements may be advised for all older vegetarians.

Lacto-ovo-vegetarians have calcium intakes that are comparable to or higher than those of nonvegetarians.[25,26] Calcium intakes of vegans, however, are generally lower than those of both lacto-ovo-vegetarians and omnivores.[26] It should be noted that vegans may have lower calcium needs than nonvegetarians because diets that are low in total protein and more alkaline have been shown to have a calcium-sparing effect.[27] Furthermore, when a person's diet is low in both protein and sodium and regular weight-bearing physical activity is engaged in, his or her calcium requirements may be lower than those of a sedentary person who eats a standard Western diet. These factors, and genetic influences, may help explain variations in bone health that are independent of calcium intake.

Because calcium requirements of vegans have not been established and inadequate calcium intakes are linked to risk for osteoporosis in all women, vegans should meet the calcium requirements established for their age group by the Institute of Medicine.[28] Calcium is well absorbed from many plant foods, and vegan diets can provide adequate calcium if the diet regularly includes foods rich in calcium.[29] In addition, many new vegetarian foods are calcium-fortified. Dietary supplements are advised for vegans only if they do not meet calcium requirements from food.

Vitamin D is poorly supplied in all diets unless vitamin-D–fortified foods are consumed. Vegan diets may lack this nutrient because fortified cow's milk is its most common dietary source. However, vegan foods supplemented with vitamin D, such as soymilk and some cereals, are available. Furthermore, findings indicate that sunlight exposure is a major factor affecting vitamin D status and that dietary intake is important only when sun exposure is inadequate.[30] Sun exposure to hands, arms, and face for 5 to 15 minutes per day is believed to be adequate to provide sufficient amounts of vitamin D.[31] People with dark skin or those who live at northern latitudes or in cloudy or smoggy areas may need increased exposure. Use of sunscreen interferes with vitamin D synthesis. If sun exposure is inadequate, vitamin D supplements are recommended for vegans. This is especially true for older persons who synthesize vitamin D less efficiently and who may have less sun exposure.

Studies show zinc intake to be lower or comparable in vegetarians compared with nonvegetarians.[16] Most studies show that zinc levels in hair, serum, and saliva are in the normal range in vegetarians.[32] Compensatory mechanisms may help vegetarians adapt to diets that may be low in zinc.[33] However, because of the low bioavailability of zinc from plant foods and because the effects of marginal zinc status are poorly understood, vegetarians should strive to meet or exceed the Recommended Dietary Allowances for zinc.

Diets that do not include fish or eggs lack the long-chain n-3 fatty acid docosahexanoic acid (DHA).

Figure 1 **Food Sources of Nutrients**

Iron	Milligrams per Serving
Breads, cereals, and grains	
Whole wheat bread, 1 slice	0.9
White bread, 1 slice	0.7
Bran flakes, 1 c	11.0
Cream of wheat, 1/2 c cooked	5.5
Oatmeal, instant, 1 packet	6.3
Wheat germ, 2 Tbsp	1.2
Vegetables (1/2 c cooked)	
Beet greens	1.4
Sea vegetables	18.1–42.0
Swiss chard	1.9
Tomato juice, 1 c	1.3
Turnip greens	1.5
Legumes (1/2 c cooked)	
Baked beans, vegetarian	0.74
Black beans	1.8
Garbanzo beans	3.4
Kidney beans	1.5
Lentils	3.2
Lima beans	2.2
Navy beans	2.5
Soyfoods (1/2 c cooked)	
Soybeans	4.4
Tempeh	1.8
Tofu	6.6
Soymilk, 1 c	1.8
Nuts/seeds (2 Tbsp)	
Cashews	1.0
Pumpkin seeds	2.5
Tahini	1.2
Sunflower seeds	1.2
Other foods	
Blackstrap molasses, 1 Tbsp	3.3

Calcium	Milligrams per Serving
Legumes (1 c cooked)	
Chickpeas	78
Great northern beans	121
Navy beans	128
Pinto beans	82
Black beans	103
Vegetarian baked beans	128
Soyfoods	
Soybeans, 1 c cooked	175
Tofu, 1/2 c	120–350
Tempeh, 1/2 c	77
Textured vegetable protein, 1/2 c	85
Soymilk, 1 c	84
Soymilk, fortified, 1 c	250–300
Soynuts, 1/2 c	252
Nuts and seeds (2 Tbsp)	
Almonds	50
Almond butter	86
Vegetables (1/2 c Cooked)	
Bok choy	79
Broccoli	89
Collard greens	178
Kale	90
Mustard greens	75
Turnip greens	125
Fruits	
Dried figs, 5	258
Calcium-fortified orange juice, 1 c	300
Other Foods	
Blackstrap molasses, 1 Tbsp	187
Cow's milk, 1 c	300
Yogurt, 1 c	275–400

Vegetarians may have lower blood lipid levels of this fatty acid, although not all studies are in agreement with this finding.[34,35] The essential fatty acid linolenic acid can be converted to DHA, although conversion rates appear to be inefficient and high intakes of linoleic acid interfere with conversion.[36] The implications of low levels of DHA is not clear. However, it is recommended that vegetarians include good sources of linolenic acid in their diet.

Figure 1 presents food sources of nutrients that are often of concern for vegetarians.

Vegetarianism throughout the Life Cycle

Well-planned vegan and lacto-ovo-vegetarian diets are appropriate for all stages of the life cycle, including during pregnancy and lactation. Appropriately planned vegan and lacto-ovo-vegetarian diets satisfy nutrient needs of infants, children, and adolescents and promote normal growth.[37] Dietary deficiencies are most likely to be observed in populations with very restrictive diets. All vegan children should have a reliable source of vitamin B-12 and, if sun exposure is limited, vitamin D supplements or fortified foods should be used. Foods rich in calcium, iron, and zinc should be emphasized. Frequent meals and snacks and the use of some refined foods and foods higher in fat can help vegetarian children meet energy needs. Guidelines for iron and vitamin D supplements and for the introduction of solid foods are the same for vegetarian and nonvegetarian infants. When it is time for protein-rich foods to be introduced, vegetarian infants can have

Figure 1 Food Sources of Nutrients *(continued)*

Zinc	Milligrams per Serving
Breads, grains, and cereals	
Bran flakes, 1 c	5.0
Wheat germ, 2 Tbsp	2.3
Legumes (1/2 c cooked)	
Adzuki beans	2.0
Chickpeas	1.3
Lima beans	1.0
Lentils	1.2
Soyfoods (1/2 c cooked)	
Soybeans	1.0
Tempeh	1.5
Tofu	1.0
Textured vegetable protein	1.4
Vegetables (1/2 c cooked)	
Corn	0.9
Peas	1.0
Sea vegetables	1.1–2.0
Dairy foods	
Cow's milk, 1 c	1.0
Cheddar cheese, 1 oz	0.9
Yogurt, 1 c	1.8

Vitamin D	Micrograms per Serving
Fortified, ready-to-eat cereals, 3/4 c	1.0–2.5
Fortified soy milk or other nondairy milk, 1c	1.0–2.5

Vitamin B-12	Micrograms per Serving
Ready-to-eat breakfast cereals, 3/4 c	1.5–6.0
Meat analogs (1 burger or 1 serving according to package)	2.0–7.0
Fortified soymilk or other nondairy milks, 8 oz	0.2–5.0
Nutritional yeast (Red Star Vegetarian Support Formula, formerly T6635[a]), 1 Tbsp	4.0

Linolenic Acid	Grams per Serving
Flax seed, 2 Tbsp	4.3
Walnuts, 1 oz	1.9
Walnut oil, 1 Tbsp	1.5
Canola oil, 1 Tbsp	1.6
Linseed oil, 1 Tbsp	7.6
Soybean oil, 1 Tbsp	0.9
Soybeans, 1/2 c cooked	0.5
Tofu, 1/2 c	0.4

Sources: Package information and data from: Pennington J. *Bowe's and Church's Food Values of Portions Commonly Used.* 16th ed. Lippincott-Raven; 1994. *Provisional Table on the Content of Omega-3 Fatty Acids and Other Fat components in Selected Foods, 1988.* Washington, DC: U.S. Dept of Agriculture: 1988: Publication No. HNIS/PT-103. Hytowitz DB, Matthews RH. *Composition of Foods: Legumes and Legume Products.* Washington, DC: U.S. Dept. of Agriculture; 1986. Agriculture Handbook No. 8–16.

[a]Red Star Yeast and Products, a division of Universal Foods Corp, Milwaukee, Wisc.

pureed tofu, cottage cheese, and legumes (pureed and strained). Breast-fed vegan infants should receive a source of vitamin B-12 if the mother's diet is not supplemented and a source of vitamin D if sun exposure is inadequate.

Vegetarian diets are somewhat more common among adolescents with eating disorders than in the general adolescent population; therefore, dietetics professionals should be aware of young clients who greatly limit food choices and who exhibit symptoms of eating disorders.[38] However, recent data suggest that adopting a vegetarian diet does not lead to eating disorders.[39] With guidance in meal planning, vegetarian diets are appropriate and healthful choices for adolescents.

Vegetarian diets can also meet the needs of competitive athletes. Protein needs may be elevated because training increases amino acid metabolism, but vegetarian diets that meet energy needs and include good sources of protein (e.g., soyfoods, legumes) can provide adequate protein without use of special foods or supplements. For adolescent athletes, special attention should be given to meeting energy, protein, and iron needs. Amenorrhea may be more common among vegetarian than nonvegetarian athletes, although not all research supports this finding.[40,41] Efforts to maintain normal menstrual cycles might include increasing energy and fat intake, reducing fiber, and reducing strenuous training.

Lacto-ovo-vegetarian and vegan diets can meet the nutrient and energy needs of pregnant women. Birth weights of infants born to well nourished vegetarian women have been shown to be similar to birth-weight norms and to birth weights of infants of nonvegetarians.[42] Diets of pregnant and lactating vegans should be supplemented with 2.0 micrograms and 2.6 micrograms, respectively, of vitamin B-12 daily and, if sun exposure is

Figure 2 **Food Guide Pyramid for Vegetarian Meal Planning**

Fats, Oils, and Sweets
Use sparingly

candy
butter
margarine
salad dressing
cooking oil

Milk, Yogurt, and Cheese Group **0–3 servings daily***	**Dry Beans, Nuts, Seeds, Eggs, and Meat Substitutes Group** **2–3 servings daily**
milk—1 cup yogurt—1 cup natural cheese—1 1/2 oz *Vegetarians who choose not to use milk, yogurt, or cheese need to select other food sources rich in calcium. For a list of calcium-rich foods, please see Figure 1.	soy milk—1 cup cooked dry beans or peas—1/2 cup 1 egg or 2 egg whites nuts or seeds—2 Tbsp tofu or tempeh—1/4 cup peanut butter—2 Tbsp
Vegetable Group **3–5 servings daily**	**Fruit Group** **2–4 servings daily**
cooked or chopped raw vegetables—1/2 cup raw leafy vegetables—1 cup	juice—3/4 cup dried fruit—1/4 cup chopped, raw fruit—1/2 cup canned fruit—1/2 cup 1 medium-size piece of fruit, such as banana, apple, or orange

Bread, Cereal, Rice, and Pasta Group
6–11 servings daily

bread—1 slice
ready-to-eat cereal—1 oz
cooked cereal—1/2 cup
cooked rice, pasta, or other grains—1/2 cup
bagel—1/2

limited, with 10 micrograms vitamin D daily.[43,44] Supplements of folate are advised for all pregnant women, although vegetarian women typically have higher intakes than nonvegetarians.

Meal Planning for Vegetarian Diets

A variety of menu-planning approaches can provide vegetarians with adequate nutrition. Figure 2 suggests one approach. In addition, the following guidelines can help vegetarians plan healthful diets.

- Choose a variety of foods, including whole grains, vegetables, fruits, legumes, nuts, seeds and, if desired, dairy products and eggs.
- Choose whole, unrefined foods often and minimize intake of highly sweetened, fatty, and heavily refined foods.
- Choose a variety of fruits and vegetables.
- If animal foods such as dairy products and eggs are used, choose lower-fat versions of these foods. Cheeses

and other high-fat dairy foods and eggs should be limited in the diet because of their saturated fat content and because their frequent use displaces plant foods in some vegetarian diets.

- Vegans should include a regular source of vitamin B-12 in their diets along with a source of vitamin D if sun exposure is limited.
- Solely breast-fed infants should have supplements of iron after the age of 4 to 6 months and, if sun exposure is limited, a source of vitamin D. Breast-fed vegan infants should have vitamin B-12 supplements if the mother's diet is not fortified.
- Do not restrict dietary fat in children younger than 2 years. For older children, include some foods higher in unsaturated fats (e.g., nuts, seeds, nut and seed butters, avocado, and vegetable oils) to help meet nutrient and energy needs.

References

1. Knutsen SF. Lifestyle and the use of health services. *Am J Clin Nutr.* 1994;59(suppl):1171S–1175S.
2. Key TH, Thorogood M, Appleby PM, Burr ML. Dietary habits and mortality in 11,000 vegetarian and health conscious people: results of a 17-year follow up. *BMJ.* 1996; 313:775–779.
3. Franklin TL, Kolasa KM, Griffin K, Mayo C, Badenhop DT. Adherence to very low fat diet by a group of cardiac rehabilitation patients in the rural southeastern United States. *Arch Fam Med.* 1995; 4:551–554.
4. Gould KL, Ornish, D, Scherwitz L, Brown S, Edens RP, Hess MJ, Mullani N, Bolomey L, Dobbs F, Armstrong WT, Merritt T, Ports T, Sparler S, Billings J. Changes in myocardial perusion abnormalities by positron emission tomography after long-term intense risk factor modification. *JAMA.* 1995; 274:894–901.
5. Janelle KC, Barr SI. Nutrient intakes and eating behavior scores of vegetarian and nonvegetarian women. *J Am Diet Assoc.* 1995; 95:180–189.
6. Jacob RA, Burri BJ. Oxidative damage and defense. *Am J Clin Nutr.* 1996; 63(suppl):985S-990S.
7. Thorogood M, Mann J, Appleby P, McPherson K. Risk of death from cancer and ischaemic heart disease in meat and non-meat eaters. *BMJ.* 1994; 308:1667–1670.
8. Fraser GE, Lindsted KD, Beeson WL. Effect of risk factor values on lifetime risk of and age at first coronary event. The Adventist Health Study. *Am J Epidemiol.* 1995; 142:746–758.
9. Roberts WC. Preventing and arresting coronary atherosclerosis. *Am Heart J.* 1995; 130:580–600.
10. Melby CL, Toohey ML, Cedrick J. Blood pressure and blood lipids among vegetarian, semivegetarian and nonvegetarian African Americans. *Am J Clin Nutr.* 1994; 59:103–109.
11. Beilin LJ. Vegetarian and other complex diets, fats, fiber, and hypertension. *Am J Clin Nutr.* 1994; 59(suppl):1130–1135.
12. Dwyer JT. Health aspects of vegetarian diets. *Am J Clin Nutr.* 1988; 48(suppl):712–738.
13. Mills PK, Beeson WL, Phillips RL, Fraser GE. Cancer incidence among California Seventh-day Adventists, 1976–1982. *Am J Clin Nutr.* 1994; 59(suppl):1136S–1142S.
14. Almendingen K, Trygg K, Vatn M. [Influence of the diet on cell proliferation in the large bowel and the rectum. Does a strict vegetarian diet reduce the risk of intestinal cancer?] *Tidsskr Nor Laegeforen.* 1995; 115(18):2252–2256.
15. Steinmetz KA, Potter JD. Vegetables, fruit and cancer. II. Mechanisms. *Cancer Causes Control.* 1991; 1:427–442.
16. Messina MJ, Messina VL. *The Dietitian's Guide to Vegetarian Diets: Issues and Applications.* Gaithersburg, MD: Aspen Publishers; 1996.
17. Adlercreutz H, van der Wildt J, Kinzel J, Attalla H, Wahalla K, Makela T, Hase T, Fotsis T. Lignan and isoflavonoid conjugates in human urine. *J Steroid Biochem Mol Biol.* 1995; 59:97–103.
18. *Cancer Facts and Figures—1994.* Atlanta, Ga: American Cancer Society; 1994.
19. Barbosa JC, Shultz TD, Filley SJ, Nieman DC. The relationship among adiposity, diet and hormone concentrations in vegetarian and nonvegetarian postmenopausal women. *Am J Clin Nutr.* 1990;51:798–803.
20. Pagenkemper J. The impact of vegetarian diets on renal disease. *Top Clin Nutr.* 1995; 10:22–26.
21. Barsotti G, Morelli E, Cupisti A, Meola M, Dani L, Giovannetti S. A low-nitrogen, low-phosphorus vegan diet for patients with chronic renal failure. *Nephron.* 1996; 74:390–394.
22. Young VR, Pellett PL. Plant proteins in relation to human protein and amino acid nutrition. *Am J Clin Nutr.* 1994; 59(suppl 5):1203S–1212S.
23. Craig WJ. Iron status of vegetarians. *Am J Clin Nutr.* 1994; 59(suppl):1233S–1237S.
24. Helman AD, Darnton-Hill I. Vitamin and iron status in new vegetarians. *Am J Clin Nutr.* 1987; 45:785–789.
25. Slatter ML, Jacobs DR, Hilner JE Jr, Caan BJ, Van Horn L, Bragg C, Manolio TA, Kushi LH, Liu D. Meat consumption and its association with other diet and health factors in young adults: the CARDIA study. *Am J Clin Nutr.* 1992; 56:699–704.
26. Tesar R, Notelovitz M, Shim E, Dauwell G, Brown J. Axial and peripheral bone density and nutrient intakes of post-menopausal vegetarian and omnivorous women. *Am J Clin Nutr.* 1992; 56:699–704.
27. Remer T, Manz F. Estimation of the renal net acid excretion by adults consuming diets containing variable amounts of protein. *Am J Clin Nutr.* 1994; 59:1356–1361.
28. National Academy of Sciences, Institute of Medicine. *Dietary Reference Intakes for Calcium, Phosphorus, Magnesium, Vitamin D and Fluoride.* Washington, DC: National Academy Press; 1997.
29. Weaver CM, Plawecki KL. Dietary calcium: adequacy of a vegetarian diet. *Am J Clin Nutr.* 1994; 59(suppl):1238S–1241S.
30. Henderson JB, Dunnigan MG, McIntosh WB, Abdul-Motaal AA, Gettinby G, Glekin BM. The importance of limited exposure to ultraviolet radiation and dietary factors in the aetiology of Asian rickets: A risk-factor model. *QJM.* 1987; 63:413–425.
31. Holuck MF. Vitamin D and bone health. *J Nutr.* 1996; 126(suppl):1159S–1164S.
32. Freeland-Graves JH, Bodzy PW, Epright MA. Zinc status of vegetarians. *J Am Diet Assoc.* 1980; 77:655–661.
33. Lei S, Mingyan X, Miller LV, Tong L, Krebs NF, Hambidge KM. Zinc absorption and intestinal losses of endogenous zinc in young Chinese women with marginal zinc intakes. *Am J Clin Nutr.* 1996; 63:348–353.
34. Sanders TAB, Roshanai F. Platelet phospholipid fatty acid composition and function in vegans compared with age- and sex-matched omnivore controls. *Eur J Clin Nutr.* 1992; 46:823–831.

35. Conquer JA, Holub BJ. Dietary docosahexaenoic acid as a source of eicosapentaenoic acid in vegetarians and omnivores. *Lipids.* 1997; 32:341–345.
36. Emken EA, Adolf RO, Gulley RM. Dietary linoleic acid influences desaturation and acylation of deuterium-labeled linoleic and linolenic acids in young adult males. *Biochim Biophys Acta.* 1994; 1213:277–288.
37. Sanders TAB, Reddy S. Vegetarian diets and children. *Am J Clin Nutr.* 1994; 59(suppl):1176S–1181S.
38. O'Connor MA, Touyz SW, Dunn SM, Beaumont PJV. Vegetarianism in anorexia nervosa? A review of 116 consecutive cases. *Med J Aust.* 1987; 147:540–542.
39. Janelle KC, Barr SI. Nutrient intakes and eating behavior scores of vegetarian and nonvegetarian women. *J Am Diet Assoc.* 1995; 95:180–189.
40. Pedersen AB, Bartholomew MJ, Dolence LA, Aljadir LP, Netteburg KL, Lloyd T. Menstrual differences due to vegetarian and nonvegetarian diets. *Am J Clin Nutr.* 1991; 54:520–525.
41. Slavin J, Lutter J, Cushman S. Amenorrhea in vegetarian athletes. *Lancet.* 1984; 1:474–1475.
42. O'Connell JM, Dibley MJ, Sierra J, Wallace B, Marks JS, Yip R. Growth of vegetarian children: The Farm Study. *Pediatrics.* 1989; 84:475–481.
43. Food and Nutrition Board, Institute of Medicine. *Nutrition During Pregnancy.* Washington, DC: National Academy Press; 1991.
44. Food and Nutrition Board, Institute of Medicine. *Nutrition During Lactation.* Washington, DC: National Academy Press; 1991.

FRAME the DEBATE

Form at end of book

Issue 3: Is vegetarianism really healthful?

Why I Am Not a Vegetarian

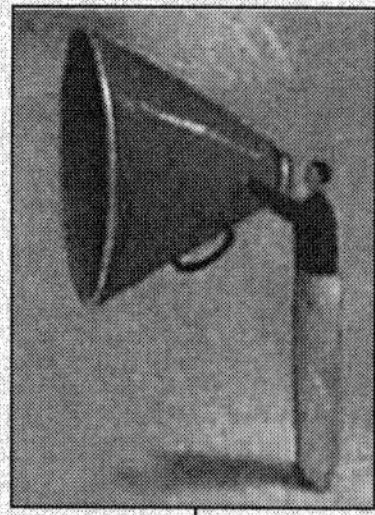

William T. Jarvis

ACSH advisor William T. Jarvis, Ph.D., is a professor of public health and preventive medicine at Loma Linda University, founder and president of the National Council Against Health Fraud, and coeditor of The Health Robbers: A Close Look at Quackery in America *(1993). This article is an adaptation of one published by Prometheus Books (Amherst, New York) in the November/December 1996 issue of* Nutrition & Health Forum *newsletter.*

Vegetarianism has taken on a "political correctness" comparable to the respectability it had in the last century, when many social and scientific progressives advocated it. Today, crusaders extol meatless eating not only as healthful but also as a solution to world hunger and as a safeguard of "Mother Earth." The Physicians Committee for Responsible Medicine (PCRM) aggressively attacks the use of animal foods and has proposed its own food-groups model, which excludes all animal products.

I disclaimed vegetarianism after many years of observance. Although the arguments in favor of it appear compelling, I have learned to be suspicious, and to search for hidden agendas, when I evaluate claims of the benefits of vegetarianism. Vegetarianism is riddled with delusional thinking from which even scientists and medical professionals are not immune.

Don't get me wrong: I know that meatless diets can be healthful, even desirable, for some people. For example: (a) Men with an iron-loading gene are better off without red meat, because it contains heme iron, which is highly absorbable and can increase their risk of heart disease. (b) Because vegetarian diets are likely to contain less saturated fat than nonvegetarian diets, they may be preferable for persons with familial hypercholesterolemia. (c) Vegetables contain phytochemicals that appear protective against colorectal cancer. (d) Homocysteinemia (elevated plasma homocysteine) approximately doubles the risk of coronary artery disease. Several congenital and nutritional disorders, including deficiencies of vitamins B6 and B12 and folic acid, can cause this condition. Since folic acid occurs mostly in vegetables, low intakes of the vitamin are less likely among vegetarians than among nonvegetarians. (e) Some people find that being a vegetarian helps to control their weight. Vegetarianism tends to facilitate weight control because it is a form of food restriction; and in our overfed society, food restriction is a plus unless it entails a deficit of some essential nutrient.

However, one need not eliminate meat from one's diet for any of the foregoing reasons. Apparently, it is ample consumption of fruits and vegetables, not the exclusion of meat, that makes vegetarianism healthful.

Dog Day Afternoon?

The term "vegetarian" is misleading, for it is not a name for people who favor vegetable consumption, but a code word for those who *dis* favor or protest the consumption of animal foods. The neologism *anticarnivorist* better characterizes the majority of those who call themselves vegetarians. I call myself a "vegetable enthusiast," because I strongly encourage eating lots of vegetables, including legumes, whole grains, and fruits. I believe that these foods are desirable not only because of their high nutrient density and low caloric density, but also because of aesthetic and gustatory factors. Being a vegetable enthusiast doesn't entail rejecting the use of meat or animal products.

Most people who categorize vegetarians identify at least five different kinds, based on which types of animal food they consume: *Semivegetarians* consume dairy products, eggs, fish, and chicken; *pesco-vegetarians* consume dairy products, eggs, and fish; *lacto-ovo-vegetarians,* dairy products and eggs; *ovo-vegetarians,* eggs; and *vegans,* no animal foods except honey. From a behavioral standpoint, I categorize vegetarians as either pragmatic or ideologic. A *pragmatic vegetarian* is one whose dietary behavior stems from objective health considerations (e.g., hypercholesterolemia or obesity). Pragmatic vegetarians are rational, rather than emotional, in their approach to making lifestyle decisions. In contrast, vegetarianism is a "matter of principle" for *ideologic vegetarians;* its appropriateness is a given.

One can spot ideologic vegetarians by their exaggerations of the benefits of vegetarianism, their lack of skepticism, and their failure to recognize (or their glossing over of) the potential risks even of extreme vegetarian diets. Ideologic vegetarians make a pretense of being scientific, but they approach the subject of vegetarianism more like lawyers than scientists. Promoters of vegetarianism gather data selectively and gear their arguments toward discrediting information that is contrary to their dogma. This approach to defending a position is suitable for a debate, but it cannot engender scientific understanding.

Because of the influence of my Seventh-Day Adventist (SDA) environment, I practiced vegetarianism for many years. My wife and I even tried to give up consuming all animal products, but this didn't work. We sometimes muse aloud about the morning we put soymilk on our breakfast cereal. We ended up eating the cereal with a fork because we found the mixture repulsive. We had another unforgettable experience when we ate with a group of vegetarian hippies in the Oregon woods. We were there at their request to advise them on vegetarian eating. They had already prepared the worst-looking vegetarian stew I have ever seen or tasted. It consisted of raw peanuts and a variety of half-cooked vegetables. After eating it, I had heartburn for hours. Digestive distress is legendary among SDAs.

Reasons for adopting vegetarianism can be very personal. Some years ago I shared a podium for several days with a vegetarian. It became clear from our informal conversations that he was not religious; so I asked him why he had opted for vegetarianism. He told me a touching story about having been a lonely boy whose closest companion was his pet dog. He said that, peering into the dog's eyes one day, he had come to see the animal as a fellow being. Soon he had applied this view to all animals, and since he could not bear the thought of eating his dog, he could no longer eat other animals.

North by Northwest

Darla Erhardt, R.D., M.P.H., listed five vegetarian postulates: (1) All forms of life are sacred, and all creatures have a right to live out their natural lives. (2) It is anatomically clear that God did not design humans to eat meat. (3) Slaughter is repugnant and degrading. (4) Raising animals for meat is inefficient and misuses available land. (5) Animal flesh is unhealthful because it contains toxins, virulent bacteria, uric acid, impure fluids, and the wrong kinds of nutrients.[1] I find all of these axioms flawed:

1. The belief that all life is sacred can lead to absurdities such as allowing mosquitoes to spread malaria, or vipers to run loose on one's premises. Inherent in the idea that all life is sacred is the supposition that all forms of life have equal value. The natural world reveals hierarchies in the food chain, the dominance of certain species over others. And most creatures in the wild die (usually the victim of a predator) long before they have reached the genetic limit on their longevity.

2. The multifarious dietary practices of human populations belie the notion that humans are designed to be vegetarians rather than omnivores. For example, Australian aborigines consume insect larvae and reptiles, Eskimos eat raw meat, and traditional Hindus are vegetarians.

The first SDA physician, John Harvey Kellogg (1852–1943), was a vegetarian zealot. Alonzo Baker, Ph.D., his former private secretary, told me of an incident that occurred circa 1939: Kellogg awakened him in the middle of the night and ordered him to board the morning train for Cleveland. There, Weston Price, D.D.S., who had just returned from the mysterious high north, was to give a report on Eskimo dietary habits. When Baker returned, he informed Kellogg of Price's finding that Eskimos ate raw meat almost exclusively (*eskimo* literally means "raw meat eater"). Kellogg accused Price of lying.

Perhaps Kellogg disbelieved Price partly because it was widely known that the 1898 Yukon gold rushers had suffered extensively from scurvy. People generally believed that Eskimos derived their vitamin C from berries the snow had preserved. In fact, Eskimos derive vitamin C from the raw meat of animals who synthesize ascorbic acid. If they had cooked their meat, they would have developed scurvy like the gold rushers. (When I visited Northwest Territories, Canada, in 1973, a Franciscan monk who raised beautiful vegetables in a greenhouse in Pelly Bay told me that the Inuits, or North American Eskimos, didn't like their taste and wouldn't eat them.)

3. Whether something is repugnant is highly individual. Hindus who will not eat animal foods readily drink their own urine for the sake of health. And what is repugnant—for example, chores such as changing a baby's diaper or caring for sick people—is not necessarily wrong. Whether such activities are degrading is a matter of opinion. That most prey are eaten while they are still alive testifies to the heartlessness of nature compared to slaughterhouses, where death is generally quick and painless.

4. The idea that animal-raising is an inefficient way to produce food is half-baked. Animals pull their weight when it comes to land-use and food-production efficiency: They graze on lands unsuitable for crop-growing, eat those portions of plants that are considered inedible (e.g., corn stalks and husks), and provide byproducts and services that ease human burdens.[2] Many nomadic populations survive on lands that lack farming potential by feeding on animals whose nourishment is coarse vegetation humans can't digest.

5. The postulate that toxins render meat unfit as food also lacks merit. Plants also contain naturally occurring toxicants, many of which are far more deadly than those of animal flesh.[3] Vegetarian evangelists who revel in portraying animal foods as unhealthful disregard the fact that those societies that consume the most animal products enjoy record longevity. They also overlook the reality that the animals they brand as diseased are herbivores whose diet consists entirely of raw vegetation. These animals develop many diseases "despite" becoming vegans after weaning.

Ideologic Vegetarianism

Much of my professional life has been spent studying health fraud, quackery, and related misinformation, and their impact on people's lives. I have discerned a recurrent sequence of behaviors: First, the prospective vegetarian eliminates reportedly unhealthful foods from his or her diet, beginning with foods that society considers "bad for you" (e.g., sugar, coffee, and white bread). Next, if concerns about food safety grow to neurotic proportions, the person scrutinizes labels and worries about ingredients indicated by terms he doesn't understand. Then he may patronize health food stores, where clerks and publications can feed his phobias. He may treat modern foods as poisonous. Finally, if he deems vegetarianism not restrictive enough, the "health foodist" may turn to veganism. In my opinion, it is at this point that vegetarianism becomes hazardous, especially for children.

The case of Sonja and Khachadour Atikian illustrates what can happen to those seduced by ideologic vegetarianism. The Atikians were from Lebanon who—because of unrelenting media barrages focusing on environmental pollution, diet, and health—became overly concerned about the safety and healthfulness of modern foods. Sonja Atikian began shopping at health food stores instead of supermarkets. Gerhardt Hanswille, a self-styled herbalist from Germany, taught classes in the rear of a health food store she patronized. Although Hanswille was not licensed to practice medicine, he saw 40 to 45 "patients" a day. He treated Ms. Atikian for a sore knee, and she took some of his courses. Hanswille taught that: (a) people should not kill animals, nor consume animal products; (b) God intended cow's milk to be food for calves, not human babies; (c) eating eggs deprives hens of fulfilling their divinely intended role as mothers; (d) people should not poison themselves or the earth with the unnatural products of modern living; (e) using herbs both as food and as medicine is God's way; and (f) the medicines of doctors are poisons. "Choose whom you will believe," said Hanswille, "me or the doctors. You can't have it both ways."

Ms. Atikian chose poorly. Except for eating fish occasionally, she followed the herbalist's advice during pregnancy. She delivered a healthy 8.2-lb girl named Loreie. Hanswille convinced the Atikians that the newborn would become a superbaby if they gave her a vegetarian diet of raw, organic foods. He dissuaded them from having the infant immunized and from continuing to see a pediatrician. And he induced them to rely on him for healthcare advice.

Four and a half months after her birth, Loreie's weight was still at the 75th percentile, but when she was 11 months old, breast-feeding—her sole source of animal food—discontinued. Fed only fruits, vegetables, and rice, she eventually stopped growing, slept more and more, and had more and more infections. As the baby's health spiraled downward, Hanswille assured the parents that her decline was merely "the poisons coming out of her body" and that she would eventually become the superbaby they desired. In 1987, 17-month-old Loreie died of bronchial pneumonia complicated by severe malnutrition. She weighed 11 1/4 lbs. The Atikians were charged with failing to provide their daughter with the "necessaries of life." Their defense was that they had truly believed they had been providing the "necessaries of life" when they followed Hanswille's advice. The judge acquitted them after the discovery that the prosecution had failed to provide important information supporting the couple's story.

Let's run through some other examples of ideologic vegetarian extremism:

- It caused mental and growth retardation in two boys underfed from birth to ages 3 and 5. Their mother had become a vegetarian, later eliminated sugar and dairy products from her diet, and eventually adopted a macrobiotic diet (see "Peculiar Vegetarianism").[4]
- Ten cases of nutritional rickets were reported among infants (most of whom were breast-fed) of strict-vegetarian mothers who had not sought medical counsel during pregnancy but had obtained advice from health food stores.[5]
- Scurvy and rickets occurred in two boys, 1 1/2 and 2 1/2 years old, whose parents were adherents of the Zen Macrobiotic diet (see "Peculiar Vegetarianism").[6]
- A 36-year-old former college professor attempted to become a "breatharian"—one who supposedly feeds on air alone—and died of malnutrition. First he became a

Peculiar Vegetarianism

Diet #7 (Diet No. 7): "Healing regimen" recommended by George Ohsawa (see "macrobiotics") in *Zen Macrobiotics: The Art of Rejuvenation and Longevity* (1965). It principally involves restricting dietary intake (including water) to brown rice and particular kinds of tea ("as little as possible") for a period of one week to an indefinite number of months. The purported objective of diet #7 and the nine other diets of Zen Macrobiotics is to maintain balance of yin and yang.

Macrobiotics (formerly called "Zen Macrobiotics"): Quasireligious movement and health-centered lifestyle whose centerpiece is a mystical form of vegetarianism. The thrust of macrobiotic nutrition is regulation of the intake of two alleged elementary forms of energy: yin and yang. Categorizing a food as yin or yang depends largely on characteristics directly cognizable by the senses and is unrelated to nutrient content. Proponents ascribe the modern version of macrobiotics either to Ishizuka Sagen (1850–1910), a Japanese physician and author of *A Chemical Nutritional Theory of Long Life,* or to George Ohsawa (1893–1966), whose names included: Georges Ohsawa, Nyoichi (also spelled "Nyoiti") Sakurazawa, and Yukikazu Sakurazawa. The leading exponent of macrobiotics is Michio Kushi, according to whom "Natural and Macrobiotic Medicine" encompasses: (a) astrological diagnosis; (b) aura and vibrational diagnosis, allegedly based on the color, frequency, "heat," and intensity of a one's "radiating aura" and "vibrations"; (c) consciousness and thought diagnosis, a variation of so-called mind reading; (d) environmental diagnosis, whose theory posits "celestial influences"; (e) meridian diagnosis, which purportedly reveals valuable information about "internal energy flow"; (f) pressure diagnosis, which supposedly reveals "stagnation of the streaming energy"; and (g) spiritual diagnosis, an apparent variation of aura analysis (probably rei-so).

Zen Macrobiotics: Early form of macrobiotics, endorsed by Herman and Cornelia Aihara. The Aiharas were students of George Ohsawa (see "macrobiotics") and coauthored *Natural Healing from Head to Toe: Traditional Macrobiotic Remedies* (Avery Publishing Group, Inc., 1994). They also founded, in 1974, the Vega Study Center, in Oroville, California. The school teaches Zen Macrobiotics.

vegetarian, then a fruitarian, then a "liquidarian" (consuming juices only), and finally, a would-be breatharian.[7]

- A 2-month-old boy died because his mother, following the invalid recommendation for colic in Adelle Davis's *Let's Have Healthy Children,* overdosed him with potassium.[8] In a television interview, the mother said that, as she became increasingly estranged toward conventional medicine, she had adopted vegetarianism and then veganism.
- A 24-year-old woman who was head of San Jose State University's student art program died after taking an extract of pennyroyal to induce an abortion. She was described as "a strict vegetarian who was involved in holistic medicine."[9]

For the ideologist, vegetarianism is a hygienic religion. It enables believers to practice self-denial. As a religion, vegetarianism attracts the guilt-ridden. It attracts masochists because it gives guilt a boost. And it seduces the unskeptical by causing guilt and/or by instilling false guilt. Guilt leads to self-denial, even asceticism. The belief that salvation is attainable by eschewing worldly pleasures marked the asceticism of early Christian zealots. Similarly, health neurotics with medical problems seem to believe that the more they restrict their alimentary pleasures, the more their health will improve. Fasting, austere diets, enemas, and the ingestion of bitter herbs are consistent with the psychological needs of health neurotics, many of whom shun those voices of conventional medicine and public health that might disenchant them.

Of course, I don't blame ideologic vegetarianism per se *entirely* for tragedies such as those outlined above. Mental or emotional disorders apparently figure in many instances. In such cases, extremism is more to blame. This doesn't take ideologic vegetarianism off the hook, however, for it can fuel or ignite psychological problems.

Eating by the Book?

SDA vegetarianism is rooted in the Bible, according to which for food God gave humans "all plants that bear seed everywhere on earth, and every tree bearing fruit that yields seed" (Genesis 1:29). Meat is said to have become a part of the human diet after the Flood, when all plant life had been destroyed: "Every creature that lives and moves shall be food for you" (Genesis 9:3). Adventists are taught that the introduction of meat into the human diet at that time decreased the human life span from the more than 900 years of the first humans to today's "three-score and ten."

However, the Bible warns against confusing dietary practices with moral behavior:

> For the kingdom of God is not food and drink but righteousness and peace. (Romans 14:17)
>
> Let no one pass judgment on you in questions of food and drink. (Colossians 2:16)
>
> One believes he may eat anything, while the weak man eats only vegetables, let not him who eats despise him who abstains, and let not him who abstains pass judgment on him who eats. (Romans 14:2–4)

It also seems to condemn vegetarianism:

> The Holy Spirit tells us clearly that in the last times some in the church will turn away from Christ and become eager followers of teachers with devil inspired ideas. These teachers will tell lies with straight faces and do it so often that their consciences won't

even bother them. They will say that it is wrong to be married and wrong to eat meat, even though God gave these things to well-taught Christians to enjoy and be thankful for. For everything God made is good, and we may eat it gladly if we are thankful for it. (I Timothy 4:1–4, *Living Bible*)

SDA Church pioneer Ellen G. White (1827–1915) was a proponent of vegetarianism even though she did not practice it herself. Like the Grahamites of her time, she taught that gradually the earth would become more corrupted, diseases and calamities worse, and the food—particularly animal foods—unsafe. In 1902 she wrote that the time might come when the use of milk should be discontinued. Although White was an advocate of science and chiefly responsible for making SDA healthcare a science-based enterprise, clearly she did not anticipate twentieth-century advances in public health and medical science. Despite the record longevity now enjoyed by people in the developed nations, vegetarian zealots within the church caught up in the doomsday hysteria of the 1990s have decided that the time has come to give up all animal foods and are fervidly preaching veganism.

East of Eden

It is possible to provide all essential nutrients except vitamin B12 without using animal foods. On the other hand, it is possible to provide *all* essential nutrients with a diet composed only of meat. Personal dietary appropriateness—including the value of a diet as a source of essential nutrients and its value as a preventative—for oneself and one's significant others is the foremost dietary consideration of pragmatic vegetarians. In contrast, the overriding dietary consideration of ideologic vegetarians varies with the particular ideology. Typically, their motivation is a blend of physical, psychosocial, societal, and moral, often religious, concerns.

A continual problem for SDAs who espouse the "back to Eden" ideology is the absence of a non-animal food source of vitamin B12. A vegetarian registered dietitian who wrote a column for a church periodical asked me if I thought vegans could derive vitamin B12 from organic vegetables that were unwashed before ingestion. I opined that it would be better to eat animal foods than fecal residues. She agreed.

A perennial assumption among vegetarians is that vegetarianism increases longevity. In the last century, Grahamites—devotees of the Christian "hygienic" philosophy of Sylvester Graham (1794–1851)—taught that adherence to the Garden of Eden lifestyle would eventuate in humankind's reclamation of the potential for super-longevity, such as that attributed to Adam (930 years) or Methuselah (969 years). I discussed this matter 25 years ago with an SDA physician who was dean of the Loma Linda University (LLU) School of Health. Although he admitted that lifelong SDA vegetarians had not exhibited spectacular longevity, he professed that longevity of the antediluvian sort might become possible over several generations of vegetarianism. SDA periodicals publicize centenarians and often attribute their longevity to the SDA lifestyle. However, of 1200 people who reached the century mark between 1932 and 1952, only four were vegetarians.[10] I continue to ask: Where on Earth is there an exceptionally longevous population of vegetarians? Hindus have practiced vegetarianism for many generations but have not set longevity records. At best, the whole of scientific data from nutrition-related research supports vegetarianism only tentatively. The incidence of colorectal cancer among nonvegetarian Mormons is lower than that of SDAs.[11] A review of populations at low risk for cancer showed that World War I veterans who never smoked had the lowest risk of all.[12] As data accumulate, optimism that diet is a significant factor in cancer appears to be diminishing. An analysis of[13] case-control studies of colorectal cancer and dietary fiber showed that, for the studies with the best research methods, risk estimates for dietary fiber and colorectal cancer were closer to zero.[13] A pooled analysis of studies of fat intake and the risk of breast cancer that included SDA data showed no association.[14]

A meatless diet can facilitate weight control because it is a form of food restriction. But one need not eliminate meat to maintain a healthy weight, and there are many overweight vegetarians. Surely prudence and selectivity overshadow mere abstention from consuming animal products.

Daniel's Diet

According to the first chapter of the Book of Daniel, Israel's captive whiz kids— "well favored, and skillful in all wisdom, and cunning in all knowledge, and understanding science" (verse 4)—after subsisting on just vegetables and water for ten days, impressed the Babylonian king as far superior to all the magicians and astrologers "in all matters of wisdom and understanding" (verse 20). Many ideological vegetarians credit vegetables for group's physical and mental improvement (see "A 'Biblical' Alternativist Method"). A more credible proposition is that abstention from drinking wine caused the improvement, which the story ascribes to God.

In an interview on the school's Christian radio station in the mid-1970s, an LLU nutrition graduate student (who was not an SDA) claimed that vegetarianism produced superior intellects. To make her case, she stated:

Linus Pauling says that vitamin C improves intelligence. Vegetarians get more vitamin C in their diets than meat-eaters. The probable reason why George Bernard Shaw and Leo Tolstoy were brilliant was because they were vegetarians.

A "Biblical" Alternativist Method

Daniel's Diet: Alleged medical panacea and "higher way of eating" promoted by microbiologist Robert O. Young, Ph.D., author of *Colloids of Light & Life, Profiles of Microscopy, Sick & Tired,* and *One Sickness—One Disease—One Treatment* (1995). In the latter book, Young holds that mycosis, or fungal infection, or over-acidification of the body (or blood), is the only disease. He further holds that an "inverted" way of living and eating, especially excessive consumption of sugars and animal protein, causes such over-acidification. Daniel's Diet excludes all foods except avocados, lemons, limes, tomatoes, vegetables (e.g., buckwheat and soybeans), dark-green vegetable juice, tofu (bean curd), millet, "sprouted" or soaked seeds and nuts, oils, sea salt, herbal teas, specific dietary supplements (e.g., Pycnogenol®, and Liquid Lightning Oxygen-O3 (a "formula" purportedly beneficial for "oxygen deprivation"). The diet is the namesake of a Jewish "prophet" and fortuneteller of the sixth century b.c.e. According to the Book of Daniel, in the Old Testament, Daniel refused to consume meat and wine assigned to him by a Babylonian king, requested vegetables and water, and, after eating only vegetables for ten days, appeared healthier and stronger.

The interviewer agreed, extolling the health and intellect of vegetarians. That Adolf Hitler was a vegetarian went unmentioned during the interview. Also unmentioned was that Jesus Christ, Mohammed, and other eminent moralists were not vegetarians.

Animal behavioral scientists have noted that, to survive, meat-eating predators must outsmart their vegetarian prey. However, I believe that all such theories break down because of the difficulty of defining intelligence.

SDAs note that meat-eating predators such as wolves and lions have tremendous speed but lack endurance. However, Arctic sled dogs that run the 1200-mile Idadarod cover more than a hundred miles per day—a feat no horse, mule or ox can accomplish.

The idea that vegetarians have superior physical endurance was reinforced in 1974 when a group of male vegetarian runners called "the vegetarian seven" set a 24-hour distance record. This inspired an undergraduate dietetics major to seek me out as a coach for a group of seven female vegetarian long-distance runners. I asked her what their motivations were—something every coach needs to know. She said they wanted to demonstrate the superiority of a vegetarian diet. I asked who would be representing the meat-eaters. She said that, because the event would not be a standard competition, no one would represent the meat-eaters. I revealed to her that three of the male runners had not been vegetarians until training for the record-setting event but merely had pledged to become so. I also told her: that genetic factors, principally the capacity for oxygen uptake, determine distance-running ability; that whether a diet is vegetarian is inconsequential to distance-running ability; and that a 24-hour run is a perilous way to try proving vegetarian superiority. "What will you do," I inquired, "if seven meat-eating, beer-drinking atheists who are world-class runners decide to beat your record?" She got the point. And although she became an accomplished amateur runner, she didn't use her success to propagandize for vegetarianism.

John Harvey Kellogg sought to prove that vegetarians were physically superior by fielding a Battle Creek College football team, which he personally coached. According to a former player, "Brother" Wright, whenever Kellogg's players lost, he railed at them for cheating on their diets and held them captive until one would say he had broken training rules and eaten meat. Wright stated that sometimes a player would eventually lie that he had eaten meat just to get the team released. He described Kellogg's efforts as "a crusade to prove the superiority of vegetarianism." Ellen G. White's condemnation of this approach to proving SDA superiority led to a policy restricting interscholastic sports by Adventist schools.

Odorless Doo-doo?

The John Harvey Kellogg character in the 1995 film *Road to Wellville* stated that his feces had no more odor than that of "freshly baked biscuits." One evening I offered a ride home from the university to an elderly colleague, an avid vegetarian. Upon entering my car, he declared: "When I drink carrot juice, my bowel movements have no odor."

Before I could respond, he said: "Rabbits eat lots of carrots, and their feces have no odor." The thought of someone running around sniffing little piles of rabbit doo-doo almost made me laugh, but I didn't want to be disrespectful. His idea that rabbits eat many carrots intrigued me. I had raised them in my boyhood and discovered that, despite the passion for carrots shown by Bugs Bunny, real bunnies are not particularly fond of carrots. Furthermore, wild rabbits seldom would have an opportunity to eat carrots. Luckily the ride was short.

The late Pulitzer Prize-winning anthropologist Ernest Becker argued that defecation is most closely associated with humankind's animality and mortality.[15] During a Bible class at an SDA school, I was taught that people did not defecate in the Garden of Eden but utilized the food they ingested in its entirety. Apparently, foul odors did not befit Paradise. (Perhaps the persistence of the miasmatic theory of disease—the theory that diseases are due to foul-smelling emanations from the earth—well into the nineteenth century, when SDA beliefs were developed, reinforced the idea of a poopless Paradise.) I was also taught that roughage became part of the human diet after the Fall. Allegedly, this broadening of the diet to include "the herb of the field" (Genesis 3:18, King James version) occurred because humans were now under the "death sentence" caused by original sin. Whether this reportedly was a voluntary dietary change or part of the curse of being ousted from Paradise is debatable. Some versions of the Bible imply that "the herb of the field" merely meant "wild foods" (New English Version), not a new source of food.

Heavy "PETAing"

In the last century, the pacifist movement was vegetarian because of the belief that meat-eating animals were fierce and vegetarian animals were docile. The British poet Percy Bysshe Shelley claimed that the French revolution had been bloody and the English revolution bloodless because the French ate more meat than the English.[16] Such invalid notions have been discredited, but not abandoned. Some boxers still eat raw meat or drink blood before a fight to increase their aggressiveness.

People who fancy themselves morally superior often have a mission to convert humanity to their worldview. The most violent ideologic vegetarians are the animal-rights activists, who have destroyed animal research facilities and threatened researchers' lives. Animal-rights groups such as People for the Ethical Treatment of Animals (PETA) consider animals on par with humans. On April 24, 1996, PETA's Ingrid Newkirk appeared on the television newsmagazine *Day & Date* opposing sport fishing. She began her argument by seeking commiseration for suffocating fish. Then she said that fish were unhealthful food because they contained mercury and other environmental contaminants. The solution, according to Newkirk, was vegetarianism. Her opponent, a TV talk-show host, pressed her into acknowledging the PETA creed. The talk-show host described an on-air encounter she had had with another PETA representative. A scenario had been presented in which the representative's daughter needed a vital organ from a beloved household pet in order to survive. The ethical question had been whether the child's life was worth more than the pet's. The PETA representative had held that the child had no more value than the pet. Newkirk did not contest the assertion that PETA considers the life of a child no more valuable than that of a pet.

When an LLU medical team transplanted a baboon's heart into an infant whose pseudonym was "Baby Fae," animal-rights activists picketed the medical center. They seemed disillusioned with SDAs, who have no qualms about prioritizing humans over animals. In October 1992, after a pig's liver had been transplanted into a 30-year-old woman to enable her to survive until a human liver was secured, a representative of PCRM engaged in a televised debate with one of the physicians who had performed the transplant. The representative lamented that the pig's consent had not been obtained.

PCRM appears to be largely a personal forum for its leader, Neal Barnard, M.D., and is said to be substantially funded by PETA. (In fiscal year 1994, donations and grants to PCRM reportedly totaled more than a million dollars.[17] Barnard extols the longevity value of vegetarianism. He has claimed: "It's not genetics or fate that gives people long, healthy lives and cuts other people short; for those who want to take care of themselves, it all comes down to diet." The surgeon argued that pigs were killed daily for meat, including their livers. The PCRM doctor retorted that the consumption of animal fat (which is highly saturated) was responsible for most deaths in modern society. He cited a study conducted by Colin Campbell in China. Campbell had focused on the relative morbidity for certain diseases without pointing out that life expectancy in China (66 years) is lower than that in the United States (75 years).[18]

Because they consider themselves morally superior, many vegetarians exhibit no reservations against using mind-control techniques or terrorism to actualize their agenda. Mind control includes using information selectively to "educate" people about the alleged superiority of vegetarianism. It may also include traumatizing people emotionally to condition them against the use of animal foods. Early in my teaching experience, I attended a meeting of SDA secondary school health teachers where many said that they converted students to vegetarianism by taking them on field trips to slaughterhouses to witness the bloodshed. This strategy offended me even though I was a practicing vegetarian at the time. Having studied for years how people have been manipulated by cults and quacks, it is now clear to me that the slaughterhouse tactic is a form of mind control—that it is as unethical as discouraging little girls from having sex by inducing them to watch a difficult childbirth.

Terrorism involves trying to coerce people to behave in ways the perpetrators desire. In December 1994, to keep people from having turkey for Christmas dinner, self-described animal-rights terrorists claimed they had injected rat poison into supermarket turkeys in Vancouver, British Columbia. The scare caused the destruction of more than $1 million in turkeys. Apparently, the activists had not foreseen the ensuing slaughter of turkeys as replacements.

Disclosure

Research into vegetarianism by vegetarians always involves at least unconscious bias. All humans have entrenched beliefs—beliefs whose rootedness makes doing related scientific research unwise. Kenneth J. Rothman, Dr.P.H., referred to SDAs in a recent discussion of conflicts of interest in research:

> We might expect conflict of interest concerns to be raised, for example, about Seventh Day Adventists who are studying the health effects of the comparatively abstemious lifestyle of their fellow Adventists. Whereas policies at [the *Journal of the American Medical Association*] and *The New England Journal of Medicine* emphasize financial conflicts, *Science* asks authors to divulge "any relationships that they believe could be construed as causing a conflict of interest, whether or not the individual believes that is actually so." In other words, to comply with disclosure policies at *Science*, authors might need to disclose to editors their religion and sexual orientation along with their financial portfolio.[19]

Although Rothman argues for letting work stand on its own merit rather than judging cynically any possible connection to a funding source, his example makes the point that motivations more powerful than money can distort data. Science fraud can be extremely difficult to detect, because the perpetrators control the information. As Mark Twain observed, "Figures don't lie, but liars figure!"

I don't believe that *all* research done by vegetarians is untrustworthy. My experience with the ongoing Seventh-day Adventist Health Study (SDAHS), a series of studies conducted from LLU School of Public Health, has been largely positive. Its chief researcher, the late Roland Phillips, M.D., Dr.P.H., was an outstanding scientist in whose objectivity I had the utmost confidence. He recognized the problem of the influence of social expectations on SDAs responding to questions about their lifestyle. Adventist groupthink makes it likely that SDAs will underreport activities disfavored by the church community (e.g., meat-eating, coffee drinking, and imbibing) and over-report those that are approved (e.g., dining meatlessly and exercising). Phillips seemed to feel that the benefits of vegetarianism per se were limited, and that one must take account of heredity, socioeconomic status, and the total SDA lifestyle. Abstention from smoking, access to state-of-the-art healthcare, and strong social support probably are responsible for most of the health benefits SDAs enjoy. The main problem with SDA vegetarian science is how the scientific information is used. To paraphrase an old Pennsylvania Dutch saying: Among SDAs, when the news about vegetarianism and health is good, "we hear it ever"; when the news is not good, "we hear it never."

I have received numerous reports from SDA health professionals, and have personal knowledge of other cases, in which church members' overconfidence in vegetarianism prevented them from obtaining effective medical care. Some reports have involved true believers in vegetarianism who were members of physicians' families. Some denied symptoms, and their denial kept them from seeking effective intervention in time. Others rejected medical care for "natural remedies" that emphasized diet. The attitudes evidenced are consistent with those identified in cancer patients who had turned to quackery because they believed they had brought the disease upon themselves and could cure it by "natural" practices.[20] The SDA Church has bent over backward to document the benefits of the SDA lifestyle and to persuade members to adopt vegetarian diets. I would like to see the church seek earnestly to expose the harm that its vegetarian teachings have caused its members. Alas, there's the rub with ideologic vegetarianism: Objectivity always takes a back seat to proselytism.

The data suggest that most SDAs are reasonable in their approach to vegetarianism. In the 1970s, the SDAHS revealed that only one percent were vegans.[21] This may change as vegetarianism becomes more popular in the general population. SDAs tend to be overachievers. If we regard something as "good," we strive to adopt it completely. If we consider something "bad," we avoid it completely. SDA vegetarian evangelists have become more aggressive in recent years because of the widespread belief in the SDA community that doomsday is nigh.

I recall an SDA church leader's fitting reply to the question of whether he ate meat: "I eat just enough to keep me from becoming a fanatic!"

One Less "Ism"

I gave up vegetarianism because I found that commitment thereto meant surrendering the objectivity that is essential to the personal and professional integrity of a scientist. As a health educator, I feel I have an obligation to endeavor to stick to whatever unvarnished facts scientific research uncovers. I can support pragmatic vegetarianism, but I believe that crusading vegetarian ideologues are dangerous to themselves and to society.

Notes

1. D. Erhardt, "The New Vegetarians, Part One–Vegetarianism and its Medical Consequences," *Nutrition Today,* November/December, 1973.
2. R. Spitzer. *No Need For Hunger.* Danville, Ill.: Interstate Printers and Publishers, 1981.
3. National Academy of Sciences. *Toxicants Occurring Naturally In Foods.* Washington, D.C.: National Academy Press, 1973.
4. J. Wood. "Mother of Starved Children Asks Permission to Give Birth Again," *San Francisco Sunday Examiner & Chronicle,* March 27, 1983, p. A5.
5. *Journal of Nutrition Education* 1981; 13:26.

6. *Newsweek,* September 18, 1972, p. 71.
7. "Temple Beautiful Diet–Death for David Blume," (AP) *San Bernardino Sun,* October 15, 1979, p. A-3.
8. C.V Wetli and J.H. Davis. *JAMA* 1978; 240:1339.
9. *San Jose Mercury News,* August 20, 1994.
10. O. Segerberg. *Living to Be 100: 1200 Who Did and How They Did It.* New York: Charles Scribner's Sons, 1982.
11. J.L. Lyon, M.R. Klauber, J.W. Gardner, and C.R. Smart, "Cancer Incidence in Mormons and Non-Mormons in Utah, 1966–70," *N Engl J Med* 1976; 294:129–133 (p. 132).
12. J.E. Enstrom. "Cancer Mortality among Low-Risk Populations," *CA—A Cancer Journal for Clinicians* 1979; 29:352–61.
13. C.M. Friedenreich, R.F. Brant, and E. Riboli, "Influence of Methodological Factors in a Pooled Analysis of 13 Case-Control Studies of Colorectal Cancer and Dietary Fiber," *Epidemiology* 1994; 5:66–79.
14. D.J. Hunter et al. "Cohort Studies of Fat Intake and the Risk of Breast Cancer–A Pooled Analysis," *New Engl J Med* 1996; 344:356–61.
15. E. Becker. *The Denial of Death.* New York: Macmillan Publishing Co., Inc., 1973.
16. J. Whorton. "Tempest in a Flesh-Pot: Development of a Physiological Rationale for Vegetarianism," *Journal of the History of Medicine,* April 1977, pp. 119–120.
17. *Good Medicine,* Spring 1995.
18. The Population Reference Bureau, Inc., Washington, D.C., 1988.
19. K. Rothman. "Conflict of Interest: The New McCarthyism in Science," *JAMA* 1993; 269 (21):2782–4.
20. B. Cassileth et al. "Contemporary Treatments in Cancer Medicine," *Ann Intern Med* 1984; 101:105–12.
21. "Researchers Release Adventist Health Study Results," *Pacific Union Recorder,* March 12, 1979.

FRAME the DEBATE

Form at end of book

WiseGuide Wrap-Up

The relative healthfulness of the vegetarian diet has been debated in health circles for over a hundred years. Vegetarianism appears to be healthful in some ways but not in others. It may decrease risk of hypertension and lung and colorectal cancers, but some health professionals conclude that vegetarians are simply more likely than others to adopt healthier lifestyles that include exercising regularly, drinking moderately, and abstaining from smoking. Vegetarians may be at risk of increased rates of calcium- and vitamin-D-related disorders, such as osteoporosis in women, and therefore should weigh the positive and negative risk factors of vegetarianism or take food supplements.

R.E.A.L. Sites

This list provides a print preview of typical **Coursewise** R.E.A.L. sites. (There are over 100 such sites at the **Courselinks**™ site.) The danger in printing URLs is that web sites can change overnight. As we went to press, these sites were functional using the URLs provided. If you come across one that isn't, please let us know via email to: webmaster@coursewise.com. Use your Passport to access the most current list of R.E.A.L. sites at the **Courselinks** site.

Site name: Vegetarianism

URL: http://www.macalester.edu/~kwiik/Veggie/vegihome.htm

Why is it R.E.A.L.? This site features brief articles on the moral, ecological, and health benefits of vegetarianism. It also lists veggie organizations and recipes, and provides links to other vegetarian pages.

Key topics: environment, animals, eating

Try this: Select one of the three main articles on morality, environment, and health benefits of vegetarians. How well do the authors support their positions? What techniques of persuasion do they use? Are the arguments based on provable facts or emotional appeals?

Site name: Meat, Meat Eating and Vegetarianism: A Review of the Facts

URL: http://www.maf.govt.nz/MAFnet/publications/9716/9716.htm

Why is it R.E.A.L.? This site, sponsored by the faculty of veterinary science at Massey University in New Zealand, offers an overview of trends in vegetarianism and images of meat eating and vegetarianism. The authors state, "Meat is simultaneously the most exalted and the most pernicious food that we have."

Try this: Read their introduction and summary pages and the articles titled, "Reasons for Reduced Meat-eating" and "Health and Food Safety." How well do the authors support their positions? What techniques of persuasion do they use? Are the arguments based on provable facts or emotional appeals?

Section 1 Summary

The effectiveness of sunscreens may be questionable. Americans may be placing themselves at an increased risk of skin cancer from too much sun exposure or at an increased risk of vitamin deficiency from too little sun exposure.

The debate over herbal medicines centers around their effectiveness and the relative safety of herbal supplements. Specifically, proponents view them as safe alternatives to chemicals that may have deleterious side effects. Opponents of herbal supplements caution that because herbs vary in concentration of active ingredients, doses may be variable, and people may overestimate the safety of herbal supplements.

Vegetarians appear to have lowered risk of certain cancers and cardiovascular disease. This may be due to a diet that is generally lower in fat and higher in fiber than the average American diet. It also may be related to vegetarians being more likely to participate in healthful behaviors.

STAND! **section 2**

Men's Health Issues

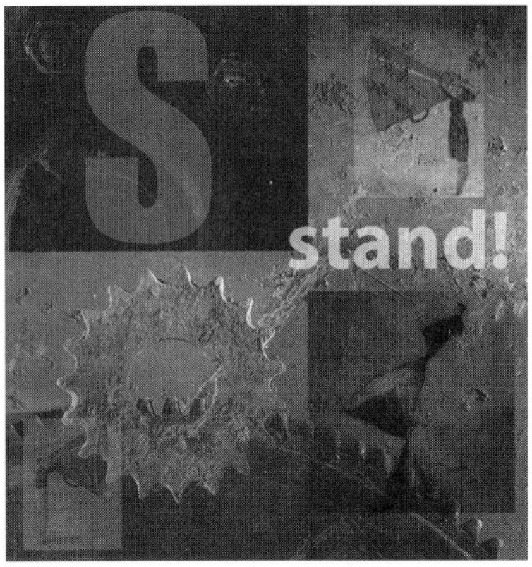

Learning Objectives

- Examine the possible drawbacks of using Viagra.
- Understand the physical and psychosocial effects and side effects stemming from the use of Viagra.
- Question the relative advantages and disadvantages of neonatal circumcision.

Introduction

Although the health-care community has not traditionally neglected men and their health problems, not until the past decade has it embraced the concept of male-specific disorders as a separate category of health concerns from general family practice. The increased awareness of men's health was heralded on May 24, 1994, when President Bill Clinton signed into law a bill that designated the week leading up to Father's Day as National Men's Health Week.

While males and females share many similarities, both genders have certain issues that are specific to their sex. Male death rates from trauma or heart disease are double that of females, male-specific prostate cancer kills upward of 30,000 males per year, and stress, depression, and suicide are responsible for more than 25,000 premature deaths among males each year. Clearly, males have major life-threatening health concerns. In addition, they have gender-specific issues that affect their quality of life, such as the role of fathers in modern society, child custody issues, stress and risk reduction, exercise, and sexuality. This section explores two issues related to male sexuality and self-esteem.

Is Viagra a Benefit or a Bane to Human Sexuality in America?

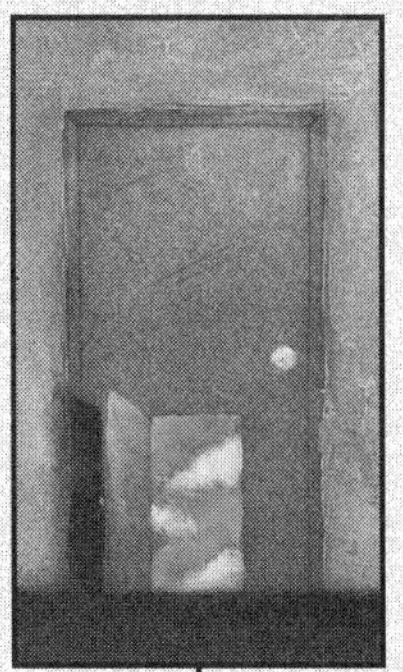

ISSUE 4

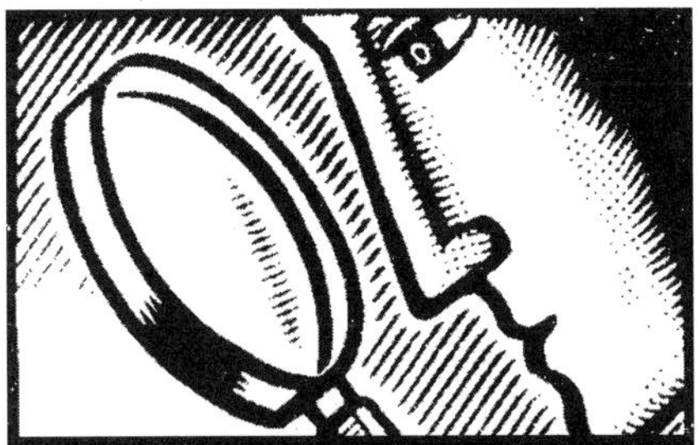

Take a Closer Look

1. List five possible side effects and/or hazards from using Viagra to treat male impotence.
2. According to Pfizer, the company that produces Viagra, what was the success rate among clinical trial participants?
3. The drug sildenafil (Viagra) was originally being tested as a possible treatment for what health problem(s)?
4. What three downfalls to Viagra use does Peterson identify in Reading 10?

WiseGuide Intro

Since its approval by the Food and Drug Administration in the spring of 1998, the anti-impotence medication Viagra has been making headlines and stirring controversy. The drug greatly improves the ability of men suffering from organic impotence to achieve and maintain penile erections. Currently, over 30 million American men suffer from impotence for medical reasons. Organic impotence, as opposed to physiological impotence, can be caused by loss of arterial elasticity, kidney dysfunction, blood pressure and heart medications, and prostate problems and urogenital surgeries. Viagra is 60 to 70 percent effective in treating organic impotence and 90 percent effective in treating psychological impotence.

Although the drug appears to be a godsend for impotent males, it is not without hazards and controversy. At least eight deaths among elderly heart patients have been attributed to the synergistic effects of Viagra and prescription drugs, such as the commonly prescribed angina medication nitroglycerin. There also is potential for misuse and abuse of Viagra by nonimpotent males who simply desire to increase their sexual responsiveness. Recently, the Los Angeles County Coroner's Office released warnings regarding the recreational use of Viagra in combination with amyl and butyl nitrates, which some gay males use to enhance orgasm.

Physicians wrote over 270,000 prescriptions for Viagra in the first few months after its release. At a price of around $10 per tablet, the cost of reimbursement by insurance companies is predicted to be in the hundreds of millions of dollars in the first few years of Viagra's general use.

Several arguments have arisen out of concerns that insurance reimbursement for Viagra might be unfair to women, since many insurance companies have policies against covering contraceptive services and goods for female subscribers. Much of the debate centers around whether sexuality and contraception are "medical conditions" and therefore part of essential health care.

In Reading 9, "The Viagra Craze," Bruce Handy reviews the uses and possible misuses of the anti-impotence drug. He addresses the purported similarities between Viagra and the release of birth control pills for women in the early 1960s and quotes several researchers and physicians. The sidebar, "The Downside of Viagra," lists some of the possible risks associated with the drug.

In Reading 10, "Viagra's Power Could Pressure Marriages," Karen Peterson discusses the backlash and disappointment that may stem from some couples' expectations that Viagra will enhance their sex lives and repair failing relationships. Peterson quotes various health-care professionals and authors of sexuality books to present viewpoints that offset the positive fervor that accompanied the release of Viagra. She suggests that, for some couples, rather than enhancing and resolving marital and relationship problems, the increase in sexual function from Viagra may actually cause more resentments, less communication, and the possibility of straying from the monogamous relationship.

Issue 4: Is Viagra a benefit or a bane to human sexuality in America?

The Viagra Craze

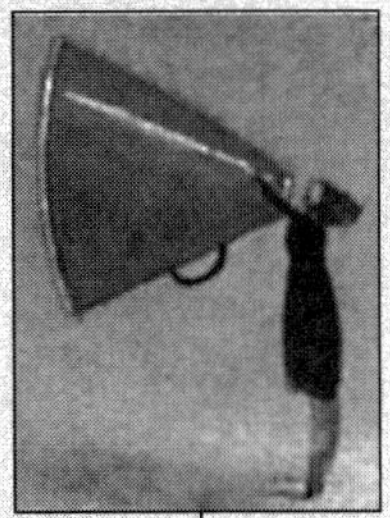

A pill to cure impotence? Afflicted men are saying Yesss! But is this the end of sex as we know it?

Bruce Handy

Besides its phony name, funny shape and unappetizing color, what's not to like about Viagra, the new pill that conquers impotence? Could there be a product more tailored to the easy-solution-loving, sexually insecure American psyche than this one? The drug, manufactured by Pfizer, went on sale three weeks ago, finally giving talk-show hosts something other than Bill Clinton and Pamela Lee to crack smarmy jokes about.

Spurred, perhaps, by just that sort of publicity, would-be patients have been besieging urologists' offices and sex clinics—men both genuinely dysfunctional and merely dissatisfied, skulking around in hopes of achieving "better" erections through chemistry. Already, a kind of Viagra connoisseurship is beginning to take hold. "The hundreds are absolutely incredible," says a very satisfied user, referring to the drug's 100-mg maximum-strength dosage, "and the effect lasts through the following morning." What else can one say but *Vrooom!* Cheap gas, strong economy, erection pills—what a country! What a time to be alive!

"We've always been waiting for the magic bullet," says Dr. Fernando Borges of the Florida Impotency Center in St. Petersburg, where he has been working with sexually dysfunctional patients for 21 years. "This," he says, "is pretty close to the magic bullet." The very day Viagra became available, Dr. John Stripling, an Atlanta urologist, churned out 300 prescriptions with the help of a rubber stamp he had had the foresight to purchase. At the Urology Health Center in New Port Richey, Fla., which participated in the drug's clinical trials, the waiting time to see a doctor for a Viagra consultation is a month. Not that this has stopped motivated patients. "We've been inundated with emergencies," says Dr. Ramon Perez. "Pain in the kidney. Blood in the urine. But when they get in here, they just want to ask us about Viagra. It's amazing. These people have been impotent for three years, and they cannot wait another few days."

Hot New Drugs

Prescriptions Dispensed during First Two Weeks on the Market

Viagra (impotence)	36,809
Propecia (baldness)	5,500
Lipitor (cholesterol reducer)	2,203
Evista (bone-density regulator)	1,624

Source: IMS Health

"It's the fastest takeoff of a new drug that I've ever seen, and I've been in this business for 27 years," says Michael Podgurski, director of pharmacy at the 4,000-outlet Rite Aid drugstore chain. After a brief lag, the drug is now being prescribed at the rate of at least 10,000 scripts a day, outpacing such famous quick starters as the antidepressant Prozac (which went on to become one of the biggest-selling drugs in America) and the baldness remedy Rogaine (which has been something of a disappointment after its initial blaze of popularity).

The run on Viagra has been abetted by the likes of David Michael Thomas, a Milwaukee, Wis., osteopath who advertises his services on the Web at *www.penispill.com* and who allegedly prescribed Viagra to some 700 patients after cursory $50 telephone examinations. At a license-suspension hearing in front of Wisconsin regulatory officials last week, Thomas agreed to stop the practice. (Normally a diagnosis of impotence involves a rigorous physical exam, blood tests and an extensive sexual history.) Other entrepreneurs have been offering prescriptions directly over the Internet.

Even supporters of the pill worry about hyped expectations. "People always want a quick fix," complains Dr. Domeena Renshaw, a psychiatrist who directs the Loyola Sex Therapy Clinic outside Chicago. "They think Viagra is magic, just like they thought the G spot worked like a garage-door opener." In the wake of fen/phen and Redux, the diet-drug treatments that were pulled from the market last year after it was learned that they could damage heart valves, caution would be advisable with Viagra. But so far the side effects seem comparatively slight and manageable: chiefly headache, flushed skin, upset stomach and curious vision distortions involving the color blue. Pfizer, leaving nothing to chance, has even requested and received the Vatican's unofficial blessing for Viagra. All in all, a happy ending for American men, their partners and especially Pfizer stockholders, who have seen the value of their shares jump nearly 60% this year alone.

Yet there's something unnerving about Viagra too, not so much on the face of it (the drug's merits appear to be manifold: doctors think it might even improve the sexual response of postmenopausal women) but in the broader philosophical implications. Is sexuality, like the state of happiness or male-pattern baldness, just one more hitherto mysterious and profound area of human-beingness that can be pharmaceutically manipulated, like any other fathomable construct of enzymes and receptors? Another looming question: Since Viagra is taken—at prices ranging from $8 to $12 a pop—not on a day-in, day-out basis but only when one actually wants to have sex, will HMOs and other insurers soon be telling us how much sex is reimbursable? Sufficient? Normal? Necessary?

And what about the impact on the freighted social interactions we euphemistically refer to as dating? "I bet that within a year, you'll see women's-magazine articles saying, 'How to Tell If It's You or Viagra,'" says James R. Petersen, who has written the *Playboy* Advisor column for the past 22 years. He adds, "I think Viagra is going to be as monumental as the birth-control pill." No less an authority than Bob Guccione, publisher of *Penthouse* magazine, believes the drug will "free the American male libido" from the emasculating doings of feminists. And not only that. According to Guccione, "the ability to have sex by older men will make them healthier and live longer. It will fool the biological clock when men are still active in the later years. It is a very significant effect of the drug that many haven't contemplated." There isn't any actual scientific evidence to back up Guccione's claims, but he does do a nice job of illuminating two important subtexts of Viagra's appeal: the chimeras of undiminishable power and perpetual youth.

Of course, the overt appeal is pretty compelling too.

In the past decade there have been great advances in the treatment of impotence, which is now seen by most therapists, in most cases, as a physiological rather than a psychological problem, rejecting the medical establishment's long-held view. The word impotence itself, like "frigidity" for women, is considered suspect in many circles; the more politically correct—or at least clinical—term is erectile dysfunction, or ED, as it is commonly abbreviated. Inspired by a 1992 National Institutes of Health Conference and landmark 1994 study on the problem, the diagnosis has been defined more broadly, from the rather strict criterion of inability to get an erection, period, to the somewhat more elastic and subjective criterion of inability to get an erection adequate for "satisfactory sexual performance." This has led to a tripling of the number of men estimated to be impotent in this country—some 30 million according to the NIH, half of whom are thought to be under the age of 65. EDis associated with age; it affects about 1 in 20 men ages 40 and up, 1 in 4 over 65.

From a drug manufacturer's point of view, this burgeoning of the potential market has coincided quite nicely with the development of pharmaceutical treatments. (At least two more impotence pills are in the pipeline from different companies.) Before Viagra, the most promising therapies involved putting gel suppositories in the urethra and injecting drugs directly into the base of the penis. The downside is not hard to grasp. "You can imagine the look most patients gave when I told them they would have to stick a small needle into the most sensitive portion of their body," says University of Chicago urologist Dr. Gregory Bales. The good news is that the erections resulting from such injections can last an hour or more, even after orgasm, though depending on one's taste and circumstances, this too could be a downside. Other treatments, which involve vacuum pumps, penile implants and penis rings, are no less awkward or, to get to the heart of the matter, no more conducive to the spontaneous, unselfconscious, beautiful sex that Calvin Klein ads imply is our daily right.

The promise of Viagra is its discretion and ease of use. Doctors recommend taking the pill an hour before sex, which might lead to some wastage among overly optimistic users but shouldn't otherwise interfere too greatly with the normal course of coital events. An even greater advantage, or at least a more naturalistic one: unlike the injectable drugs, which when efficacious produce an erection regardless of context (famously proved by Dr. Giles Brindley, a leading British impotence researcher, who once demonstrated a successful experimental treatment by dropping his trousers in front of hundreds of astonished colleagues at a conference), Viagra merely paves the way for the *possibility* of arousal. Erections must still be achieved the old-fashioned way, whether through desire, attraction, physical stimulation, the guilty thrill of an illicit affair, page 27 of *The Godfather* or what have you.

Loyola psychiatrist Renshaw offers the instructive example of a couple who came to see her the day after the man had taken Viagra for the first time: "They went to bed to wait for something to happen and fell asleep while they were waiting. They forgot to have foreplay. They expected an instant erection." The next night, after Renshaw gently reminded them about the importance of stimulation, they had intercourse for the first time in three years.

The Downside of Viagra

Viagra may help millions of men—and even some women—but it is not a sexual cure-all. It is not an aphrodisiac; it will not work in the absence of desire. Nor will it make a normal erection harder or make one last longer. It will not, in and of itself, save a marriage. In fact, there are some risks to taking Viagra that everyone, whether sexually dysfunctional or merely dissatisfied, should consider before rushing to the pharmacy:

- **Headaches** One out of 10 men in the clinical trials developed blinding headaches that grew more severe at higher doses.
- **Seeing Blue** Because the eyes contain an enzyme similar to the one on which Viagra works in the penis, about 3% of users develop temporary vision problems, ranging from blurred vision to a blue or green halo effect.
- **Blackouts** Viagra can trigger sudden drops in blood pressure, and there is a risk that men who take it in combination with nitroglycerin or other antihypertensive drugs could faint or go into shock.
- **Priapism** Although it never happened in the trials, there is a theoretical risk that men with sickle-cell anemia, leukemia or urethral inflammation could, when taking Viagra, develop priapism (defined as an erection that lasts four hours or more). Untreated, priapism can lead to tissue damage and even impotence.
- **Coital Coronaries** Sometimes impotence is an early indicator of heart disease, diabetes and some types of cancer. Taking Viagra could mask these life-threatening conditions. Men with coronary problems who have not had sex for many years should consult their doctors before putting too much strain on a weakened heart.
- **Abuse** Nobody knows the long-term effects of large doses of Viagra, especially on men who take it for the wrong reason. Although it is a relatively safe drug, there is a possibility that users will become psychologically dependent on it, unable to achieve an erection without Viagra.

—By Christine Gorman

During the drug's clinical trials, which as a rule tend to have rosier outcomes than real life, Pfizer reported a 60%-to-80% success rate, depending on the dosage (compared with a 24% success rate for placebos). The anecdotal evidence is even more compelling, if one can put up with a certain amount of crowing. Earl Macklin, a 59-year-old security guard in Chicago, has suffered from impotence on and off for 10 years as a result of diabetes. The first two times he tried Viagra, it produced minimal results; the third time he was able to have intercourse with his girlfriend for the first time in their four-month relationship. "I've been using it every day since then," he says (four days later) with a conspiratorial chuckle. "It makes me feel like I'm in my 30s again." Macklin's insurance company has notified him that it won't be reimbursing him, so, he says, "I'll limit myself to 20 pills a month."

Tom Cannata, a 43-year-old accountant from Springfield, Mass., has been taking Viagra for the past three years as a trial subject. He was suffering from partial impotence brought on, he believes, by years of bicycle riding (an activity, it should be noted, that is not universally held to be a cause of impotence). Cannata was able to achieve erections but felt that they "should have been stronger and much longer-lasting." Viagra worked for him the first time and has worked ever since. "Not only is the frequency of our sex greater," he says, "but for me it is much more intense than it was without the medication. The quality is so much better. Much firmer, stronger erections. And the orgasm is much more explosive." So pleased has Cannata been with the results that he was inspired, he says, to go out and buy a sports car not long after beginning the drug—indicating, perhaps, a soon-to-boom, Viagra-inspired market for souped-up cars, Aramis, oversize stereo equipment and other accoutrements of the virile life-style.

Some patients TIME queried had no reaction to Viagra whatsoever. Others have had more ambiguous experiences. Consider Irving Mesher, a 73-year-old retired New York City firefighter, who currently lives at a family-owned nudist resort in Pennsylvania's Pocono mountains. He describes himself as "sexually motivated" and "very active." Thanks to injection therapies (prostate-cancer treatments six years ago left him "semihard"), he has been having sex—by his account—as often as three or four times a week with several girlfriends in their 20s. Still, he was eager to try Viagra. Taking a 50-mg dose the first time, he was pleased with the results: "About as hard as it can get." However, a subsequent experiment with a 100-mg pill backfired, having no beneficial effect, as did a return to 50 mg. Mesher nevertheless plans to continue with Viagra, inspired, perhaps, by the example of his 70-year-old best friend Frank, who took the drug last week and "turned into a monster." The two are planning to invite several friends to a Viagra party.

As Mesher's story suggests, and many doctors insist, more isn't necessarily more with Viagra. Known to chemists by the less evocative name of sildenafil (the word Viagra, redolent of both "vigor" and "Niagara," had been kicking around Pfizer for years, a brand name in search of a product), the drug began life as a heart medication designed to treat angina by increasing blood flow to the heart. Sildenafil, it turned out, wasn't so good at opening coronary arteries, but happy test subjects did notice increased blood flow to their penises, a side effect brought to Pfizer's attention when the test subjects were reluctant to return their leftover pills. The medication works by suppressing the effect of the naturally occurring enzyme phosphodiesterase type 5 (PDE5), which causes an erection to subside after orgasm by breaking down the body chemical known as cyclic GMP. It is cyclic GMP that initiates the muscular and vascular changes that lead to an erection in the first place. While PDE5 is always present in the penis, cyclic GMP is produced only during arousal. The catch in impotent men is that they may not produce enough cyclic GMP to temporarily "win out" over the PDE5. Thus the efficacy of Viagra: by strong-arming PDE5, it allows a little bit of one's cyclic GMP to go a long way.

One more nugget of possibly boring but crucial biochemistry: the erectile tissue in the penis has a finite number of receptors for cyclic GMP. This means that a normally functioning man with adequate levels of the chemical shouldn't get any more bang for his buck by gobbling Viagra; the variations anyone feels in his or her sexual response are due to factors outside the drug's purview. At the same time, Pfizer hasn't done any testing of the drug on nonimpotent men to prove the point, but it's hard to imagine that biochemical nitpicking is going to stop people from experimenting. Certainly it will be hard for wet blankets and smarty-pants to compete with the siren calls coming out of sex clinics around the country from men "feeling 18 again."

"If you can have an erection naturally, you probably won't need Viagra," says Thomas Burnakis, pharmacy clinical coordinator at Baptist Medical Center in Jacksonville, Fla. "It's not going to make your erection harder or last longer. But I can guarantee you that if you walk in and say, 'Doc, I'm having trouble keeping my flag up,' most physicians are not going to insist on testing. What's to keep you from using it? Absolutely nothing. And just as with fen/phen, while a lot of doctors said they would not give that drug, a lot of clinics were prescribing it. It's going to be a moneymaking procedure. They'll give a cursory exam, charge you for that and write the prescription"—a prediction that has already been borne out on the Internet. According to Pfizer, there's no evidence that overeager users could develop a physical addiction to Viagra. But as for a psychological addiction, that is uncharted territory.

It is because of the potential for abuse and, more to the point, the traditionally seedy associations that cling to impotence remedies (witness the ads in the back of low-rent men's magazines for spurious Spanish fly, hard-on creams and the like) that drug companies have only recently turned their attention to sexual dysfunction. This would account for the tone adopted by Pfizer chairman and CEO William Steere even as he figuratively licks his chops over the potential market in "aging baby boomers." He is careful to point out that "quality-of-life drugs are gene-based just like those for serious medical conditions. In areas like impotence, aging skin, baldness and obesity, the science is just as profound as if you were working in cancer, asthma or anti-infectives." In other words, Viagra is sober stuff and not at all akin to Sy Sperling's Hair Club for Men.

Along related lines, a brochure for Pfizer employees points out that while "jokes and puns are often used in conversation about sexual health topics . . . you can redirect humorous remarks to more appropriate discussion by not joining in the humor and pointing out the seriousness of the subject matter, reminding the people with whom you speak that ED is a significant medical condition that affects the lives of millions of men and their partners." This is true, of course. It also speaks to the tricky questions of taste and exploitation that Pfizer will have to navigate in marketing the drug. So far, without an official launch or virtually any promotion, Viagra is doing fine. But why hold back? Advertisements will begin appearing in medical journals in about six weeks, followed by consumer ads this summer. A company spokesman says they will be "tasteful and emotional, emphasizing [impotence] as a couple's condition." One can imagine.

At any rate, it's an emphasis that should remind us that human sexuality is far too rich and complex for the entire subject to be balanced on the delicate fulcrum of an erection. As with the debate in psychiatry between traditional talk therapists and their more pharmacologically minded colleagues, controversy over Viagra and its cousins may well provoke a rift among sex researchers. Raymond Rosen, a professor of psychiatry at the Robert Wood Johnson Medical School in Piscataway, N.J., makes the obvious but necessary point that Viagra will not be the final word on sexual dysfunction or dissatisfaction: "There's a danger that we could lose sight of the fact that a lot of sexual problems relate to poor relationships or poor self-esteem or anxiety, depression or other factors." Or as Petersen, the *Playboy* adviser, puts it, "You can take an angry couple and give them Viagra, and then you have an angry couple with an erection." Oddly, that's reassuring.

Reported by Edward Barnes and Lawrence Mondi/New York, Wendy Cole/Chicago, Greg Fulton/Altanta and Arnold Mann/Washington.

FRAME the DEBATE

Form at end of book

Issue 4: Is Viagra a benefit or a bane to human sexuality in America?

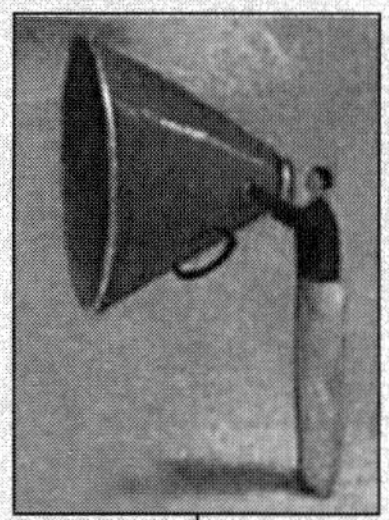

Viagra's Power Could Pressure Marriages

Karen S. Peterson

Believing that Viagra, the new pill for male impotence, will solve the sexual problems of most couples is somewhat akin to believing in the perfect orgasm, sex therapists say.

The pill can improve performance in the sexually dysfunctional male of most any age. But much of what goes awry in the bedroom—from power struggles to complacency—can't be cured by a trip to the medicine cabinet.

In fact, although Viagra will restore sexual vigor for uncounted couples, it may actually cause some relationships to expire.

Overall, the effects of Viagra will be dramatic. The drug could have one of the biggest impacts on America's sex life since the birth control pill, says pioneering sex therapist David Schnarch. "It is a bold statement to make, but it is certainly in the ballpark. Viagra will have a profound impact."

Approved by the Food and Drug Administration on March 27, Viagra increases the ability of a man to have and sustain an erection once he is sexually aroused.

Viagra is "the biggest breakthrough in the treatment for male sexual dysfunction in 30 years," says Robert Kolodny, medical director of the Behavior Medicine Institute in New Canaan, Conn.

Like the birth control pill, it will be accepted by both doctors and patients, says prominent sexologist and sociologist John Gagnon. "Doctors like giving pills to solve problems. Pills are not messy."

Viagra was tested on men with pronounced erectile dysfunction from such causes as surgery, disease and medications. But Gagnon strongly suspects that "other men who do not have really significant dysfunctions but are anxious about their erections will take it as well."

There is, however, a downside that has been ignored in the initial euphoria. "Better sexual functioning can actually destabilize a relationship," says Schnarch, author of Passionate Marriage (Holt/Owl, $12.95). Many couples have come to terms with the status quo.

"This pill may bring to the surface underlying issues that the couple is not prepared to deal with," Schnarch says. "Doctors cannot ignore this aspect of Viagra, or we (sex therapists) will get the fallout."

How can a pill lead to marital therapy? "The conjugal bed is often not just an amorous place, but a place where anger and resentment get played out in various ways," Kolodny says. "Sex is not just about physical interaction, but about emotional dynamics, too."

Viagra "gives better erections," he says. "But it does very little to address the underlying intimacy issues, communication problems, power struggles, issues of trust."

In fact, Kolodny sees a possible perversion of trust in already troubled marriages. Men whom women knew to be incapable of sex may now be in the market for adultery. "The male with new-found prowess may stray" from a dysfunctional marriage, or at least the possibility may make many wives quite nervous, says the author of *Heterosexuality* (HarperCollins, $27.50).

Old issues about which partner wants sex, when and how often can resurface. "There may be additional bids from him for greater intimacy or eroticism," Schnarch says. "His partner may feel that she can no longer fend off those demands." And she may not regard Viagra as an opportunity for the marriage to grow.

Kolodny envisions the man "already gassed up and ready to go" having taken his $10 pill. But his wife is still at her desk writing a report. She feels that her needs have not been taken into account, while he feels "he has wasted his money."

Men are already calling their doctors, says author Gail Sheehy, to say something like "I could have spent my $10 on a pizza!" Sheehy's book *Understanding Men's Passages* (Random House, $24) is due in bookstores this week.

Gagnon, co-author of *Sex in America* (Little, Brown, $22.95), does not think many women "believe good sex will come from a pill. Viagra will not produce intimacy, expressive moments, a caring for the other person. All this pill does is make the penis harder. Wow!"

On the flip side, it certainly might be the woman who has not had a full sex life for months or years who requests her partner to get Viagra. Couples may hear an "earthquake of gender," Sheehy says.

Women may see their husbands' Viagra as wives' due. "One-third of wives who work full time earn more than their husbands," Sheehy says. "That is a big social change," one that may make a woman feel she is entitled to more than snuggles.

That's exactly the type of power-and-control issue that experts say can play havoc with sex lives. And pressure on men from women to get Viagra may make men even more anxious, Schnarch says. "We have already seen that strong sexual desire from women can intimidate men," who feel the need for peak production at work and home.

Experts also say Viagra tends to influence a man's performance, not his desire to have sex. The drug still requires direct sexual stimulation by a partner seen to be "attractive and interesting," Schnarch says.

Couples who have taken each other—and impotence—for granted for years may need to learn new techniques. Others may have to look into motives as well as methods.

Schnarch recalls one woman who gained 80 pounds and believed that her change caused her husband's impotence. More important, her extra pounds let her hide from a more basic question: Did she really want to stay with him, whether he was impotent or not? What would happen if she lost the weight and he regained his sexual stamina?

"There is a lot of 'couples work' that has to be done to make this work," Sheehy says. "And the best place to do it is at home."

Experts emphasize that Viagra really will be magical for many committed, caring couples whose sex lives have been put on hold for years.

Tolman Geffs, 64, or Orange County, Calif., participated in a clinical trial of the drug while it was tested by the FDA. He has been taking Viagra a year.

"This drug is no flash in the pan," Geffs says. "I call it my nighttime vitamin. I just take a pill every evening and let life take its course. If we feel intimate, fine. If not, that is not a problem."

Married in 1990, Geffs says, "I thought I'd finally found this warm, close relationship I've always wanted." Then in 1995 he underwent prostate surgery, which affected his sexual performance. "It was devastating to me," he says. "Subconsciously, I feared if I'd lost my abilities to perform as a man, I would lose my mate."

No way, says his wife, Jill Geffs, 59. And now she says the pill has given them back a full sex life. "I have my macho man back."

Baby boomers facing midlife also feel very positive about the drug. "If the time comes that I need it, I would have no trouble asking for it in industrial strength," says Bill Flynn, 51, of Manassas, Va.

"I've been amazed by the number of men my age with an interest in it," says Dennis M. Taylor, 51, of Helena, Mont. "The fear of impotency must be really pervasive in my generation. We invented the sexual revolution in the '60s, and we are also in the greatest denial about aging."

But Taylor also worries that his generation seeks a magic bullet for sexual problems. "It is not just your ability to achieve an erection that allows a full, loving relationship with your partner."

Schnarch agrees. He also worries a little about the ethics of "producing sexual wonder pills." While Viagra will be a gift to men with true erectile problems, "are we doing other men a favor if it gives them expectations of bionic performance and perfection?"

A true marriage or long-term commitment," he says, "includes letting one's true self be known, including one's limitations."

FRAME the DEBATE

Form at end of book

WiseGuide Wrap-Up

The drug sildenafil was released to the prescription drug market as Viagra in September 1998. Since then, physicians have been writing over 300,000 prescriptions per week. The drug enhances the effects of nitric oxide, which, in turn, enhances penile erection. Viagra carries certain liabilities, however, such as an increased risk of acute hypotension, particularly among males who may be taking nitroglycerine or other nitrate drugs. For males with no heart disease and who are not taking nitrates, the physical risks of taking Viagra are few. Some odd side effects, like seeing a blue haze, facial flushing, and headaches, are associated with Viagra.

Even though Viagra appears to be effective in helping impotent males achieve and maintain erections, it may also carry psychosocial risks. Some argue that Viagra use may hamper, rather than enhance, sexuality as some males may feel more pressure to perform. In addition, the spontaneity of personal relations may decrease as the erection becomes the focus, rather than the intimacy of the moment.

R.E.A.L. Sites

This list provides a print preview of typical **Coursewise** R.E.A.L. sites. (There are over 100 such sites at the **Courselinks**™ site.) The danger in printing URLs is that web sites can change overnight. As we went to press, these sites were functional using the URLs provided. If you come across one that isn't, please let us know via email to: webmaster@coursewise.com. Use your Passport to access the most current list of R.E.A.L. sites at the **Courselinks** site.

Site name: A Urology Opinion

URL: http://www.a-urology.com/viagra.htm

Why is it R.E.A.L.? This site contains information for health-care professionals on sildenafil. The site also provides several links to articles related to male erectile dysfunction and the prescription of Viagra.

Key topics: impotence, sildenafil, Viagra

Try this: Read the article, "Viagra, Cure or over the Falls without a Barrel?" Explore the rest of the site. Visit some of the links on the site. List and discuss three physical health issues and three psychosocial health issues regarding male sexual problems. What types of issues are at stake when counseling and treating males with erectile dysfunction?

Site name: Viagra: The Rationing Precedent

URL: http://news.bbc.co.uk/hi/english/health/newsid_260000/260460.stm

Why is it R.E.A.L.? This site reviews the controversy surrounding the proposal by Great Britain's health secretary, Frank Dobson, to limit prescriptions of Viagra by the National Health Service.

Key topics: impotence, rationing, sildenafil, Viagra

Try this: Read the article "Viagra: The Rationing Precedent," and select at least two other related story links to prepare yourself for a debate on the real and perceived need to ration Viagra. Select a "side" to the argument, and then prepare yourself to support your thesis with at least five factually supported points. Could this happen in America?

Is Routine Circumcision for Baby Boys Mutilation or Hygiene?

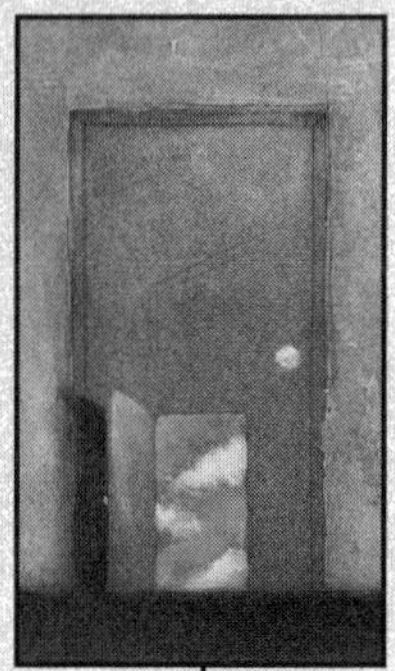

ISSUE 5

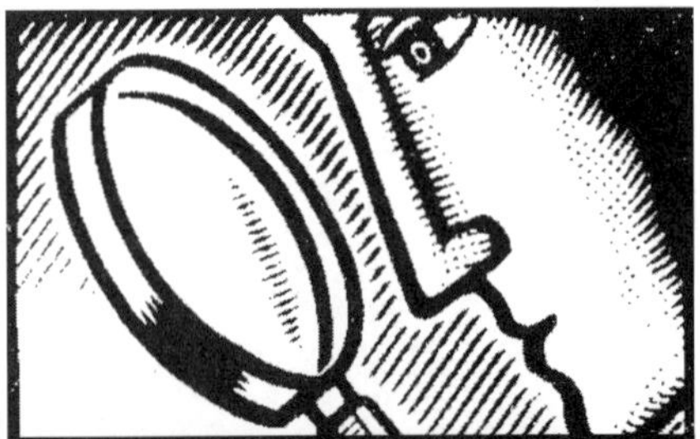

Take a Closer Look

1. According to Goldman in Reading 11, how much of the skin from the average penis is removed during circumcision?
2. According to Kellogg in Reading 11, in the past, what was circumcision of the penis supposed to prevent?
3. Use information from Reading 11 to compare the relative risk of penile cancer and sexually transmitted diseases for uncircumcised males to the risk of surgical injury from the circumcision operation.
4. What persuasion techniques does Jenkins use in Reading 11 to discredit the practice of routine circumcision?
5. In Reading 12, what are three methodological flaws that Schoen identifies in Laumann et al.'s research?
6. In Reading 12, Goldman contends that doctors with a certain personal profile favor circumcision. Describe the profile.
7. In Reading 12, what do Howe and Cold propose for testing the relative penile sensitivity of men with circumcised and uncircumcised penises?

WiseGuide Intro

Each year, 1.2 to 1.8 million newborn boys in America undergo routine penile circumcision, the removal of the foreskin from the end of the penis. The procedure is generally performed within days of birth and most often without anesthetic. The practice is widespread in the United States but not worldwide. Common reasons for the practice range from hygiene, to lowered risks of sexually transmitted diseases and urinary tract infections, to simply making a son "look like Dad." Cultural and religious dogmas may also call for circumcision—for example, Muslims and Jews may perform circumcisions as part of religious practices. Critics of the practice say that the hygienic benefits are negligible, that the risk of injury is high, and that the practice not only puts the newborn through undue pain and distress but may also reduce tactile sexual sensations and enjoyment later in adulthood.

In Reading 11, "Separated at Birth," Mark Jenkins takes an oppositional stand on routine circumcision of newborn boys. He presents arguments against performing the operation for hygienic reasons. Testimonials and quotes from circumcised men and physicians who oppose circumcision bolster Jenkins' stance. Jenkins discusses the historical and social contexts surrounding the practice. Accompanying the debate is a set of sidebars that present basic anatomy and function of the foreskin, along with a step-by-step narration of the circumcision procedure. One of the unique and intriguing arguments that Jenkins presents is that significant financial gains may be the motivation for continuing the practice of circumcision.

Reading 12, "Advantages and Disadvantages of Neonatal Circumcision," consists of the individual letters of seven doctors and a reply from Dr. Laumann and his colleagues following an article on circumcision by Laumann et al. in a previous issue of *The Journal of the American Medical Association.* The experts offer several compelling and well-supported arguments for and against routine circumcision. Most of the discussion centers around circumcision for hygienic reasons and for the prevention of sexually transmitted diseases. Issues of tradition, cultural beliefs, and scientific evidence also enter the debate.

Issue 5: Is routine circumcision for baby boys mutilation or hygiene?

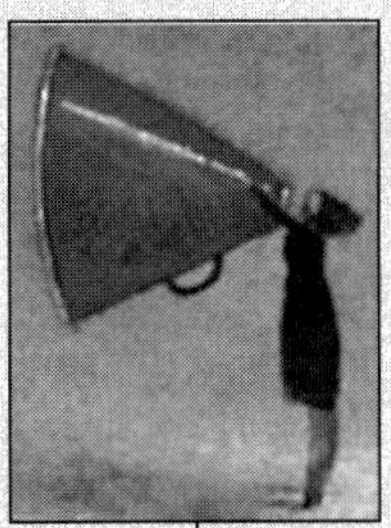

Separated at Birth

Mark Jenkins

For the typical American boy, life begins with circumcision, a painful cut to the sensitive skin on his penis. Is it necessary?

The baby, J. Hernandez, is less than a day old . . . tiny head still slightly misshapen, eyelids puffy, mouth half-open in sleep. The nurse has taken him from his mother and is carrying him to a side room in the pediatric ward. The nurse pops on a white heat lamp with her elbow, removes the child from a blue blanket, and lays him in a molded plastic form bolted to the counter. This bathtub-like shell is called a Circumstraint. There are indentations for the baby's arms and legs. The nurse binds Velcro straps around his limbs, bends the light over him and steps back. The baby is naked and spread-eagled, and he begins to cry.

Every 30 seconds a baby boy is circumcised. It is the most common surgery performed in America. It is usually done without anesthesia, and often without the consent of the parents.

"I never questioned it," says Kyle Joseph, the father of a circumcised boy. "The doctor took him away, performed the operation and brought him back. That's just the way it was done. I was circumcised; he was circumcised. I don't even remember signing a consent form."

That's typical, according to Craig Shoemaker, M.D., a North Dakota pediatrician and member of the American Academy of Pediatrics (AAP) task force on circumcision. "Many doctors do not adequately counsel parents regarding circumcision—what the risks are, what the potential benefits are, how much it costs. Performing a circumcision without such counseling is inappropriate. Some people would call it criminal assault."

Most parents don't know what circumcision really is, and yet 65 percent of them still allow doctors to do the surgery.

America is the only country in the Western world that routinely circumcises newborn boys. Eighty-five percent of the world's men are uncircumcised.

"The practice violates all seven principles of the American Medical Association's code of ethics," charges George Denniston, M.D., a Seattle physician and founder of Doctors Opposing Circumcision. "By definition, it's not even surgery. Surgery is removal of diseased tissue, or a repair of some kind."

"Nonsense," says Edgar Schoen, M.D., director of perinatal screening at Kaiser Permanente Medical Center in California, and an outspoken proponent of circumcision. "There are numerous medical reasons for it."

This pro and con argument has been raging in the medical community for almost three decades. Meanwhile, the circumcisions continue.

The doctor enters the room, scrubs his hands in the sink, and snaps on plastic gloves. The nurse passes him a package, and he opens it on the counter beside the child. Inside are several large, light blue cloth napkins; some squares of gauze; a squeeze-tube of Betadine (an antiseptic ointment); and an assortment of stainless-steel utensils: a pair of scissors, two hemostats (small, needle-nose pliers), a heavy metal clamp attached to a hollow cone, a scalpel handle, and a scalpel in a sterile packet.

If you're like most American men, you're circumcised. But you probably haven't given it any thought since junior high school, when you first noticed that not every kid in the locker room looked the same. In fact, if you're single or childless now, you may think that it's purely a father/son issue of little concern to you. Think again.

"Circumcision removes one-third to one-half of the skin on the penile shaft," says Ronald Goldman, Ph.D., executive director of the Circumcision Resource Center in Boston and author of *Circumcision: The Hidden Trauma.* "The average circumcision cuts off what would grow into about 12 square inches of sexually sensitive skin."

According to Canadian pathologist John Taylor, M.B., the foreskin is one of the key erogenous zones of the male body. Its 240 feet of nerves and 1,000 nerve endings are similar to those on the fingers and lips.

"The fact is," says Goldman, "when it comes to sex, circumcised men don't know what they're missing."

Separated at Birth, Mark Jenkins. MEN'S HEALTH, July/August 1998. Reprinted by permission of the author.

But a few do. Increasingly, men who were circumcised as adults (for various medical reasons) are speaking out against circumcision, providing firsthand accounts of sex before and after.

"I had ample sexual experience, and I was quite happy as an intact male," says Rick Thomas, who was circumcised on advice of his doctor at age 26. "After my circumcision, that pleasure was utterly gone. On a scale of 10, the uncircumcised penis experiences pleasure of at least 11 or 12; the circumcised penis is lucky to get to 3. If men who were circumcised at birth knew the loss of pleasure they would experience, they would storm the hospitals and not permit their sons to undergo this."

Douglas McArthur, a 55-year-old locksmith for Pennsylvania who was also circumcised as an adult, reports similar problems. "Sex before circumcision was like driving a luxury car with automatic transmission," he explains. "I used to just glide along. Sex now is like driving a tiny, powerless compact with a manual transmission. It takes a lot of work to get anywhere. My penis has lost 90 percent of its sensitivity."

Only in the last decade have scientists devoted in-depth studies to the structure and function of the foreskin. The foreskin is a complex, two-layer organ similar to the eyelid; it's designed to protect the head of the penis from abrasion and infection. Its surface represents 50 percent of all penile skin, and folds around the opening of the penis. Its inside surface is composed of a soft mucosa that secretes antibacterial and antiviral lubricants called *smegma,* which further protect the glans from friction and infection. Because the glans is sheathed in this moist envelope, it retains its sensitivity. During sex, the foreskin glides along the penile shaft, providing lubrication and stimulation.

Says one spouse of her uncircumcised husband: "There's a big industry in this country selling lubricants and jellies to enhance sex, but they're unnecessary for those of us lucky enough to have married an uncircumcised man. An intact man's glans is naturally moist and juicy."

The doctor swabs the baby's testicles and penis with antiseptic-soaked gauze, then lays one cloth over his torso, another over his legs, and a third, with a small hole in the middle, over his genitals. He pops the tiny penis through the hole. The baby is still crying. The nurse mentions that babies feel safest in the fetal position. She says they hate having their arms held away from their bodies. The parents are not in the room. The nurse shuts the door.

Outside of the Jewish community, where it's a religious rite, circumcision was practically unheard of in America until 1870, when Lewis Sayre, M.D., claimed to have cured a 5-year-old boy of paralysis by stretching out his foreskin and snipping it off. For the next two decades, Dr. Sayre and his associates crusaded for circumcision, claiming it could cure hip-joint disease, epilepsy, hernia, convulsions, elephantiasis, poor eyesight, tuberculosis, and rectal prolapse, among other things. This was all disproved, of course, and circumcision would probably have vanished from the American medical scene had its backers not found a compelling new way to sell it: as a cure for masturbation.

To the publicly puritanical but privately lascivious Victorians, masturbation was the root of numerous social maladies and physical illnesses, including blindness and even insanity. Naturally, they believed, if circumcision could prevent masturbation, it would prevent other diseases as well.

Doctors of the time reported that "removal of the protective covering of the glans tends to dull the sensibility" of the penis and "thereby diminishes sexual appetite." In 1888, John Harvey Kellogg, M.D., of cereal fame, summed up the medical profession's opinion and gave justification for the next 60 years of foreskin removal. "A remedy for masturbation which is almost always successful in small boys is circumcision. The operation should be performed by a surgeon without administering an anesthetic, as the pain attending the operation will have a salutary effect upon the mind."

The doctor snaps the scalpel blade onto the handle, then places it beside the baby. Lifting the hemostat, which resembles a sharp-tipped pair of pliers, he begins. Holding the penis in one hand, he moves the point of the hemostat through the hole at the end of the foreskin. The foreskin is tightly attached to the glans, like a fingernail to a finger. The doctor begins pushing the point between the foreskin and glans. The operation is similar to running a razor blade underneath the fingernail. The baby bucks on the plastic form, in obvious pain.

By the end of World War II it was clear that circumcision was not stopping men from masturbating; but, by then, the procedure was institutionalized. It had become the norm for white, middle-class American men. The uncircumcised were often recent immigrants or African-Americans. Probably as a result of racial prejudice, the uncircumcised penis was viewed as unhygienic and unclean.

But this, too, turns out to be false.

"The uncircumcised penis is self-cleaning," explains Robert Van Howe, M.D., a pediatrician from Wisconsin who has been studying the causes of circumcision for 20 years. "Every time you urinate, you flush out the preputial cavity. The hygiene issue was just another excuse. Since its inception, circumcision has been a surgery looking for a rationale. First it was disease, then masturbation, then hygiene; now it's back to disease." In 1971 the American Academy of Pediatrics (AAP) stated that circumcision was medically unnecessary. At the time more than 80 percent of American baby boys were circumcised. Then in 1989, the AAP released a new position paper that equivocated: "Newborn circumcision has potential medical benefits, as well as disadvantages and risks." Still, by the following year, the rate was down to 59 percent.

Dr. Schoen chaired the AAP task force that made that reversal. He still stands by the position, claiming that the foreskin is the genital equivalent of the appendix, and that newborn circumcision is "a preventive health measure analogous to immunization."

"The most important health benefit of circumcision is the decreased risk of urinary-tract infections," explains Dr. Schoen, citing a well-known 1985 study, which he says has since been "over-whelmingly confirmed" by other studies. But Martin Altschul, M.D., a pediatrician and M.I.T.-trained mathematician, has reexamined the evidence and finds it fraught with problems.

"The whole body of research on this issue is a how-to-lie-with-statistics classic," argues Dr. Altschul. "Depending on how you collect the data, you can get almost any result you want." Dr. Altschul's own research also found that many of the urinary-tract infections in uncircumcised boys were "attributable to congenital anomalies." Recently, several studies have suggested that neonatal circumcision may actually increase the infection rate.

Dr. Schoen cites two other medical benefits of circumcision, namely decreased risks of developing penile cancer and contracting sexually transmitted diseases, such as HIV and syphilis.

"You're more likely to be struck by lightning than to suffer from penile cancer," counters Dr. Van Howe. "Japan, Norway, Finland, and Denmark all have lower rates than the United States, and they don't circumcise their boys."

In fact, in 1996, representatives of the American Cancer Society wrote a letter to the AAP in which they pointed out that "fatalities caused by circumcision accidents may approximate the mortality rate from penile cancer." The letter also stated the "Perpetuating the mistaken belief that circumcision prevents cancer is inappropriate."

"Penile cancer is extremely rare—less than one case for every 100,000 men," adds Dr. Altschul. "It's preposterous to even suggest that because we have some minuscule risk of disease, we should cut off the foreskin of every little boy."

"Breast cancer in women is common," says Dr. Denniston, "more common than the all purported health risks of the foreskin combined. Does that justify cutting off all breasts at puberty?"

What about circumcised men and STDs? A recent study published in the *Journal of the American Medical Association* found that circumcised men did have a lower incidence of syphilis and HIV. But they had a higher rate of infection with herpes, hepatitis, and chlamydia. Overall, the study authors wrote, "We found no evidence of a prophylactic role for circumcision, and a slight tendency in the opposite direction."

"The bottom line," says Dr. Denniston, "is that the alleged benefits of circumcision don't approach the risks."

The child struggles against the straps. The foreskin is attached firmly to the glans, and it's difficult to pry loose. The doctor scrapes the point of the hemostat in a circular motion around the glans, tearing the skin off the head of the penis. The child continues to buck on the plastic form. This is why the Circumstraint is bolted to the counter.

- **July 3, 1991; Oakland, California:** While circumcising a 12-hour-old baby, the doctor cuts off one-third of the glans. The severed head is "reattached," but the child is disfigured. A court awards the minor plaintiff $256,000.
- **September 12, 1992; San Diego, California:** During a circumcision, a doctor cuts off a boy's glans. The doctor claims that since there is "no apparent loss of function," he met the standard of care. A jury awards the minor plaintiff $36,400 in damages.
- **July 18, 1995; Houston, Texas:** A 5-year-old boy goes into a coma while being circumcised. He dies a week later.

"The complication rate for circumcision varies from 2 to 6 percent," says Dr. Van Howe. "The average male will have more health problems from being circumcised than from being left alone."

Some medical professionals believe that circumcision for other than religious purposes would disappear from America if it weren't covered by insurance. This is what happened in England, where the circumcision rate prior to World War II was roughly equivalent to that in the United States. After the war, British doctors could find no compelling evidence to continue the surgery, and it was dropped from the list of covered services. Within a decade, the circumcision rate dropped from 50 percent among the working class and 85 percent among the upper class to less than half a percent in both.

"Why is this procedure still covered by HMOs and health-insurance companies? The simple answer is, because parents want it," says Patricia Wald, M.D., regional coordinating chief of pediatrics for Kaiser Permanente Medical Center in southern California. There, doctors counsel parents so they're making an informed decision, and don't perform the operation unless asked. "We cover it as a courtesy. But to me it's cosmetic surgery, like ear piercing."

Circumcision is estimated to be a $400 million business in America. The average cost of the procedure ranges from $50 to $350, with $115 being the average. The usual insurance reimbursement to doctors is around $95.

Dr. Van Howe claims that a busy doctor can generate $25,000 a year from circumcisions alone. But Dr. Shoemaker disputes the contention that money alone lies behind the practice.

"After you counsel the parents appropriately and do the procedure," Dr. Shoemaker explains, "it's not a profitable use of time."

The foreskin is still attached to the glans, and the doctor must rake the hemostat around the head of the penis several times. The baby is shrieking now, his face red, his eyes squeezed shut.

Circumcision is the only surgery in America routinely performed without anesthesia. Sixty-four to 96 percent of circumcised infants endure the procedure with nothing to deaden the pain. Until recently, doctors often told parents they didn't feel the same pain as adults.

"I didn't know what circumcision really was when I consented to have my three sons circumcised," says Marilyn Milos, founder and executive director of the National Organization of Circumcision Information Resource Centers (NOCIRC). "My doctor told me it was necessary, that it didn't hurt, and that it took only a moment to perform—like cutting the umbilical cord, I thought."

Ten years after her last son was born, Milos went back to school to become a registered nurse. As a student, she was asked to assist at a circumcision. "To see a part of a baby's penis being cut off—without an anesthetic—was devastating." Later, while working as a nurse, she made a videotape of the procedure and called it *Informed Consent.*

"Parents had no idea what was happening to their baby boys," she explains. "The point was to show them what circumcision really entailed." The hospital, Marin General in California, refused to allow expectant parents to view the tape. "They said it was too much for parents to see. I said, 'Then perhaps it's too much for babies to experience.' "

In 1985, Milos founded NOCIRC. "It's all such an unspeakable cover-up. The doctors are in denial, so the hospitals are in denial, so the parents are intentionally, illegally uninformed. Circumcision is the worst fraud in American medical history." Recent studies support Milos' gut reaction to unanesthetized circumcision. A recent issue of the *Journal of the American Medical Association* reported that "newborns . . . who did not receive an anesthetic suffered great distress during and following the circumcision, and they were exposed to unnecessary risk (from choking or apnea)." The report goes on to say that the skill of the surgeon did not reduce the pain, and that infantile amnesia (the "he-won't-remember-it-anyway" argument) can't justify it.

But even if doctors did use anesthesia, the reduction in pain would have to be measured against other concerns, such as the danger of using potent painkillers on day-old babies.

Then there is the question about how long the hurt lasts. "Circumcision causes such traumatic pain in newborns that it may have damaging effects upon the developing brain," says James Prescott, Ph.D., director of the Institute of Humanistic Science in Long Beach, California. A psychologist who has written extensively on childhood trauma and its long-term effects, Prescott says the stress of circumcision damages the neural systems that mediate genital pleasure. In effect, he says, the baby's brain is encoded to associate pain with pleasure. In fact, the pain is so severe that it's not unusual for babies to go into a kind of shock, suddenly becoming silent and ceasing to struggle.

The foreskin is finally separated from the glans. Using a second hemostat, the doctor runs the point up inside the foreskin, clamps it to constrict blood flow, moves the hemostat a quarter inch, takes up the scissors and slices the skin along the clamp line.

Ten years after Milos founded her organization, 24 nurses at the St. Vincent Hospital in Santa Fe, New Mexico, declared themselves "conscientious objectors to infant circumcision." Later, several of them formed Nurses for the Rights of the Child. "Our goal is to protect unconsenting infants and children from surgical alteration of their genitals," says co-founder Mary Conant.

Two years ago attorney J. Steven Svoboda, a former Human Rights Fellow at Harvard Law School, founded Attorneys for the Rights of the Child. "Our position is that circumcision is medical malpractice," he explains. "The medical profession, which has perpetuated this tragic disfigurement of baby boys' genitals, will now be challenged by an organization of legal professionals."

The courts are already considering cases. On July 22, 1995, a jury in Montgomery, Alabama, found Jackson Hospital and Clinic guilty of negligence in a case where a newborn was mistakenly circumcised against his mother's wishes. The minor plaintiff was awarded $65,000.

Suddenly the baby is quiet . . . mouth open, but no sound; body rigid. The foreskin is splayed open and bleeding. The doctor tears a hole in the skin and forces a hollow cone up inside the foreskin. The baby begins screaming again, straining at the straps. The stainless-steel cone keeps the glans from being cut off. Using both hands, the doctor places a heavy clamp over the child's penis, which protrudes through a hole in the clamp. The doctor tightens the clamp, picks up the scalpel, and in one smooth, practiced motion, circles it around the foreskin.

Most of the world's leading medical establishments have come out against this surgery. "Circumcision of newborns should not be routinely performed," says the Canadian Paediatric Society. "To circumcise . . . would be unethical and inappropriate," says the British Medical Association. The Australasian [Australia and New Zealand] Association of Paediatric Surgeons states: "Neonatal male circumcision has no medical indication. It is a traumatic procedure performed without anesthesia to remove a normal, functional and protective prepuce."

The AAP is expected to publish its new position on circumcision sometime this year. "This is just my opinion," says task-force member Dr. Shoemaker, "but I think the Academy is going to say there's not enough medical evidence to recommend routine circumcision—but that there's also not enough evidence to say it shouldn't be done at all." If this happens, the position paper will again be subject to interpretation, and it will be of little guidance.

Kent Kleppinger, M.D., a pediatrician who performs circumcisions, says, "I tell parents circumcision is cosmetic surgery. It isn't difficult to dissuade the mothers, but the fathers generally override their decisions. They want their boys to look like other boys in the locker room. They want their boys to look like them."

Like father, like son. This may be one of the hidden reasons why infant boys are still circumcised in America. But Shell Thompson, an editor for a national outdoor magazine and father of two boys, finds the "locker-room argument" specious. "I was a fat kid, a tub boat. I was teased unmercifully when I was a teenager. But so were the skinny kids and the kids with acne and the kids with red hair. At that age, boys will find something to pick on, no matter what's between their legs."

Thompson was circumcised as an infant but chose not to circumcise his boys, a decision that is becoming increasingly common. Rates for circumcision are dropping all over the country. On the West Coast they're already down to 34 percent. By the time a baby born today takes his first junior-high shower, he may be in the minority if he's circumcised.

It may all come down to the basic human rights of the child. In 1996, the Canadian Medical Association approved a code of ethics that instructs doctors to "refuse to participate in or support practices that violate basic human rights." This suggests that, in the case of circumcision, parental preference should not override the child's physical rights to his body.

Margaret Somerville, professor of law and medicine at McGill University in Montreal and founding director of the Centre for Medicine, Ethics and Law, recently raised the hair on the necks of all North American pediatricians by declaring circumcision "technically criminal assault."

"Once you decide that circumcision is not medically necessary, you take away the therapeutic intent. Take away therapeutic intent, and circumcision becomes an unjustified wounding," she says.

Leo Sorger, M.D., writing in *ObGYN News,* is even more explicit: "Circumcision causes pain, trauma, and a permanent loss of protective and erogenous tissue. Removing normal, healthy, functioning tissue [for no medical reason] . . . violates the United Nations Universal Declaration of Human Rights (Article 5) and the United Nations Convention on the Rights of the Child (Article 13)."

In September 1996, the United States Congress passed a law banning the mutilation of female genitalia. "Americans are horrified by female genital mutilation," says attorney Svoboda, "but they somehow don't recognize the routine torture going on in their own culture." He acknowledges that a clitoridectomy is a more serious and detrimental surgery than circumcision, but he argues that "human-rights law doesn't say if you cut off four toes, it's a human rights violation, but if you cut off only three, it's okay. That's not how human-rights law works. If it's wrong, it's wrong. Involuntary circumcision is wrong."

The foreskin is peeled away like the rind of an orange. The baby is still crying. After several minutes, the doctor removes the clamp, pops off his gloves, and leaves. The nurse quickly applies an antiseptic ointment and returns the trembling child to his parents.

FRAME the DEBATE

Form at end of book

Issue 5: Is routine circumcision for baby boys mutilation or hygiene?

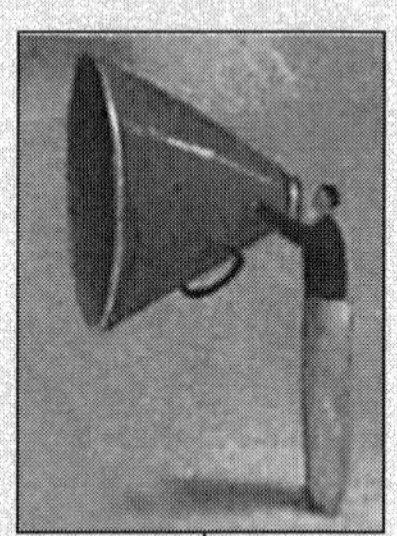

Advantages and Disadvantages of Neonatal Circumcision

To the Editor

The article by Dr. Laumann and colleagues[1] supports the conclusions of the 1989 American Academy of Pediatrics (AAP) Task Force on Circumcision (of which I was the chair) that newborn circumcision has potential benefits as well as risks. The authors present new information that indicated circumcised men had slight benefit in terms of sexual satisfaction and less likelihood of sexual dysfunction. This complements a 1988 survey of women that demonstrated female sexual preference for circumcised men.[2]

Although the subjective survey method reported by Laumann et al. is valid for the issue of sexual satisfaction, it is not applicable for studying sexually transmitted diseases (STDs). As the authors point out, self-reported STDs will be underreported because patients with STDs may be asymptomatic, and the diagnosis carries a social stigma. Relying on the memories of men ranging in age from 18 to 59 years on this sensitive topic is not justified. Further, it is not valid to group all 7 listed STDs. The mechanism of infection of the individual STDs can vary (e.g., transfusions and intravenous drug use as well as sexual transmission for hepatitis B and human immunodeficiency virus [HIV] infection). The incubation periods before symptoms are apparent vary widely among the individual STDs (e.g., days for gonorrhea, months or years for HIV), which can make recall unreliable. Moreover, laboratory testing usually is required for diagnosis. The risk of drawing conclusions on STDs from this study, which has a relatively small sample size (353 uncircumcised men) and lack of objective data, is exemplified by the paucity of the HIV data. Epidemiological studies during the past decade indicate that uncircumcised men have a significantly greater risk of acquiring HIV infection than do circumcised men.[3–6] These studies, as well as published evidence on other STDs, are unjustifiably trivialized by the unwarranted general conclusion that there is no significant difference in risk for STDs between circumcised and uncircumcised men.

Edgar J. Schoen, M.D.
Kaiser Permanente Medical Center
Oakland, California

Appreciation is expressed to the Medical Editing Department, Kaiser Foundation Research Institute, who provided editorial assistance.

References

1. Laumann EO, Masi CM, Zuckerman EW. Circumcision in the United States: prevalence, prophylactic effects, and sexual practice. *JAMA.* 1997; 277:1052–1057.
2. Williamson ML, Williamson PS. Women's preferences for penile circumcision in sexual partners. *J Sex Educ Ther.* 1988; 14(2):9–12.
3. Simonsen JN, Cameron DW, Gakinya MN, et al. Human immunodeficiency virus infection among men with sexually transmitted diseases: experience from a center in Africa. *N Engl J Med.* 1988; 319:274–278.
4. Cameron DW, Simonsen JN, D'Costa LJ, et al. Female to male transmission of human immunodeficiency virus type 1: risk factors for seroconversion in man. *Lancet.* 1989; 2:403–407.
5. Moses S, Plummer FA, Bradley JE, Ndinya-Achola JO, Nagelkerke NJD, Ronald AR. The association between lack of male circumcision and risk for HIV infection: a review of the epidemiological data. *Sex Transm Dis.* 1994; 21(4):201–210.
6. Caldwell JC, Caldwell P. The African AIDS epidemic. *Sci Am.* 1996; 274(3):62–68.

(JAMA. 1997; 278:201)

To the Editor

Dr. Laumann and colleagues[1] conclude that circumcision provides no preventive medical benefit, thus reviving an ongoing controversy. While issues related to the risk of childhood urinary tract infection with and without circumcision may be debatable, the authors have been

Advantages and Disadvantages of Neonatal Circumcision. JOURNAL OF THE AMERICAN MEDICAL ASSOCIATION (Letters to the Editor), July 16, 1997, Volume 278, p. 203.

blinded to the medical benefits of circumcision for adults. Indeed, only 1 week following the report by Laumann et al., Royce et al. reported that "male circumcision consistently shows a protective effect against HIV infection," with an 8-fold increased rate of HIV disease among uncircumcised men.[2] Royce et al. further report a greater incidence of HIV in sexual partners of uncircumcised men and speculate that the abundance of Langerhans cells in the foreskin may be a contributing factor and that the presence of a foreskin actually may increase infectiousness.

Periodic arguments against circumcision have been supported by a variety of evidence, much of which has been directed toward the "inhumanity" of such procedures. While data from studies such as Royce et al. should help to restore this paper-churning debate to its proper perspective, the findings of Leumann et al. that sexual dysfunction was less common in circumcised men inadvertently adds weight to the medical argument.

Irvin R. Berman, M.D.
Southeast Georgia Regional Medical Center
Brunswick

References

1. Laumann EO, Masi CM, Zuckerman EW. Circumcision in the United States: prevalence, prophylactic effects and sexual practice. *JAMA.* 1997; 277:1052–1057.
2. Royce RA, Sena A, Cates W, Cohen MS. Sexual transmission of HIV: current concepts. *N Engl J Med.* 1997; 336:1072–1078.

(JAMA. 1997; 278:201)

To the Editor

Dr. Laumann and colleagues[1] conclude that with respect to STDs "there is no evidence of a prophylactic role for circumcision and a slight tendency in the opposite direction." However, the authors did not consider one important aspect of the relationship, if any, between male circumcision and the risk of STDs including cervical cancer in their female partners. Hunter et al.[2] found that women whose partners are uncircumcised are at increased risk of STDs, including HIV. Human papillomavirus (HPV), which plays an important role in the pathogenesis of cervical cancer,[3] also is sexually transmitted, although men are frequently asymptomatic. Several studies have shown that women whose sexual partners are uncircumcised are at increased risk of cervical cancer secondary to HPV.[4,5] These findings deserve further examination and, if confirmed, would be important information for parents and physicians to consider in deciding whether to circumcise or recommend circumcision of male infants.

Lainie Friedman Ross, M.D., Ph.D.
University of Chicago
Chicago, Illinois

References

1. Laumann EO, Masi CM, Zuckerman EW. Circumcision in the United States: prevalence, prophylactic effects, and sexual practice. *JAMA.* 1997; 277:1052–1057.
2. Hunter DJ, Maggwa BN, Mati JK, Tukei PM, Mbugua S. Sexual behavior, sexually transmitted diseases, male circumcision, and risk of HIV infection among women in Nairobi, Kenya. *AIDS.* 1994; 8:93–99.
3. Cannistra SA, Niloff JM. Cancer of the uterine cervix. *N Engl J Med.* 1997; 334:1030–1038.
4. Agarwal SS, Sehgal A, Sardana S, Kumar A, Luthra UK. Role of male behavior in cervical carcinogenesis among women with one lifetime sexual partner. *Cancer.* 1993; 72:1666–1669.
5. Viladoms Fuster JM, Leira Juanos J. Human papillomavirus in the male. *Acta Urol Esp.* 1989; 13:343–346.

(JAMA. 1997; 278:201–202)

To the Editor

Circumcision depends on the perpetuation of American cultural beliefs that support it. One way to justify inflicting pain and harm on others is to believe that otherwise more pain and harm will follow. Using this strategy to defend circumcision requires minimizing or denying the harm caused by circumcision and producing medical claims about protection from potential future pain and harm. Circumcision advocates claim that the surgery has prophylactic effects. Laumann et al.[1] provide another response to this belief.

For some people, claims of medical benefits are sufficient justification for circumcision partly because circumcision is a surgical procedure that is done on someone else. Using medical claims and studies to defend circumcision may be an unconscious way for some physicians to avoid the emotional discomfort of questioning their own circumcision. A survey of primary care physicians showed that circumcision was supported more often by physicians who were older, male, and circumcised.[2]

Full and open debate on the circumcision issue is necessary, particularly regarding long-term effects and ethical considerations, but this debate has not yet occurred. Even with full debate, the overwhelming pain and harm of circumcision cannot be proven to many circumcision advocates because people tend to avoid new information that strongly conflicts with their beliefs.

Thus far, the feelings of those who must live with the decision—the infants—generally have been ignored. The fact that infants can't physically resist and stop the procedure makes it easy to dismiss their feelings. Of course, adult feelings are not so easily dismissed. A preliminary survey of 75 men suggests that the more men know about the important functions of the prepuce, the more likely they are to be dissatisfied about being circumcised.[3] Now that an increasing number of men are learning about the prepuce and expressing this dissatisfaction, clinicians must acknowledge that it is impossible to predict how a male infant will feel about his circumcision when he is older. A prudent course would be to allow men to make the decision about circumcision for themselves when they reach adulthood.

What prevents the adoption of such a new policy is the reluctance to acknowledge such a mistake and all that it implies. This avoidance of guilt helps to explain the tenacity with which some people defend existing circumcision policies,[3] and the ongoing denial requires the continued acceptance of cultural beliefs. More than new studies, clinicians will need courage to change. The children of the future are depending on it.

Ronald Goldman, Ph.D.
Circumcision Resource Center
Boston, Massachusetts

References

1. Laumann EO, Masi CM, Zuckerman EW. Circumcision in the United States: prevalence, prophylactic effects, and sexual practice. *JAMA.* 1997; 277:1052–1057.
2. Stein M. Marx M, Taggert S, et al. Routine neonatal circumcision: the gap between contemporary policy and practice. *J Fam Pract.* 1982; 15:47–53.
3. Goldman R. *Circumcision—The Hidden Trauma: How an American Cultural Practice Affects Infants and Ultimately Us All.* Boston, Mass: Vanguard Publications; 1997.

(JAMA. 1997; 278:202)

To the Editor

Dr. Laumann and colleagues[1] conclude that data from the National Health and Social Life Survey do not lend clear support to either side in the circumcision debate. However, by demonstrating that circumcision does not reduce the risk of contracting STDs, the authors may have knocked another prop out from under a medical procedure that already depends on the frailest of support. Moreover, their finding that removal of the foreskin alters patterns of sexual behavior over a lifetime casts further doubt on the appropriateness of circumcising infants too young to give informed consent.

Circumcision is an invasive procedure that is not essential to an infant's welfare and virtually always can be deferred with little or no risk. The finding that circumcision has significant impact in later life adds further credibility to the view that a decision regarding circumcision should be postponed until a man can choose for himself. In 1995, the AAP Committee on Bioethics[2] stressed the importance of involving children in decisions concerning their health care. The committee counseled physicians to view children as persons in their own right, with interests distinct from those of their parents.

Neonatal circumcision subjects male infants to an operation that they may well reject if they were old enough to consider its advantages and disadvantages. A number of studies, such as that of Taylor and colleagues,[3] have provided evidence that the foreskin is a complex structure that performs important sensory functions. The summary ablation of this structure prior to the age of consent infringes on one of the most basic human rights, namely, the right to physical integrity.

Although the courts have traditionally emphasized the importance of the family, the rights of parents to govern their children are by no means unrestricted. In a society founded on respect for the individual, it is clearly in the interest of a child to participate, whenever possible, in decisions concerning his or her own body.

Circumcision is an irreversible procedure that confers few, if any, prophylactic benefits and appears to have long-term effects on sexual behavior. Hippocrates advised his followers to treat patients conservatively. Perhaps it is time that infant males born in America were once again treated in accordance with a principle that has formed a cornerstone for the practice of medicine since ancient times.

Dennis Harrison
Vancouver, British Columbia

References

1. Laumann EO, Masi CM, Zuckerman EW. Circumcision in the United States: prevalence, prophylactic effects, and sexual practice. *JAMA.* 1997; 277:1052–1057.
2. AAP Committee on Bioethics. Informed consent, parental permission, and assent in pediatric practice. *Pediatrics.* 1995; 95:314–317.
3. Taylor JR, Lockwood AP, Taylor AJ. The prepuce: specialized mucosa of the penis and its loss to circumcision. *Br J Urol.* 1996; 77:291–295.

(JAMA. 1997; 278:202)

To the Editor

I read with great anticipation the article on circumcision in the United States,[1] after hearing the press release about this article on the news. However, I not only was sorely disappointed in the results and conclusions in this study, but must say that I have never read an article that had so many generalities, such as "slight tendency," "slightly less likely," "may have," "it seems unlikely," "results escape easy interpretation," "cast doubt," and "may reflect attitudes." I found the article to be highly unscientific and probably more suitable for publication in a journal of sociology or perhaps psychology than in a medical journal.

Perhaps the most obvious example was a comment by the authors that "Results may also have been affected by the possibility that some respondents did not know whether they had been circumcised." I rest my case.

John E. Pipas, M.D.
Syracuse, N.Y.

References

1. Laumann EO, Masi CM, Zuckerman EW. Circumcision in the United States: prevalence, prophylactic effects, and sexual practice. *JAMA.* 1997; 277:1052–1057.

(JAMA. 1997; 278:202)

To the Editor

That the article by Dr. Laumann et al.[1] documented differences in the sexual practices of men with regard to circumcision status is not surprising. Surgical removal of the prepuce results in the loss of the majority of fine-touch neuroreceptors found in the penis,[2] leaving only the exposed glans, which is innervated with free nerve endings that can only sense deep pressure and pain.[3]

A hypothesis is needed to explain the findings of Laumann et al. in light of the known neurohistology. We suggest that a penis with foreskin and its full complement of neuroreceptors may make heterosexual coitus more satisfying, thereby making the man less likely to seek out alternate forms of stimulation. The only portion of the prepuce remaining in a man with surgically altered genitalia is the remnant between the corona and the scar. While there are some fine-touch receptors in this tissue, the most sensitive portion of the prepuce at the tip is removed in even the most moderate circumcision.[2] The remaining prepuce and any remaining portions of the frenulum can be preferentially stimulated by masturbation and oral sex, whereas the sensation of deep pressure dominates during heterosexual coitus. The imbalance from not having the input from the missing fine-touch receptors may make the experience less satisfying, causing a man with an incomplete penis to supplement his sexual experiences with other forms of stimulation.

To date, the effect of circumcision on sexual function has not been carefully studied. In rodent studies, removal of the prepuce resulted in marked changes in the mechanics of copulation,[4] the hormonal response of the female partner, and aggressive behavior. In humans, behavioral alterations have been demonstrated in the pain response of circumcised infants.[5] Unfortunately, studies of men circumcised as adults have had too few subjects or differences in sensation were not well documented. Testing penile vibratory thresholds has demonstrated that men experience increasing thresholds with age, while those with premature ejaculation have low thresholds regardless of age.[6] Application of this technique could be used to demonstrate if a sensation difference exists between circumcised and uncircumcised men.

Robert S. Van Howe, M.D.
Marshfield Clinic—Lakeland Center
Minocqua, Wisconsin

Christopher J. Cold, M.D.
Marshfield Clinic
Marshfield, Wisconsin

References

1. Laumann EO, Masi CM, Zuckerman EW. Circumcision in the United States: prevalence, prophylactic effects, and sexual practice. *JAMA.* 1997; 277:1052–1057.
2. Taylor JR, Lockwood AP, Taylor AJ. The prepuce: specialized mucosa of the penis and its loss to circumcision. *Br J Urol.* 1996; 77:291–295.
3. Halata Z, Munger BL. The neuroanatomical basis for the protopathic sensibility of the human glans penis. *Brain Res.* 1986; 371:205–230.
4. Lumia AR, Sachs BD, Meisel RL. Sexual reflexes in male rats: restoration by ejaculation following suppression by penile sheath removal. *Physiol Behav.* 1979; 23:273–277.
5. Taddio A, Katz J, Ilersich AL, Koren G. Effect of neonatal circumcision on pain response during subsequent routine vaccination. *Lancet.* 1997; 349:599–603.
6. Xin ZC, Chung WS, Choi YD, Seong DH, Choi YJ, Choi HK. Penile sensitivity in patients with premature ejaculation. *J Urol.* 1996; 156:979–981.

(JAMA. 1997; 278:203)

In Reply

Collectively, the letters commenting on our article on circumcision are a microcosm of the highly contentious state of opinion on the wisdom of mass neonatal circumcision in the United States. Most of the authors make useful reference to other studies that bear on evaluating the impact of circumcision on such issues as penile sensitivity, sexual satisfaction, and transmission of other diseases to sex partners (e.g., cervical cancer) and that we could not examine because of the limitations on clinical data gathering imposed by a broad-based population survey such as ours.

However, we take strong exception to Dr. Schoen's observation that the survey method is simply inapplicable because of its invalidity for studying STDs. We acknowledged in our article the limitations of self-reported STDs from a lay population, especially with respect to underreporting because of selective recall, lack of awareness and of diagnosis of asymptomatic disease, and the avoidance of social stigma. We found that 17% of the men reported that they had been informed of medical diagnoses of specific STDs, and that such experiences were associated with risk factors, such as numbers of partners, condom use, and military service, that the literature would lead us to expect.[1,2] Moreover, lacking a plausible mechanism that links the presence or absence of a foreskin with a differential ability to recall and report medically diagnosed STD experiences, we fail to see the significance of Schoen's remarks regarding our findings.

Drs. Berman, Ross, and Schoen refer to studies claiming a prophylactic effect of circumcision against HIV transmission in African populations as inconsistent with our findings for the United States. Our study, however, does provide evidence that there are strongly associated social and behavioral covariates with circumcision status that include social background characteristics, such as age, education, race/ethnicity, and sexual practices and preferences. In short, circumcision is a marker for a complex array of social and behavioral characteristics that are known to be implicated in STD transmission. It is certainly the case that circumcision in Africa also is heavily influenced by social factors, such as tribal affiliation and religion (e.g., Islam),[3] and these factors have important implications for sexual practices and partner choice. Without rigorous, systematic control for cofactors relevant to the particularities of the African context, the prophylactic status of the presence or absence of the foreskin remains an open question.

Edward O. Laumann, Ph.D.
Christopher M. Masi, M.D.
Ezra W. Zuckerman, M.A.
University of Chicago
Chicago, Illinois

References

1. Holmes KK, Anders M, Sparling P, Wiesner PJ. *Sexually Transmitted Diseases.* 2nd ed. New York. NY: McGraw-Hill Book Co; 1990. [In-text reference not available.]
2. Laumann EO, Michael RT, Gagnon JH, et al. Sexually transmitted infections. In: *The Social Organization of Sexuality: Sexual Practices in the United States.* Chicago, Ill: University of Chicago Press; 1994:376–441.
3. Paige KE, Paige JM. *The Politics of Reproductive Ritual.* Berkeley: University of California Press; 1981.

(JAMA. 1997; 278:203)

FRAME the DEBATE

Form at end of book

WiseGuide Wrap-Up

Rates of neonatal circumcision have decreased over the past decade. Currently, the National Center for Health Statistics reports that 34.2 percent of baby boys are circumcised in America. Part of this decrease may come from parents weighing the relative benefits of circumcision (such as reduced risks of cancer and certain sexually transmitted diseases) against the possible health risks of the procedure (such as surgical pain, surgical injury, and decreased sexual sensation). While the debate among health-care providers continues, all appear to recognize the need for full disclosure between physician and parents regarding the benefits and risks of the procedure.

R.E.A.L. Sites

This list provides a print preview of typical **Coursewise** R.E.A.L. sites. (There are over 100 such sites at the **Courselinks**™ site.) The danger in printing URLs is that web sites can change overnight. As we went to press, these sites were functional using the URLs provided. If you come across one that isn't, please let us know via email to: webmaster@coursewise.com. Use your Passport to access the most current list of R.E.A.L. sites at the **Courselinks** site.

Site name: Medical Benefits from Circumcision

URL: http://www-personal.usyd.edu.au/~bmorris/circumcision.shtml

Why is it R.E.A.L.? This site supports the practice of male circumcision and provides an extensive review of the literature with numerous references to medical literature. The author states, "Interestingly, the physical difficulties experienced by the uncircumcised may explain why the word for uncircumcised in Hebrew means 'obstruction' or 'to impede' . . . . "

Key topics: circumcision, male, penis, sexually transmitted diseases

Try this: Read the article at this site. How well does the author support his various theses? What strategies does he use to persuade readers to his point of view? What are the main strengths of his arguments? What weaknesses do you see? Select two powerful quotes from this article, and be prepared to discuss their merits.

Site name: National Organization to Halt the Abuse and Routine Mutilation of Males

URL: http://www.noharmm.org/

Why is it R.E.A.L.? This site showcases arguments against the routine circumcision of neonatal males. The site provides links to a variety of papers that take a strong stance against circumcision. The authors state, "Circumcision of healthy infants and children is not in their best interests."

Key topics: circumcision, male, penis, sexually transmitted diseases

Try this: Read at least three of the articles linked to this site. How well do the authors support their theses? What strategies do they use to persuade readers to their points of view? What are the main strengths of their arguments? What weaknesses do you see? Select two powerful quotes from one of the articles, and be prepared to discuss the merits of the quotes.

Section 2 Summary

The subject of male impotence has traditionally been taboo in America. With the release of Viagra, a pharmaceutical treatment for impotence, the subject has become front-page fodder in newspapers and magazines, and on television news. While Viagra seems promising and proponents herald it as the male equivalent of the "pill" in liberating male sexuality, debate has emerged over the physical and psychosocial consequences of the use and misuse of this drug.

Over the past four decades, most American men were routinely circumcised out of tradition, hygiene considerations, and concerns over appearances. Recently, however, this widespread practice has been questioned. Evidence supports the need for parental and physician consultation, including thorough exploration of the benefits and liabilities of circumcision.

STAND! **section 3**

Women's Health Issues

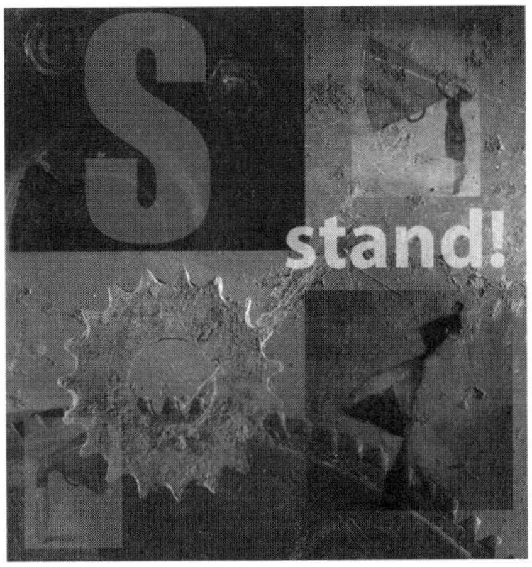

Learning Objectives

- Increase understanding of women's health issues, particularly as they relate to the aging process.
- Become informed on the controversy surrounding the use of hormones in prevention of heart disease in women.
- Question the efficacy of mammograms as an early detector of breast cancer in women.

Introduction

In the past two decades, women have become more vocal in the health marketplace and health-care system. Proponents of women's health issues stress the need for research and investigation into gender-specific cancer rates, mental health problems such as depression, the differences in aging-related health issues such as menopause, and increased risks of osteoporosis and breast and cervical cancers. Breast cancer alone will claim the lives of 44,000 women this year. The health goals for the nation outlined in Healthy People 2000 called for a reduction in breast cancer deaths to no more than 20.6 per 100,000 and the rates of uterine cancer to no more than 1.3 per 100,000. Early screening, proactive medicine, and positive health behavior are the most significant factors in meeting these goals.

Contemporary physicians and health-care providers recognize the need for a distinct approach to women's reproductive and health issues separate from that of men and pediatrics. This section deals with two controversial issues: the need for and effectiveness of hormone replacement therapy for women and the recommendations for breast cancer screening.

Is Hormone Therapy for Women Safe, Effective, and Healthful?

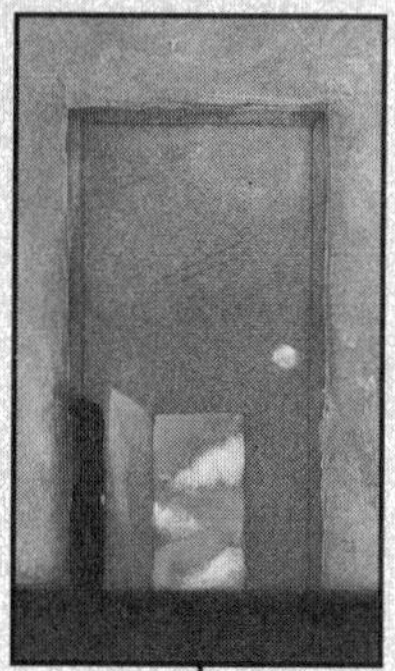

ISSUE 6

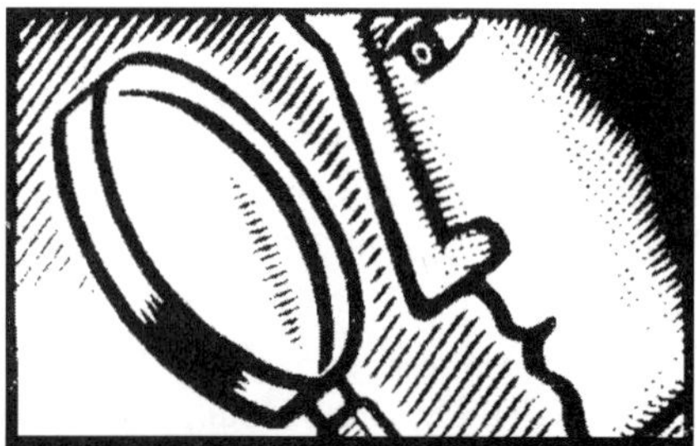

Take a Closer Look

1. According to Love in Reading 13, what are women aged 35 to 75 most likely to die from?
2. According to Reading 14, physicians prescribe estrogen replacement therapy to reduce the risks of which four diseases in menopausal women?
3. According to Northrup in Reading 15, breast cancer can result from uncontrolled cell division and what else?
4. What does progesterone do to help prevent breast cancer?

WiseGuide Intro

The average American woman reaches menopause in her late forties to mid-fifties. Menopause is associated with hot flashes, night sweats, and sleep and mood disorders, including personality changes and depression. Most of these changes are believed to be due to a sudden drop in the female hormone estrogen. Hormone replacement therapy (HRT) has been shown to relieve some of these symptoms. HRT may also help to prevent heart disease, osteoporosis, colon cancer, and perhaps, Alzheimer's disease. Critics note, however, that HRT may increase a woman's risk of having breast and cervical cancers, as well as blood clots, which are often associated with stroke.

Reading 13, "Love's Labor Lost?" profiles Dr. Susan Love, a controversial surgeon turned women's health advocate. Dr. Love is diametrically opposed to HRT for women as a "cure" for menopause because she believes that HRT may actually be placing women at a higher risk of breast cancer. She is also concerned about the lack of hard scientific evidence supporting the prophylactic effects of HRT in regard to heart attack.

Reading 14, "Hormone Replacement Therapy: Weighing the Benefits and Risks," is a good overview of the pros and cons of HRT. For the past thirty years, doctors have prescribed the hormones estrogen and progesterone to women at the age of menopause to help reduce hot flashes and depression, as well as to lower the risk of heart attack. Research indicates, however, that, although HRT may help prevent heart disease, it may at the same time increase the risk of breast cancer among certain women. The difficulty that physicians have now is wading through seemingly contradictory research that demonstrates HRT as both helping and hurting women's health.

Physician Christane Northrup has been on the cutting edge of controversy surrounding the re-examination of conventional treatment regimens in women's health, such as hormone replacement therapy. In Reading 15, "Is Progesterone Good for Your Breasts?," Dr. Northrup favors the use of progesterone in the prevention of breast cancer. She uses an analogy of a tree, its trunk, and leaves to explain the growth cycle of breast tissues, their reactions to estrogen and progesterone, and their propensity to abnormal cancerous growth. Studies on the effects of progesterone creams on breast tissue growth are reviewed favorably in this reading. Dr. Northrup endorses progesterone supplementation to make up for the decreased progesterone production as women age. She concludes with specific recommendations regarding the use of progesterone creams.

R E A D I N G 1 3

Issue 6: Is hormone therapy for women safe, effective, and healthful?

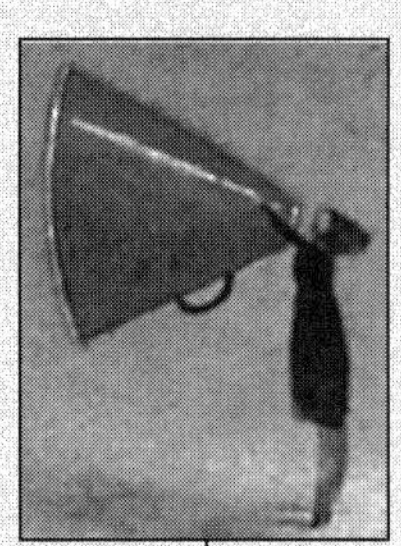

Love's Labor's Lost?

Critics say best-selling author Dr. Susan Love has gone too far in her warnings about estrogen and breast cancer. Are they right?

Rosie Mestel

Rosie Mestel is a contributing editor.

I like Susan Love. For someone who's a medical media star, with two popular books under her belt and a jam-packed itinerary of speaking engagements, she's personable and unpretentious and not in any visible hurry to get this pesky interview over with. Plus, she's funny.

We're ensconced in a small medical library at the University of California at Los Angeles, surrounded by books on blood and guts and bones; and one minute she's cackling over the prospect of Rosie O'Donnell playing her in an upcoming movie, the next she's up on her feet, hamming it up as a hopelessly humpbacked crone creaking along with her walker. Then she's describing what it's like when two cohabiting women—in this case Love and her life partner, Helen Cooksey—approach menopause together. "We're flashing asynchronously," she says. "It doesn't help." ("These are not hot flashes I'm having; they're power surges," declares the button on her lab coat.)

Love thinks a lot about the changes she's going through right now, such as her decision to resign as director of the Revlon-UCLA Breast Center and end her nearly two-decade career as a breast surgeon. "I was beginning to burn out," she says. "My options were either to become less attached to the patients or to stop, and I didn't *want* to become less attached." Then there's her brand-new career. Love is in business school, immersed in the world of budgets and payrolls with the hope of whipping health maintenance organizations into shape.

"HMOs could be great for improving health care," she reckons. "For the first time they make doctors accountable for how much they charge and what treatments they prescribe. But I think in order to take advantage of them we need people who are bilingual, who speak business as well as medicine."

Yet there's more going on her than reformer's zeal and physician's burnout. To Love's mind, menopause itself brings a whole new perspective on life. "You see a lot of women changing their careers and doing things differently around their fifties," she says. "It's a time when you reevaluate, when you ask, Where am I, and what am I going to do with the other half of my life?"

Whatever Love decides to do, it'll probably make a wave or two; she's never been a toe-the-line, button-your-lip kind of gal. Not in her private life—she and Cooksey waged (and won) a four-year battle in the courts so that Cooksey could become a legal parent to Love's biological daughter—and certainly not in her professional life. She shook up colleagues with her views on mastectomies. We're doing way too many of them, she said, in cases where less invasive measures would be just as effective. She coined the phrase "slash, burn, and poison" to describe state-of-the-art breast cancer treatment. She's argued against the standard breast self-exam. "It teaches women to see the breast as an enemy," she writes in *Dr. Susan Love's Breast Book.* She's fought fiercely alongside political activists to get more money for breast cancer research. And she's been a passionate advocate for patients.

Still, abrasive as some people find her, Love has earned plenty of respect. Her ideas on mastectomy are deemed radical no longer, and her book won accolades from medics and lay readers alike.

Now she's turned to menopause, galvanized not only by her own hot flashes but by a growing conviction: that the medical establishment is leading American women seriously astray.

Menopause, she says, is a natural stage of life that doctors and drug companies have transformed into a disease—and promised to cure with powerful, potentially dangerous hormones. True, taking estrogen after menopause may help keep bones strong and hearts healthy (and *may* is the operative word, Love insists). But there are other routes to those gains—plus mounting evidence that estrogen increases the odds of breast cancer. "I really felt that we were overestimating the benefits and underestimating the risks," Love says. "Here we were, with this train rushing down the tracks, and no one was standing up and saying, 'Wait. We don't have all the facts yet.' "

So Love jumped in to wave some red flags. She's been giving talks and writing in the newspapers, and in 1997 she hit the bookstores again, this time with *Dr. Susan Love's Hormone Book,* 348 pages on the pros and cons of hormone replacement therapy.

There's no question that women are listening. Her book is selling like crazy, her talks are packed, and her take-charge message seems to resonate with many women who are anxious about the Change but chary of committing to decades of popping pills.

This time, though, professional accolades are thinner on the ground. Many a physician and hormone researcher takes issue with her stance. They say that she gets facts wrong, that the facts she gets right she distorts, that by shining a spotlight on breast cancer she is scaring women away from a remedy that could lengthen their lives. Love's critics were particularly annoyed by her editorial last year in the *New York Times,* which left readers with a clear message: Whoa! Don't let the drug companies sell you down the river on *this* one.

By shining a light on breast cancer, many experts say, Love is scaring women away from a remedy that could lengthen their lives.

Over at Case Western Reserve University in Cleveland, professor of reproductive biology Wulf Utian read Love's essay and got mightily riled. "It seemed to me it was a piece designed to sell books," he says, "that it was more related to marketing than to a concern for women's health." At the Harvard School of Public Health epidemiologist Meir Stampfer was steamed by the mistakes it contained. "Either she had made an egregious error or hadn't done her homework properly," he says. "Hormone replacement therapy is a highly charged issue, and there's plenty of room for disagreement. But we should at least have the basic facts right."

So what, exactly, is Love saying? Is she guiding middle-aged women to safe harbor or steering them onto the rocks?

First off—one might as well get this out of the way—Love has no problem with short-term use of hormones to treat hot flashes. There's no evidence that taking estrogen for five years or less does anything significant to breast cancer risk. Her beef is with long-term therapy, and it's here that she and her critics butt heads. Their main charge: She's playing up estrogen's risks while downplaying its benefits. This is how *they* see the hormone trade-off.

Item one: Coronary heart disease kills six times more women than does breast cancer. Item two: Studies suggest a woman's breast cancer risk increases by only 2.3 percent for every year she's on estrogen. Item three: Studies suggest taking hormones can slash a woman's odds of developing heart disease in half. Thus, say estrogen defenders, replacing the hormone is well worth doing for someone at no special risk for breast cancer.

Yet Love takes issue with this seemingly clear-cut formula. Here's what she wrote in her book and in the *New York Times* that so irked so many: "In women younger than age 75 there are actually three times as many deaths from breast cancer as there are from heart disease."

Love's point was that, yes, heart disease may be the bigger killer, but different diseases strike at different times, and breast cancer comes knocking earlier. "Most women aged 50 know someone who's died of breast cancer; they do not know someone with heart disease," she says. Does it make sense for a 50-year-old woman to take action to reduce a future threat if she's thereby raising a more immediate one?

The trouble is, Love's "three times" calculation is wrong. The truth is precisely the other way around. Three times more women between the ages of 35 and 75 die from heart disease than from breast cancer.

Did Love accidentally flip the numbers? That's what Stampfer assumed when he read her essay and fired off a letter to the *New York Times* correcting her. Malcolm Gladwell, a writer at the *New Yorker,* was less charitable. Last June he lambasted Love for her mistake, lumping her in with the touchy-feely alternative medicine crowd but suggesting she's all the more dangerous because of her academic respectability.

Love says she didn't do a switcheroo. She says she got her numbers from the Nurses' Health Study at Harvard, which has tracked more than 121,000 women on all manner of wellness issues. Keep in mind that these nurses aren't representative of the U.S. population: They are healthier to begin with and therefore have a lot less heart disease. But Love felt justified in looking at this group, she says, because she thought it closely mirrored the kind of woman likely to be thinking about hormones.

Critics have problems with this explanation. Apart from the responsibility issues—why didn't she fess up to what she was doing instead of leaving the impression that her numbers applied to *all* women?—she seems to assume only healthy women take hormones.

What's more, says Stampfer, the nurse study doesn't even support her claim. Many of the women Love looked at were still in their fifties. When a new analysis was done a couple of years later, after more of the women had reached their early seventies or died, the number of deaths from heart disease was roughly the same as the number from breast cancer. By the time *all* the women either die or turn 70, Stampfer says, the heart disease mortality will have way outstripped that of breast cancer.

Murky, all this, but rather a tempest in a teacup? Not so, insists Nananda Col, a physician at Boston's New England Medical Center and author of her own menopause book, *A Woman Doctor's Guide to Hormone Therapy*. Polls show many women already think—incorrectly—that breast cancer is their biggest long-term health threat. They don't need any encouragement. Several months ago a patient of Col's—diabetic, sedentary, seriously overweight, not good at keeping her blood sugar in line—came into Col's office after reading Love's writings and announced that she wasn't taking hormones anymore. "Her risk for heart disease was tremendous; her chances of living long enough to develop breast cancer were very small. And all she could think about was breast cancer," says Col.

Today Love regrets the whole numbers affair, if only because it eclipsed her point. Breast cancer *does* strike younger women, and that's one reason women fear it more. The average age for a first heart attack is 73; for a breast cancer diagnosis, it's 65. "You can't just look at the global statistics," Love insists. "A lot of those heart deaths are at very old ages." The death of a younger person—who would argue?—is more tragic.

In any case, Love has other bones to pick. No one, she says, has *proven* that hormones spare us from heart disease. For one thing, most studies to date are of women taking estrogen alone, whereas today's standard regimen is estrogen plus progestin (to protect against the heightened risk of uterine cancer). So far the findings on the effectiveness of combination therapy have been mixed.

In addition, the largest studies have pretty much all looked at women who had already decided whether or not to take hormones (scientists call these observational studies). Real proof comes from clinical trials, where researchers enlist a bunch of people, randomly divide them, then give one group the drug and the other a placebo. Any difference the drug makes will show up when the two groups are compared at the end of the study. Until such a trial is completed—a huge one, the Women's Health Initiative, is under way right now—how does anyone know the slashed heart risk was due to the estrogen? Maybe the women who opted to take estrogen were healthier as a group to begin with, due to differences in diet, exercise, or something else. Estrogen may have had nothing to do with it.

"It's a good argument," says Stampfer, "but you can't just stop there. You have to ask, How much could the differences explain the benefits? Well, we've looked at smoking, hypertension, diabetes, obesity, cholesterol, dietary fat—on and on. My conclusion is that after accounting for these differences you still have about a 40 percent reduction in risk."

For the record, Love says she's not out-and-out against hormones. She just thinks there are safer ways to protect your heart and bones.

Critics also see something lopsided in the way Love argues her points. On the heart data she's tough as nails. On the cancer data she's practically soft; she calls those figures definitive, in fact. But it so happens that breast and heart data come from the same kind of studies—observational ones, the type that can't provide the final answer on HRT. Isn't she being a tad disingenuous?

No, says Love. She argues that the breast studies, if anything, underestimate the cancer risk. She explains: Many women who opt for hormone therapy do so because of intense menopausal symptoms. That means they have less natural estrogen, Love says, and therefore a lower risk for breast cancer. Besides, the level of risk that's acceptable for a preventive therapy—particularly one for illnesses large numbers of women are unlikely to get—should be much lower than that for a drug that cures disease. "I feel, conservatively, that we should not be putting women on a drug for 30 years until we can prove, one, that it's not dangerous, and, two, that it works."

In any case, she adds, whatever estrogen's heart benefits end up to be, there's a much safer, low-tech way to keep your heart healthy, by God: Clean up your act! If only we could eat right, exercise, and quit smoking, studies suggest, we would stamp out a mind-boggling 80 percent of all heart disease.

Love is trying her darnedest to do it herself. She's lifting weights and doing aerobics. She's eating less fatty food, and she's taking vitamins. She's also working soy and flaxseed into her diet, because both contain estrogen-like chemicals that may rein in cholesterol, counter bone loss, and possibly control hot flashes.

Hats off to Love for her efforts, say critics, but does she have any idea how hard it is to convince most people to do likewise? "I spend 90 percent of my time trying to get patients to eat better, to exercise, to stop smoking, says Col. "But it's just not easy to get people to do it. This naive idea that everybody could be risk factor-free reflects the fact that Love has never practiced primary care."

But Love thinks most doctors don't try hard enough. "We'll say, 'Well of course you should exercise and eat healthy, and here's your prescription.' But how often do we say, 'We think exercise is the most critical thing you can do in your life, so let's look at your schedule and figure out how you can do it'? And how many people do we send to a nutritionist?"

It's a classical standoff, but even though Love and Col sound diametrically opposed, they actually agree on the essentials. If you're interested in protecting your heart, they say, taking hormones shouldn't be the first line of attack. If you just can't stick to a clean-up-your-act regimen, however, HRT might be a good idea. Neither choice rules out the other.

But enough already about the heart. Estrogen's also supposed to protect our bones. What does Love have to say about that? On this she is more persuaded—but not what you'd call *persuaded.*

Love does believe that estrogen helps prevent the bone loss that typically accelerates at menopause and can set the stage for dangerous, debilitating fractures. That's because in this case scientists have done some of those super-duper clinical trials, and they found that estrogen does keep women's bone density up. Analyses of medical records, meanwhile, show that women taking estrogen have half the fracture rate of nonusers.

Love's complaint is that because of these findings doctors want to put *every* 50-year-old woman on hormones, even though not everyone with low bone density will end up with osteoporosis. "This is a bit like telling someone with high cholesterol that he or she has heart disease," she wrote in the *New York Times.*

That's silly talk, say bone experts. Low bone density is a powerful predictor of fractures down the road. What does Love want? For women to wait until they fall down and bust a hip before tending to the health of their skeleton? "That's like waiting to treat high blood pressure until somebody has a stroke," says bone specialist Clifford Rosen, chief of medicine at St. Joseph Hospital in Bangor, Maine. One-fifth of all hip fractures kill. If they don't, they often mean life with a walker or in a wheelchair—or, worse, life in a nursing home.

Again, Love counters, let's look at when those fractures are happening. Average age: 79. Do we really need to start taking drugs in our fifties? Maybe not: A recent study found that the bones of women who began HRT after 60 were nearly as dense as those of women who'd been taking estrogen since menopause.

For the record, Love says she's not out-and-out against hormones. Here's what she advises. If hot flashes or other menopausal symptoms are making you miserable, take them for a while. Then, if you're seriously losing bone or your heart disease risk is through the ceiling—or if fractures and heart attacks loom large in your family history—hormone therapy in the early years after menopause might make sense. But if the situation isn't drastic, do the good, clean-up-your-act routine. Monitor your progress, and consider hormones if the picture clouds somewhere down the line. Love admits that she herself could change her mind and start popping hormones tomorrow should her cholesterol readings suddenly skyrocket.

Put in those terms, Love's views don't seem outrageous. But if they still come across that way, the reason is easy to spot. From the outset her tone was combative, her charges incendiary. Her writing is chockablock with big-bad-drug-company rhetoric. Pharmaceutical companies, as far as Love is concerned, don't care if your heart and bones are in tip-top shape; they want *all* women to go on hormones at menopause. And they're leaning on doctors to push those "magic little pills" on more and more women.

Physicians, too, are subjected to her withering glare. She questions the motives of OB-GYNs, going so far as to charge them with putting women on hormones just to keep them as patients. "Once you stop having babies, you don't often need to see a gynecologist unless you're on hormone therapy," she writes in her book. She also thinks too many doctors still subscribe to the idea that menopausal women are "sick failures." She reserves a special slam for the American College of Obstetricians and Gynecologists. As she tells it, the group recommends that every postmenopausal woman be on replacement hormones for the rest of her life.

Such talk fits right in with the world-view of some particularly angry women. "These are drugs, not penny-candy panaceas to toss off to the worried well who have been seduced by drug company propaganda," writes one member of an Internet support group where Love's hormone book holds Bible-like stature.

Of course there's not the teensiest bit of doubt that drug companies do want us using their products. And women have had plenty of cause to be angered by the condescending attitudes of old-school physicians. But Love's easy dismissal of doctors seems just that—too easy.

For one thing, there is no such blanket statement by ACOG. The society's technical bulletin clearly outlines both risks and benefits of estrogen therapy, and states that it isn't right for all women. Furthermore, says Col, "The literature, scant though it is, doesn't support the notion that most doctors are recommending hormone therapy to most patients."

Nationally, around 35 percent of women opt to take hormones during menopause, but only 15 percent are still on them at age 65 and only 7 percent at age 80. The numbers of prescriptions *are* going up, but that doesn't mean we're in the middle of a stampede.

I really do like Susan Love. I like that she genuinely cares about women and that she wants us to have a say in what happens to us. I like, too, her candor in admitting that as a breast surgeon she is bound to have a bias.

And I like that she has the courage to get out there and speak her mind.

"Susan shakes things up," says Laura Esserman, director of the breast care center at the University of California at San Francisco. "And that's good. I think, frankly, if she hadn't raised a stink, people wouldn't be as receptive to exploring different options for menopause."

If some people read her message as an evil-hormone diatribe, Love isn't entirely to blame. "I think women see in it what they want to," she says. "When I give talks, sometimes a woman will come up to me afterward and say, 'Your book is wonderful; it helped me make the decision to take hormones.' Then another will come up and say it supported her decision not to. When you write a book, you try to be as even as you can, but once it's out there people are going to use the information however they want to.

Okay, so she isn't *entirely* to blame. Still, I can't help feeling disappointed by the way she shades her message—with numbers that aren't quite kosher and association statements that don't quite exist, with inflammatory grandstanding about drug companies and patronizing pill-happy physicians. Love does come down harder on the science that points to estrogen's favorable effects. And she may well be scaring some women away from a drug that might help them.

Perhaps the take-home message is just what Love wants to stress: that the hormone decision is personal, not to be dictated by a doctor but made by each individual with the very best information she can get. Which simply means, to get the full picture, she shouldn't listen only to Susan Love.

FRAME the DEBATE

Form at end of book

R E A D I N G 1 4

Issue 6: Is hormone therapy for women safe, effective, and healthful?

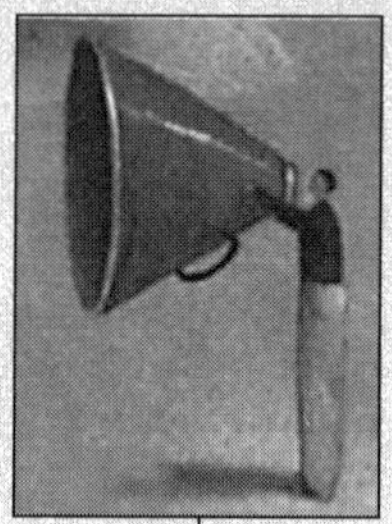

Hormone-Replacement Therapy:
Weighing the Benefits and Risks

"The elimination of menopause is perhaps the most important technical advance by which women may equip themselves for an enduringly feminine role in modern life. . . . Thanks to hormone therapy, [women] may look forward to prolonged well-being and extended youth."

So wrote a gynecologist named Robert Wilson in 1966 in his best-selling book, *Feminine Forever,* a watershed publication credited as the driving force behind the subsequent surge in hormone use among women going through "the change." While Dr. Wilson argued that menopause was a deficiency disease "curable" with the hormone estrogen, today the pendulum has begun to swing the other way.

One of this year's best-sellers, *Dr. Susan Love's Hormone Book,* urges women to think twice before jumping on the estrogen bandwagon. "Menopause is not a disease," according to Dr. Love, "it's a natural stage in a woman's life."

No wonder the topic sparks so much controversy. At the same time that the estrogen-replacement formulation Premarin has become the most widely prescribed drug in the United States, many women wonder whether they should start hormone-replacement therapy (HRT), while others ponder if they should stop using it.

The steady stream of news reports about the pros and cons of estrogen compounds the dilemma. Most research suggests that HRT increases the risk of breast cancer, yet it has also been shown to stave off osteoporosis, and it may prevent heart disease.

Many postmenopausal women wonder if they should start taking hormones; others ponder if they should stop using them.

A recent report from the ongoing Nurses' Health Study at Harvard, which ranks as the largest, most comprehensive look at the impact of hormone therapy to date, tips the scales in favor of the treatment for some women. Although the study doesn't provide the final word on HRT, it does shed light on some of the important health concerns postmenopausal women should consider.

A Balancing Act

When estrogen replacement therapy came on the scene in the 1960s, it was hailed as a "cure" for the health problems that begin during the menopausal years, when the body's production of estrogen wanes. It was thought that replenishing dwindling hormone supplies would remedy everything from hot flashes to sexual problems to depression. In the mid-1970s, however, a troubling side effect surfaced: the rate of uterine cancer rose substantially among women taking estrogen. Doctors didn't know at the time that estrogen taken alone promotes the growth of cancerous cells in the *endometrium,* the inner mucous membrane of the uterus. It was later discovered that the hormone progesterone curbs the cell growth that estrogen triggers. Today most women take both estrogen and progestin (synthetic progesterone) to protect against uterine cancer.

But the worries didn't end there. A body of evidence gathered during the past three decades has implicated HRT as a culprit in breast cancer. Estrogen is also suspected to increase the risk of gallstones and blood clots originating in the deep veins of the legs.

On the other hand, a strong case for the benefits of HRT has been built over the years. It is firmly established that estrogen helps alleviate short-term symptoms of menopause, such as hot flashes, vaginal dryness, and sleep disturbances. When it comes to longer term use, investigators have found that estrogen significantly reduces a woman's chances of developing osteoporosis, the bone-thinning disease that can set the stage for serious fractures. A wealth of research also points to HRT as a defender against cardiovascular disease. Some evidence suggests HRT may reduce the risk of colon cancer as well.

In addition, preliminary studies have shown that estrogen might enhance memory and other mental functions, possibly by preventing damage to brain cells and boosting their capabilities. A recent report from the Baltimore Longitudinal Study of Aging, begun in 1978, found that women who took estrogen at any time during their postmenopausal years had about half the risk of developing Alzheimer's disease as those who had not taken the hormone.

Piecing through the Evidence

Despite the research, experts have been hard-pressed to make firm recommendations about HRT for a number of reasons. For one, HRT users as a group tend to be leaner, more physically active, and better educated than women who don't take hormones. These women typically start out with fewer risks for heart disease, such as high blood pressure. Thus, scientists find it difficult to determine whether women who use HRT are protected against certain diseases because they take hormones or because they are healthy to begin with. Also unclear is whether HRT users see their doctors more regularly than other women, giving them a better shot at early diagnosis and treatment of disease.

Another hitch is that many studies evaluate the pros and cons of HRT based on use at only one point in time. That approach fails to factor in how long and how continuously hormones were taken before the research began.

The latest report from the Nurses' Health Study speaks to some of those issues. In this ongoing investigation, begun in 1976, the researchers examined the impact of long-term HRT use in more than 60,000 nurses. They looked at length and continuity of hormone use and how this affected the women's death rates. They also studied women who used estrogen alone or in an estrogen/progesterone combination and adjusted their data to account for smoking, weight, exercise, and other lifestyle habits.

Overall, the researchers found that the death rate among HRT users was 37% lower than that of women who had never taken hormones, primarily because the hormones appeared to protect women against heart disease. Indeed, the risk of dying of cardiovascular disease was 53% lower in the HRT group. The researchers found, however, that women must continue taking hormones throughout their postmenopausal years to reap the full cardiovascular benefits. In those who stopped taking estrogen, its protective effects weakened and eventually disappeared after five years.

Women who benefited most from HRT were those with cardiovascular risk factors such as a family history of heart disease, obesity, high blood cholesterol, or smoking: they had nearly a 50% drop in their death rate, compared to an 11% reduction in women at lower risk of cardiovascular disease. The dark side to the report, however, is that the death rate from breast cancer among those on HRT for at least 10 years was 43% higher than in non-users.

Daunting as the 43% figure may be, statistically speaking, HRT still appears to promote longevity. Contrary to popular belief, heart disease kills about six times as many women as does breast cancer during the postmenopausal years.

Consider that approximately 1 in 200 women aged 70 to 74 will die of heart disease annually, whereas only 1 in 850 will succumb to breast cancer. Thus, if a 70-to-74-year-old HRT user's yearly risk of dying of breast cancer increases by 43%, she still has only about a 1-in-590 chance of dying from the illness. This is still much better than the 1-in-200 risk of death from cardiovascular disease. Of course, genes and lifestyle influence an individual woman's risk of breast cancer, heart disease, and osteoporosis. And statistical calculations can't begin to address any one woman's medical background and personal preferences.

Women who have been diagnosed with breast cancer are often advised to avoid or discontinue HRT because of the concern that estrogen may promote a recurrence of the cancer. This advice is controversial, however, in light of recent evidence supporting the safety of HRT for certain women with a history of breast cancer. Those with liver disease are also discouraged from using HRT because estrogen alters liver function and may put undue stress on the organ. Also, women are often steered away from HRT if they have had deep-vein blood clots. Those with unexplained vaginal bleeding, uterine fibroids, endometriosis, gallbladder disease, or migraine headaches need to consider that HRT may exacerbate these conditions.

More Than One Option

Judging from the Nurses' Health Study and other recent research, a sound alternative for many postmenopausal women is to take HRT for the first year or two of menopause if short-term symptoms such as hot flashes and sleep disturbance are problematic. HRT could then be resumed sometime after age 60, when the risk of both heart disease and bone fractures begins to rise. Indeed, a recent study from the University of California, San Diego, found that women who began HRT after age 60 and continued for an average of 9 years had bone mineral density levels that were similar to those of women who took hormones for an average of about 20 years. Thus, putting off HRT until a woman's 60s is one way she can reap some of the benefits while minimizing her exposure to estrogen, thereby curbing the risk of breast cancer.

Women may soon have another option besides estrogen. Testing is under way on a class of drugs called *selective estrogen receptor modulators* (SERM), which experts hope will confer the bone-building, cardiovascular benefits of estrogen without raising the risk of breast or uterine cancer. Within the next year, raloxifene, the first SERM earmarked for HRT, is expected to be approved by the U.S. Food and Drug Administration. Women should bear in mind, however, that hormones are not the be-all and end-all to preventing heart disease and fractures. Staying active, maintaining a healthful weight, not smoking, and eating a balanced, low-fat diet confer protection against cardiovascular disease and may even help fight breast cancer. And exercising and consuming ample calcium help prevent osteoporosis.

Whatever women decide about HRT, they should probably revisit the issue with their physician at routine check-ups to discuss new research findings. For those in whom breast cancer ranks as an overriding concern, HRT may not be the right choice at this point. Women with a high risk of osteoporosis or heart disease, however, may have the most to gain from estrogen therapy.

FRAME the DEBATE

Form at end of book

Issue 6: Is hormone therapy for women safe, effective, and healthful?

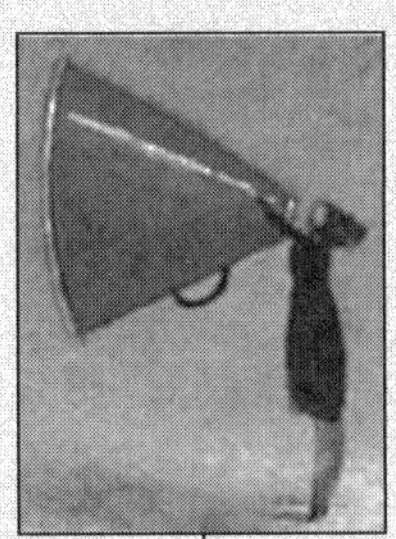

Is Progesterone Good for Your Breasts?

Christane Northrup

I recently received a letter from a man concerned about his wife's breast health. She had switched from estrogen replacement therapy (Premarin) to a natural progesterone skin cream. As a result, her breast pain and tenderness had gone away, as did her headaches. What's more, she had almost complete relief from her hot flashes. Still, he was concerned about a possible connection between progesterone and breast cancer, and wanted reassurance that his wife was on the right track.

I wouldn't be surprised to hear that you share this concern. There is much confusion and anxiety surrounding this topic—and not even the experts agree on it. I want to allay any concerns you may have about progesterone use and reassure you that progesterone can be a powerful ally in promoting breast health. In fact, I use a 2% progesterone skin cream myself regularly.

Progesterone: Unsung Hormonal Heroine?

A "quiet" hormone known for maintaining pregnancy and associated with receptiveness, progesterone is often shaded from the limelight by its more outgoing cousin, estrogen. Yet a recent review of the literature strongly suggests that progesterone may actually *decrease* the risk of cancer developing in estrogen-sensitive areas such as breast, cervical and uterine tissues. Progesterone does *not* enhance undifferentiated cell growth, which is at the heart of the controversy. Let's take a closer look to see why this is so . . .

In healthy breast tissue (as in other areas of our bodies), nature in her wisdom has created a balance between growth of new cells and death of cells no longer needed—a sort of biologically planned obsolescence called *apoptosis.* Breast cancer is one of the outcomes that can arise in the presence of—

1. Excessive, uncontrolled cell division beyond what is healthy and balanced; and
2. Lack of a normal, healthy programmed cell death (apoptosis) in a timely manner.

As with all our bodily processes, the signals that direct growth, development and apoptosis are embedded in our genetic code. You're going to be hearing a lot about this cutting edge research in the general media in the months to come, but I wanted you to have the research and facts now, so you will not be afraid to use hormones appropriately.

How Hormones Affect Your Breasts

Estrogen causes breast cells known as *ductal tissue* to divide and grow. Progesterone, on the other hand, causes breast cells to differentiate into *lobular cells*—nature's preparation for milk production if pregnancy were to happen. If pregnancy does not occur, these lobular cells simply undergo programmed cell death—they cannot go backward in time. In other words, a lobular cell is not capable of growing into a cancer cell.

David Zava, Ph.D., director of Aeron LifeCycles Laboratory, who has researched the effects of hormones on breast tissue for many years, likens different types of breast tissue to the corresponding parts of a tree. Estrogen makes the trunk and branches (ductal, structural tissue) grow, while progesterone (lobular cells) makes the leaves grow from the ends of the branches. Once a tree cell becomes a leaf, it can never go back to being a trunk or a branch. It simply grows up, matures and eventually dies at the end of its life cycle (apoptosis). This is not true with the trunk or branches, however. Their cells can grow at any time into an infinite number of branches.

In a similar fashion, unopposed estrogen has the capacity to create infinite amounts of growth of breast tissue—including cancerous growth. Progesterone, in

Is Progesterone Good for Your Breasts? Christane Northrup. HEALTH WISDOM FOR WOMEN, December 1997. Reprinted by permission.

contrast, cordons off the cells and directs their growth into a more differentiated and benign form, just like the leaves on the tree.

A Little Progesterone Goes a Long Way

The scientific literature strongly suggests that women with enough progesterone to balance their estrogen are at decreased risk for breast cancer. In one study, infertile women with progesterone deficiencies were shown to have a 5.4 times greater risk for premenopausal breast cancer compared to a control group. And in a 1995 study in which transdermal progesterone was placed directly on the skin of the breast itself, researchers found that progesterone inhibited breast cell proliferation. The dosages used were approximately the same as when a woman is using a cream such as Fem-Gest or Pro-Gest—a 2% progesterone cream at recommended dosages (one quarter to one half teaspoon once or twice per day anywhere on the skin).

Another study showed that women who had physiologically adequate levels of progesterone for their life stage at the time of breast cancer surgery had a decreased risk of recurrence than women with low levels. My recent review of the literature on progesterone and breast cancer found "... substantial documentation that progestogens not only reduced the rate of spread of breast cancer, but may even be responsible for reducing the incidence of new cases."

These studies confirm my own clinical experience with prescribing progesterone cream over the last 20 years. My confidence is backed up by the experience of many of my colleagues, particularly John Lee, M.D., and Joel Hargrove, M.D., both pioneers in the use of natural hormones; and the work of David Zava, Ph.D., a biochemist who has done significant research on the effects of estrogen and progesterone.

Estrogen and Progesterone: Fine-Tune Your Ideal Balance

So, getting back to the husband concerned about progesterone and breast cancer, you probably know what I told him: "Your wife is on the right track."

And if any of the following ring true, you may also be courting estrogen excess or an estrogen/progesterone imbalance:

- irregular or heavy menstrual periods
- body fat percentage greater than 28%
- sedentary lifestyle
- polycystic ovarian syndrome
- fibroid uterine tumors
- breast tenderness
- a low-fiber, high-fat diet
- HRT with estrogen only.

If you see yourself here, I recommend that you balance high estrogen levels with progesterone, especially during perimenopause, when you are most likely to start skipping ovulations due to low progesterone levels. Remember, it's convenient and easy to test with my at-home Wisdom Hormone Support Program. To order your kit ($129 plus $4.95 S&H), please call Phillips Products & Services at 800/705–5559.

For many of you, simply rubbing one quarter to one half teaspoon of a 2% progesterone cream such as Fem-Gest* into the palms of your hands twice per day will bring up your progesterone levels and ease your symptoms. However, some of you will do better with individually formulated hormone replacement therapy to address more persistent symptoms of perimenopause, such as hot flashes, night sweats and irritability.

In addition, I recommend the following to further balance your progesterone and estrogen levels:

- Restore balance into your life via meditation, yoga or other spiritual practice.
- Exercise! A recent study in the *New England Journal of Medicine* showed that women who exercise at least four hours per week have a 36% less chance of getting breast cancer than those with sedentary lifestyles. Even more recent research confirms that cancer risk is closely correlated with weight gain. Exercise keeps your weight down and modulates your body's estrogen production. Every little bit counts—start with 30 minutes twice per week and move up gradually. Bottom line: get some progesterone cream, and get moving!

References

Badwe, RA, et al, Timing of surgery during menstrual cycle and survival of premenopausal women with operable breast cancer. *The Lancet,* Vol. 337, May 25, 1991, pages 1261–1264.

Chang, KJ, et al, 1995, Influences of percutaneous administration of estradiol and progesterone on human breast epithelial cell cycle in vivo, *Fertility and Sterility,* Vol. 63, pages 705–791.

Cowan, AD, et al, 1961, Breast cancer incidence in women with a history of progesterone deficiency, *American Journal of Epidemiology,* Vol. 114,(2) pages 209.

Drife, JO, Breast Development in Puberty, *Ann N.Y. Acad. Sci.* Vol. 464, pages 58–65, 1986.

*Available from Doctor's Preferred, Inc. 800/304–1740, ext. 2743E.

What You Need to Know About Progesterone

Progesterone is essential to the normal and healthy functioning of your body, no matter what your age. To understand how important progesterone is, it might help to review how this often forgotten hormone affects you at different times during your life—from your teenage years through your 80s and beyond.

During your childbearing years, estrogen causes eggs to mature and be released each month. The spot on the ovary where the egg is released, called the *corpus luteum,* becomes a tiny factory for making progesterone. Its job is to get the uterus ready for pregnancy. If fertilization occurs, the corpus luteum will continue to produce progesterone until the placenta takes over. If the egg is not fertilized, after several days, the production of progesterone falls dramatically, which triggers the shedding of the lining of the uterus, or menstruation. *For premenopausal women, having adequate levels of progesterone is vital for normal functioning of the reproductive system. But, what about for those of us approaching menopause or even past it?*

As you come closer to menopause, estrogen levels actually increase relative to progesterone levels, forcing a hormone imbalance. This disparity can affect the way we feel every day and can put you at risk for hormone-related diseases like breast cancer and osteoporosis. Without adequate levels of progesterone you might experience some or all of these common symptoms, including hot flashes, decreased sex drive, vaginal dryness, mood swings, weight gain, night sweats and fatigue.

So, progesterone actually promotes a feeling of well-being or balance and its effects can go far beyond keeping symptoms at bay. In fact, here's a short list of just some of the good things that progesterone does for your body:

- protects against breast fibrocysts
- acts as a natural diuretic
- helps use fat for energy
- acts as a natural antidepressant
- helps thyroid hormone function
- normalizes blood clotting
- restores libido
- normalizes blood sugar levels
- restores proper cell oxygen levels
- protects against endometrial and breast cancer
- stimulates the production of bone
- balances the effects of estrogen.

Dulbecco, R, et al, Cell types and morphogenesis in the mammary gland. *Proc Natl. Acad. Sci. USA,* Vol. 79, pages 7346–7350, Dec. 1982.

Longacre, T. and Bartow, S. A, Correlative morphologic study of human breast and endometrium in the menstrual cycle, *The American Journal of Surgical Pathology,* Vol. 10(6), pages 382–393, 1986.

Mauvais-Jarvis, et al, Antiestrogen action of progesterone in breast tissue, *Hormones Res.* 28, pages 212–218, 1987.

Mohr, PE, et al, Serum progesterone and prognosis in operable breast cancer, *Brit. J. Cancer,* 1996.

Shizhong, BU, et al, 1997, Progesterone induces apoptosis and upregulation of B53 expression in human ovarian carcinoma cell lines, American Cancer Society, 1944–50.

Weinberg, RA, 1996, How cancer arises. *Scientific America,* Sept. 96, pages 62–70.

Wren, Barry and John A. Eden, Do progestogens reduce the risk of breast cancer?, A review of the evidence, *Menopause: The Journal of the North American Menopause Society,* 1996, Vol. 3, No. 1, pp. 4–12.

FRAME the DEBATE

Form at end of book

WiseGuide Wrap-Up

Hormone replacement therapy (HRT) for women may reduce the annoying symptoms of menopause, such as hot flashes, night sweats, and sleep problems, and also may reduce the risk of osteoporosis, cardiovascular disease, and heart attack among women. Despite these apparent benefits, HRT may also increase a woman's risk of certain cancers, blood clots, and gallstones. Some experts also express concern that HRT is part of a harmful outlook that does not view menopause as a natural aging process for women but as a medical condition that requires treatment.

R.E.A.L. Sites

This list provides a print preview of typical **Coursewise** R.E.A.L. sites. (There are over 100 such sites at the **Courselinks**™ site.) The danger in printing URLs is that web sites can change overnight. As we went to press, these sites were functional using the URLs provided. If you come across one that isn't, please let us know via email to: webmaster@coursewise.com. Use your Passport to access the most current list of R.E.A.L. sites at the **Courselinks** site.

Site name: Menopause

URL: http://bewell.com/hic/menopause/index3.asp

Why is it R.E.A.L.? This site gives a brief overview of signs, symptoms, and treatments for menopause.

Key topics: menopause, hormone replacement therapy, estrogen

Try this: Read the article at this site, and write three factual statements about menopause and women's health. Write three discussion questions that deal with the emotional, spiritual, and social aspects of menopause. Consider how menopause affects women's health and lifestyles.

Site name: Health by Web MD, Menopause

URL: http://content.health.msn.com/topic_summary/1370

Why is it R.E.A.L.? This site provides several good articles on the physical and psychosocial health aspects of menopause.

Key topics: aging, hormone replacement, menopause, women's health

Try this: Visit this site and read the articles "Estrogen and Other Hormone Therapies," "Hormone Replacement Therapy for Menopause," and "Postmenopausal Hormone Prophylaxis" and one other article from the list. From what you see presented by Web MD, do you feel that menopause is no longer viewed as a natural part of aging but rather as a medical problem worthy of medical treatment?

Are Mammograms for Younger Women Necessary?

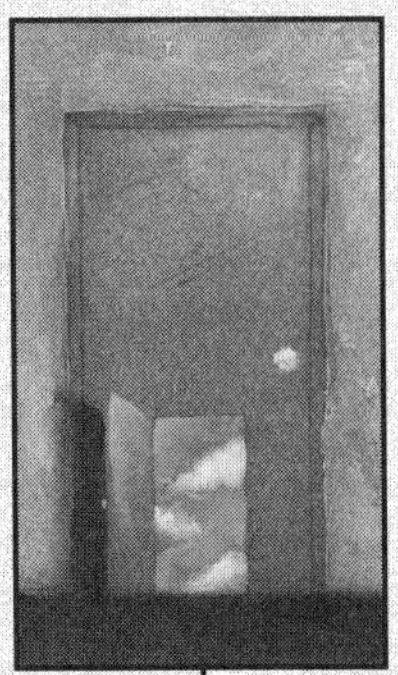

ISSUE 7

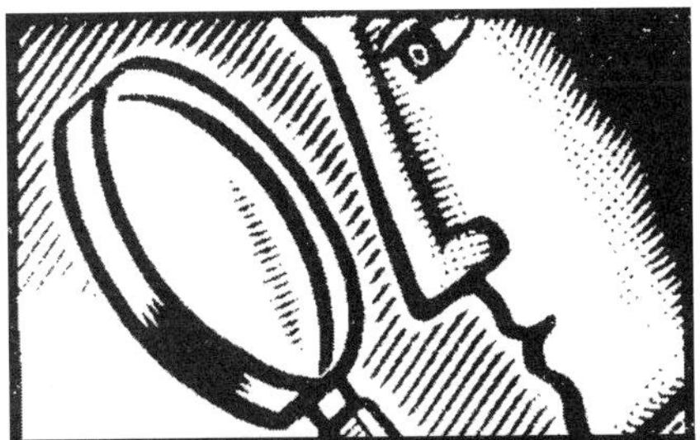

Take a Closer Look

1. What did Swedish studies discover about middle-aged women who screened positively for breast cancer using mammography?
2. How do the American Cancer Society and the National Cancer Institute differ in their recommendations regarding mammography?
3. According to *Consumer Reports* (Reading 17), at what age should women receive a baseline mammogram?
4. About how much does the breast cancer death rate stand to drop as a result of regular mammograms?
5. What is the major problem with mammograms?
6. According to Paykel and Wolberg in Reading 18, what is the major methodological fault in most current medical studies on mammograms and the occurrence of breast cancer?
7. According to Ritter in Reading 19, what disease carries a higher risk of death among women than breast cancer?

WiseGuide Intro

Breast cancer is the second leading cause of cancer death among women ages 40 to 55 behind lung cancer. It is the first leading cancer in terms of incidence. The American Cancer Society estimates that 178,700 new cases of breast cancer will be diagnosed in 1998 and will account for 43,900 deaths in the United States. Mammography has been widely used in recent years as a screening and diagnostic tool in the battle against breast cancer among women. The two leading cancer organizations in the United States—the National Cancer Institute and the American Cancer Society—are currently at odds with one another over not the effectiveness of mammography for screening breast cancer but the age recommendations for beginning routine mammograms.

Reading 16, "Hard-Won Consensus on Screening Younger Women," reviews the conclusions of the meeting of the National Institutes of Health Consensus Development Panel in January 1997 regarding the efficacy of mammography for detecting breast cancer in women ages forty to fifty. The panel concluded that it did not support the practice of administering routine mammograms for women in their forties. The reading describes the reactions of the National Cancer Institute and the National Cancer Advisory Board to this conclusion.

In Reading 17, "The Mammogram Debate," *Consumer Reports* provides an objective overview of the debate over the need and effectiveness of administering breast cancer screening mammograms to women under age fifty. The reading presents important statistics on the incidence of both cancerous and benign breast tumors and suggests some decision-making considerations.

In Reading 18, "Concerns about Recommending Routine Screening Mammograms for Women Ages 40 to 49," Jacquelyn Paykel and William Wolberg discuss some of the financial and diagnostic problems associated with early routine mammograms. They also present the hypotheses that screening and diagnostic mammograms for breast cancer should be administered based on patients' menopausal status and not their chronological age and that mammograms may actually be a causative factor in some cases of breast cancer.

In Reading 19, "Deceiving Numbers: Breast Cancer Risk Often Overestimated," reporter Jim Ritter points out that the often-cited statistic of "one in nine women will get breast cancer" may be misleading. He quotes an article from the *New England Journal of Medicine* and an expert from the American Cancer Society regarding the proliferation of inflated statistics on the actual risks of breast cancer. Ritter is concerned that cancer advocacy groups may use truthful statistics but often do not place them in perspective, which may cause over- and under-estimation of relative risks for younger and older women, respectively.

Issue 7: Are mammograms for younger women necessary?

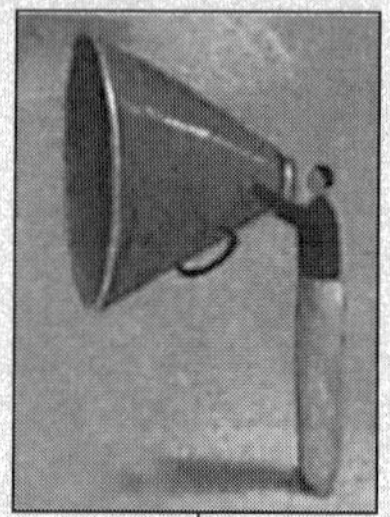

Hard-Won Consensus on Screening Younger Women

A Consensus Development Panel convened by the National Institutes of Health (NIH) met in January to review new worldwide clinical trial results examining the benefit of screening mammography in women aged 40 to 49. The report of the expert Panel stated that it could not recommend regular screening in this age group, thus triggering a cascade of concern, controversy and activity by other organizations agreeing or disagreeing with the NIH Panel.

On March 27, the National Cancer Institute (NCI), a co-sponsor of the NIH Conference, announced its support of mammography screening in this age group, stating that women in their 40's should be screened "every one to two years." The NCI position brings to a close four years of contentious disagreement among public health agencies, and will hopefully relieve widespread confusion among women and their doctors about who should be screened, how often, and which authority to believe.

New clinical trial data which originated in Sweden, reported in March 1996, prompted Dr. Richard Klausner, the NCI's Director, to request a Consensus Development Conference. In this established NIH mechanism, a panel of experts is appointed to review data and then answer predetermined questions about important medical subjects of controversy or emerging advances (see *NABCO News,* October 1996). Swedish national screening studies with up to 15 years of follow-up demonstrated with statistical certainty that women 40 to 49 whose breast cancers were found by mammography died of breast cancer at a lower rate than women diagnosed in a control group with no screening.

At the January 1997 Conference, a 14-member Panel of radiologists, clinicians, statisticians and consumers heard two days of presentations on the benefits and drawbacks of screening mammography for women in their 40's. In addition to the Swedish data, collected in five separate county studies and demonstrating a mortality benefit from regular mammography of up to 44 percent, updated results were presented from other U.S. and Canadian studies as well as from expert radiologists' large screening databases. Also reviewed were several meta-analyses that combined worldwide trials in order to reach a statistically-determined overall result; these found that regular screening mammography of average risk women in their 40's reduces breast cancer mortality by about 17 percent. Included in the Swedish results were data showing a number of breast cancers that emerged in the interval between screens (18 to 24 months in most studies), suggesting that the mortality benefit from mammography could increase with an annual screening interval.

More qualitative information at the Conference included two opposing consumer viewpoints—one downplaying the importance of screening younger women and the other characterizing it as crucial—as well as demographic information showing that the maturing "baby boom" cohort will result in a larger number of women younger than age 50 than those in their 50's being diagnosed with breast cancer this year. The limitations of regular mammography in young women set forth included the challenges of imaging dense breast tissue. Dense tissue can be opaque when x-rayed, making it more difficult to find breast cancer on a mammogram (a false negative) or producing abnormal screening results with follow-up biopsy showing no cancer (a false positive), plus the attendant anxiety, discomfort and expense. Several presentations offered reassurance that radiation risk from regular use of current screening mammography technology is negligible.

Given the nature of the data presented to the Panel, the very vocal and impassioned audience of practitioners, advocates and members of the media were taken aback by the negative and inconclusive tone of the Panel's written statement, presented at a press conference on the third and final day. There, a reporter asked Dr. Klausner (who was present for the entire Conference) for his reaction to the Panel statement. He expressed his concern with the statement's "lack of balance," suggesting that it understated screening benefits while overemphasizing its risks.

Following Dr. Klausner's expressed concern, the National Cancer Advisory Board (NCAB) formed a special subcommittee to study the issue and make recommendations to the NCI. Dr. Jeanne Petrek, a Panel member who is a surgical oncologist at Memorial Sloan-Kettering Cancer Center in New York, resigned from the Panel saying that she disagreed with its statement, and several other Panel members began formulating a statement of "minority opinion."

The American Cancer Society (ACS), which had recommended mammography starting at age 40, then "every year or two" until 50, released its statement in strong opposition to the Panel, and subsequently convened its own expert workshop to review the data once again and recommend changes to its own screening guidelines. On March 23, the ACS issued a statement changing its recommended screening guidelines to annual screening mammography starting at age 40. In the days that followed, several prominent breast cancer organizations, including NABCO, expressed their intention to adopt the new ACS guideline in all education and outreach efforts.

Some advocates dismiss the focus on mammography as peripheral to the search for breast cancer's prevention and cure. However, in February both the U.S. House of Representatives and the Senate issued resolutions calling for the NCI to further study the benefits of mammography and issue guidelines to screen women in their 40's. Sen. Arlen Specter (R-PA), Chair of the powerful Senate Appropriations Subcommittee overseeing NCI, separately expressed his strong support of screening women starting at age 40.

On March 27, the NCAB issued its report recommending screening mammography every one to two years, both for women in their 40's and for women 50 and older, and the NCI announced its immediate acceptance of these recommendations. In addition, the Institute adopted the guidance that high-risk women should seek expert advice about how often they should be screened, possibly starting at an earlier age.

This announcement changes NCI's position from its 1993 policy of no stated breast cancer screening guidelines to one that matches in spirit, if not in frequency, the positions of most leading national organizations. This consensus was highlighted by a second, notable NCI statement supporting screening mammograms for women also released on March 27, this one issued jointly by NCI and ACS.

FRAME the DEBATE

Form at end of book

Issue 7: Are mammograms for younger women necessary?

The Mammogram Debate

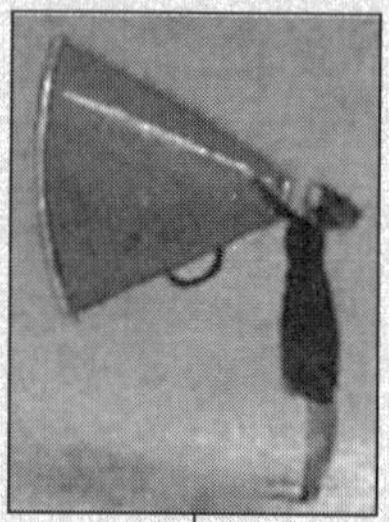

Conflicting medical advice is nothing new. But seldom is the conflict this vivid. Breast cancer is the leading cause of death among women in their 40s. The American Cancer Society says that women should start being regularly screened for breast cancer, using mammograms, when they turn 40. Yet the National Cancer Institute says routine screening need not start until age 50. Each has several other medical groups endorsing its position.

There was hope that the conflict might be resolved recently, when the head of the National Cancer Institute called a high-level "consensus conference" of independent experts to take another look at the evidence and reconsider the matter. No such luck. The conference ended without a firm conclusion on the value of mammograms for this age group. The panel recommended instead that a woman in her 40s discuss the risks and benefits of mammography with her doctor. Then she "should decide for herself whether to undergo mammography."

Why the Puzzle?

Mammography is basically an X-ray technique for imaging breast tissue that looks for dense spots or tiny specks of calcium that might be signs of early cancer. If a suspicious spot turns out (after it's sampled and examined) to be cancerous, surgery stands a good chance of removing all the cancerous cells before they can multiply and spread elsewhere in the body.

When women from 50 on up routinely obtain mammograms, the procedure spots breast cancer often enough and early enough to markedly reduce the chance of dying from the disease. And everyone agrees that the widespread use of mammography makes little sense in women under 40 (except for one "baseline" image made at about age 35).

It's the transition age group that's at issue. There aren't as many cases of cancer to be caught, and mammography has a more difficult time spotting the tumors in a younger woman's denser breast tissue. So the evidence for its effectiveness is fuzzy. It's hard to decide exactly when screening becomes beneficial for enough women for it to be deemed worthwhile.

What to Consider

Here are the pros and cons. Women in their 40s certainly do get breast cancer (more than 30,000 cases are diagnosed per year in the U.S.) and mammography certainly catches some of those cancers. The incidence of breast cancer approximately doubles from age 40 to age 49, so mammography increases in value as the decade progresses. And mammography can detect cancers earlier, when they are more curable and when a patient has more treatment options, such as breast-conserving lumpectomy rather than mastectomy.

Furthermore, there's some evidence that, in the long run, mammography saves lives in this age group. The evidence has not been strong, in large part because few studies of mammography were designed to answer that question, and possibly because the studies didn't track women long enough. But the benefit may be a reduction in breast-cancer deaths of as much as 30%.

The major risk of mammography is false alarms, which can cause anxiety for a woman and her family and sometimes lead to surgery. Mammograms find abnormalities that 9 times out of 10 turn out to be harmless. But sometimes that's not clear until after biopsy, or, in rare cases, lumpectomy or mastectomy.

Another often-cited risk is that a mammogram can overlook a tumor, so a woman will be given false assurance that she has no cancer. If it leads a woman to skip self-examination, professional exams or mammograms for several years, it is a problem. Otherwise, going a year or two between screenings with an undiscovered lump is not as bad as going the entire decade with no examination at all. One theoretical risk is that the X-ray itself may slightly increase the chance of cancer.

Consumer Reports Recommendations

There's no question about the value of mammography for women over 50. But for those in their 40s, the sometimes emotional debate over a national recommendation is likely to persist. Meanwhile, the decision will remain a personal one.

CR's medical consultants have long believed, and still do, that women in their 40s should have mammograms every year or two. It's important to be aware that mammography is not flawless, and to be aware that an abnormal finding may well turn out to be harmless. But those drawbacks are not reasons to shun a potentially life-saving procedure.

For Better Results

To improve your chance of an accurate mammogram:

- Use a facility with a radiologist on site, so if additional views are needed you won't have to be called back.
- Make sure there's no powder or deodorant on your skin. They can leave white flecks on the image.
- Tell the technologist if you're using hormone replacement therapy, which can make your breasts denser.

FRAME the DEBATE

Form at end of book

Issue 7: Are mammograms for younger women necessary?

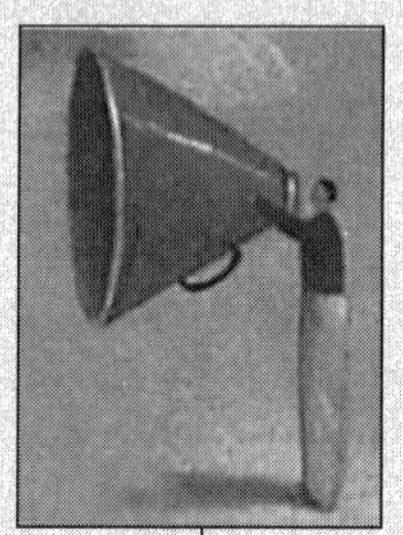

Concerns about Recommending Routine Screening Mammograms for Women Ages 40 to 49

Jacquelyn Paykel and William H. Wolberg

Ms. Paykel is a fourth-year medical student at the University of Wisconsin. William Wolberg is a professor in the Department of Surgery, Medical School, University of Wisconsin.

The controversy concerning the usefulness of screening mammography in younger-than-50 women continues. In general, two factors are consistently overlooked that should bear heavily on screening recommendations, particularly as they pertain to national policy. First, understanding why screening is more beneficial *after* as opposed to *before* age 50; second, assessing the societal cost of routine screening in younger women.

Pivotal to this discussion—and unavailable from any of the current studies—is the menopausal status of the patients being screened. Biological age is more important than is chronological age. At the time of menopause, the ovaries cease to produce estrogen. Lacking bodily estrogen, the breast glandular tissue involutes, and cancerous nodules become more apparent by mammogram. Therefore, screening is going to be as advantageous to a woman who is postmenopausal at age 48 as it is to a woman at age 55 or older. The reported screening studies have been conveniently designed based on the subjects' date at birth (age), rather than on the appropriate standard which is the menopausal status of the subject. Furthermore, women who started to receive mammograms before age 50 continued to receive them after their fiftieth birthday. Not only was the menopausal status ignored, but any beneficial effect of screening before 50 could not be distinguished from that occurring after 50.

Some otherwise undetectable cancers are found by mammography in younger-than-50 women. Women in this age group who have been mammographically diagnosed become strong advocates for screening. However, the radiation given with mammograms undoubtedly causes some cancers particularly in younger women when the breast is under estrogen stimulation. What is unclear is whether mammograms result in curing more cancers than they cause in this age group. The available data indicate that there is a close trade off.

However, now that screening mammograms have been recommended for younger-than-50 women, the societal cost of routine screening in 40 to 49 year old women should be considered. The average cost of a screening mammogram in the United States is $125. The National Census Bureau states that there are currently 20,050,000 women in the 40 to 49 age range. Simple arithmetic reveals that if every woman in this age group in the United States obtained a screening mammogram this year the total cost would be 2.5 billion dollars. To put this into perspective, the entire 1997 budget for the National Cancer Institute is 2.15 billion dollars. Of this amount only one seventh ($300 million) is allocated for breast cancer research. At this rate, less money is allocated by the NCI to research *all* cancers than it would cost for all women ages 40 to 49 to receive a screening mammogram this year. This does not include the amount spent on further diagnostic tests necessary to rule out cancer in the 10% of mammograms falsely considered to harbor cancer. The inescapable conclusion is that recommending screening in 40 to 49-year-olds is a relatively costly step that is based on contro-

Concerns about Recommending Routine Screening Mammograms for Women Ages 40 to 49, Jacquelyn Paykel and William H. Wolberg. Reprinted by permission.

versial data. Equating tax dollars spent for governmentally funded research with HMO/insurance carrier dollars spent for mammograms seems like comparing apples and oranges. Remember that both tax dollars and third party health care dollars come from the same pocket . . . yours.

Breast cancer will claim 44,000 lives this year. However, scare tactics designed to victimize women, such as "One of eight women will develop the disease some time during their lives," are used by some. Such a figure would be valid only if all women live to age 90. Half that number, one of fifteen, is more realistic. Furthermore, only a third of women who develop breast cancer will die of breast cancer. These numbers are substantial but they are inadequate to cause panic. Hence, a cost-benefit analysis seems in order . . . $2.15 billion for screening versus $300 million for research.

In our opinion, the answer lies beyond screening mammograms particularly in younger women. Lest we be criticized for advocating a policy that is detrimental to women's health, note that despite a 30% reduction in breast cancer deaths in women age 50 to 69, screening mammography did **not** improve overall survival (i.e., death from all causes) in the extensive Swedish trials. If the war against breast cancer is to be won, the focus of funding in this country must go beyond spending society's money on mammograms in order to provide better funding to explore new means of diagnosis, treatment and prevention.

FRAME the DEBATE

Form at end of book

READING 19

Issue 7: Are mammograms for younger women necessary?

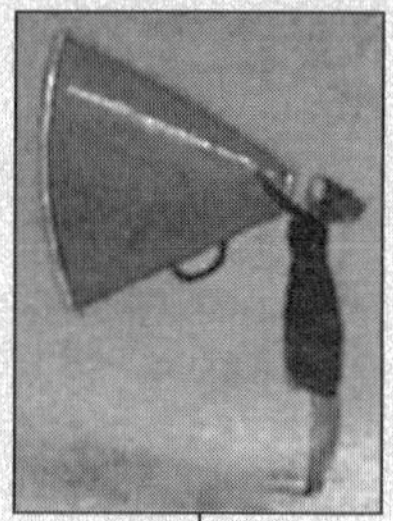

Deceiving Numbers:
Breast Cancer Risk Often Overestimated

Jim Ritter

It's one of the most commonly quoted statistics in medicine: One in nine women will get breast cancer.

The figure pops up repeatedly in medical journals and the media. While accurate, the statistic can "distort the public's perception of the risk," according to a recent report in the *New England Journal of Medicine.*

The statistic refers to a woman's cumulative risk of getting breast cancer if she lives past age 85. But in any given decade, her risk is far lower.

A woman has a 1-in-250 chance of getting breast cancer in her 30s, a 1-in-77 chance in her 40s, a 1-in-43 chance in her 50s, a 1-in-38 chance in her 60s and a 1-in-42 chance in her 70s.

Other diseases take a similar or higher toll. In a group of 1,000 women, the potential years of life they can expect to lose because of breast cancer totals 463, compared to 1,553 years lost to cardiovascular disease and 460 years lost to lung cancer.

Statistics should be put in context so that women do not become "disproportionately frightened" by breast cancer or overlook other preventable causes of illness and death, said the report, written by three Canadian breast cancer experts.

Breast cancer advocacy groups often quote the one-in-nine statistic "because it would draw attention to the cause," said Debbie Saslow of the American Cancer Society.

"We avoid using it," she said. "We make efforts to explain why it is misleading. . . . We do not want women to be more afraid of breast cancer than they need to be."

A woman's risk of getting breast cancer increases with age. More than 75 percent of all cases occur in women older than 50, Saslow said.

Younger women tend to overestimate their risk, and older women tend to underestimate their risk, she said.

FRAME the DEBATE

Form at end of book

WiseGuide Wrap-Up

Mammograms for women ages fifty and older appear to be one of the most effective tools for early detection of breast cancer. Mammograms may help to lower breast cancer death rates up to 30 percent among middle-aged to senior-aged women. The controversy lies in determining when mammography becomes an effective tool for early detection of breast tumors. Pre-menopausal women's breasts are often too dense for mammograms to effectively detect small, cancerous tumors, and this is the primary reason why health-care providers are divided on this issue. One side holds to the traditional recommendation of yearly or biannual mammograms for all women ages forty to forty-nine. Others recommend that only a baseline mammogram be performed at age thirty-five and that regular mammograms be delayed until age fifty. Is it safer and more cost effective to begin mammograms early—at an age when they may not be as effective—and risk "false alarms"? Or is it better to delay regular mammograms until women enter the high-risk age group when detection by mammogram is more probable, even though this may mean missing some of the younger-age-of-onset cases?

R.E.A.L. Sites

This list provides a print preview of typical **Coursewise** R.E.A.L. sites. (There are over 100 such sites at the **Courselinks**™ site.) The danger in printing URLs is that web sites can change overnight. As we went to press, these sites were functional using the URLs provided. If you come across one that isn't, please let us know via email to: webmaster@coursewise.com. Use your Passport to access the most current list of R.E.A.L. sites at the **Courselinks** site.

Site name: Breast Cancer

URL: http://www3.cancer.org/cancerinfo/main_cont.asp?st=wi&ct=5

Why is it R.E.A.L.? This site offers a detailed description of breast cancer epidemiology that should help you to become more informed on the incidence, physiology, and health concerns of breast cancer.

Key topics: breast cancer, mammograms

Try this: After reading the article on breast cancer at this site, describe breast cancer etiology in your own words (do not copy from the article). What is the incidence of breast cancer? Who is most at risk? Explore the American Cancer Society site, and collect information on two other sex-specific cancers for women and for men. Compare the rates of breast cancer with other types of cancer. Be prepared to defend whether or not you believe breast cancer concerns are overrated or underplayed in the media compared to other types of cancer.

Site name: Decisions, Decisions: The Fortysomething Mammography Mess

URL: http://www.acsh.org/publications/priorities/0903/decisions.html

Why is it R.E.A.L.? The article at this site addresses whether or not early mammograms are effective enough to warrant their use. The article comes from a web site dedicated to critically evaluating scientific and pseudo-scientific assumptions, hoopla, and hyperbole found in today's media. Dr. London states, "Screening transforms symptomless people into patients."

Key topics: breast cancer, mammograms

Try this: Read the article. How well does Dr. London present both sides of the argument? What strategies does he employ to persuade readers to his point of view? Prepare yourself to argue the relative economics of third-party payment for mammograms if (1) they are started as early as age thirty-five or (2) they are delayed until age fifty. Bear in mind the costs of multiple mammograms versus breast cancer treatments.

Section 3 Summary

In recent years, the health education specialty called "women's health" has emerged. Health educators and health-care practitioners in this area are most concerned with issues that directly affect women's health, such as sex-specific cancers, osteoporosis, pregnancy, menopause, and women's sexuality. Among current women's health issues are the topics of mammograms in breast cancer reduction and hormone replacement therapy to reduce the deleterious effects of menopause and the pernicious onslaught of osteoporosis. Both issues carry relative risks versus benefits and financial considerations.

STAND! **section 4**

Human Sexuality

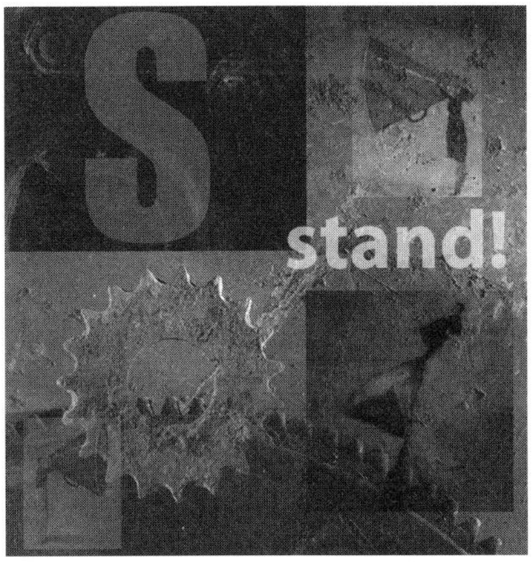

Learning Objectives

- Explore the place of values in sex education.
- Review the practicality of federal grant provisions for abstinence-based sex education programs.
- Consider the relative gains and losses of contraception-based and abstinence-based sex education programs.

Introduction

Few specialties in education garner as much controversy as health education, and few health topics are surrounded by as much controversy as sex education. Nearly everyone—from parents to teachers to school administrators—has an opinion on how and what should be included in or omitted from sex education curricula.

The only point that all sides agree on is that American teenagers are sexually active. According to the Centers for Disease Control and Prevention, 54 percent of high school students report having had sexual intercourse. This rate may be the indirect result of sex education, or it may be suppressed by sex education. Everyone agrees that teenagers face problems of sexually transmitted diseases and adolescent pregnancies at rates unseen in any other generation in America. All agree that something must be done to slow these upward trends. The problem, however, lies in reaching a consensus on how to best approach the issue.

Since the 1970s, contraception-based sexuality programs have dominated in most school districts. These programs focus on providing thorough and complete information on all areas of human sexuality, including pregnancy prevention and prevention of sexually transmitted diseases, all in as value-free an environment as possible. For the most part, contraception-based programs focus on the premise that providing students with complete and value-free knowledge allows them to make informed and healthful decisions regarding their sexual behavior. Proponents of contraception-based sex education accept that some teens are going to be sexually active to varying degrees and that correct and complete information may be the only way to help them avoid sexually transmitted diseases and pregnancies.

In recent years, however, many school districts and communities have questioned this guiding premise and called for approaches to sex education that emphasize abstinence as the only surefire way of preventing sexually transmitted diseases and adolescent pregnancies. The premise driving abstinence-based sex education programs is not new. Historically, parents, clergy, and community have taught most Judeo-Christian teens in America that sexual activity is something to be avoided until marriage. Many school health programs followed this same value-based model until the so-called "Sexual Revolution" of the late 1960s and 1970s, when most established values regarding human sexuality were challenged.

Contemporary abstinence-based sex education programs may or may not be based on Judeo-Christian values and doctrine. Private schools are more likely to adopt strong moral messages regarding sexuality, while public schools are more likely to adopt abstinence-based programs with subtler (but not entirely value-free) doctrines. Proponents of abstinence-based programs argue that contraception-based programs send the wrong message to teens and may, in fact, promote sexual activity. Research supports the contention that teens who participate in abstinence-based sex education programs have lower rates of sexually transmitted diseases, pregnancies, and promiscuity. This section presents arguments on both sides of the sex education debate.

What Type of Sex Education Program Is Most Effective in Preventing Pregnancies and Sexually Transmitted Diseases?

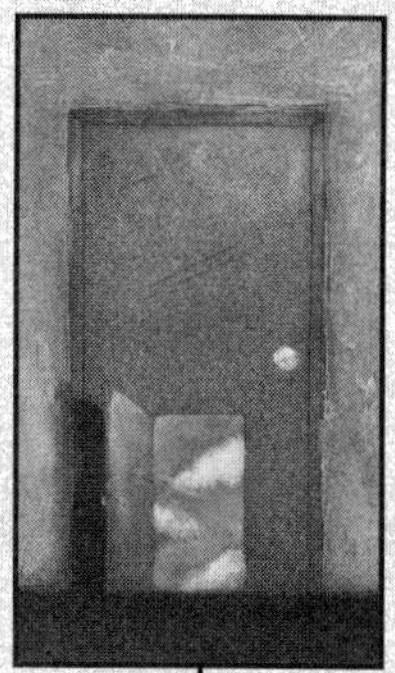

ISSUE 8

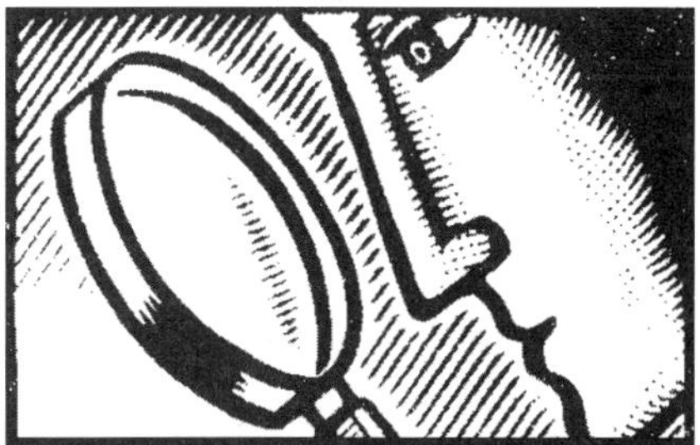

Take a Closer Look

1. In Reading 20, Whitehead describes four tenets of modern comprehensive sex education orthodoxy. Describe three of the four.
2. In Reading 20, Whitehead specifically criticizes the "Learning about Family Life" curriculum. Describe at least three major points of contention she makes regarding the curriculum.
3. According to the National Survey of Young Men and the National Survey of Family Growth, both quoted in Reading 20, have the numbers of sexually active teens actually increased in the past decade?
4. How is race a factor in age of first intercourse?
5. Does being religious make a difference in early sexual activity?
6. In Reading 21, what effect did a California abstinence-only initiative have on teen sexual intercourse?
7. From Reading 21, identify two or three SIECUS guidelines on abstinence for each of the following age groups: (a) nine to twelve years old, (b) twelve to fifteen years old, and (c) fifteen to eighteen years old.

WiseGuide Intro

Teen pregnancies have increased steadily in the past two decades and now represent 54.4 out of every 1,000 live births in America. Currently, the rates of sexually transmitted diseases and HIV among young Americans have reached all-time highs. Nearly all health education professionals consider sex education a core part of a comprehensive school health curriculum. All types of school sex education programs have the underlying goals of helping students understand reproductive anatomy and physiology, develop healthy adult sexuality, and avoid sexually transmitted diseases and unwanted or unplanned pregnancies.

For the past twenty years, contraception-based programs have prevailed in public schools. These programs center on two hypotheses: first, that teens should be given full and complete information regarding sexuality, reproduction, contraception, and disease prevention; and second, that all information should be given free of values and with the underlying assumption that, despite efforts to curtail them, many teens will choose to have sex and are best served if they have complete information. Critics of this approach tend to favor the abstinence-based programs that emphasize discouraging adolescents from having sex or placing themselves in difficult situations. Proponents of the abstinence-based approach generally feel that contraception-based programs actually encourage teens to become sexually active or, at the very least, send mixed messages regarding sexuality.

In Reading 20, "The Failure of Sex Education," Barbara Dafoe Whitehead argues that comprehensive and contraception-based sex education programs fail to lower adolescent rates of pregnancy and sexually transmitted diseases. She points out that, despite the popularity of contraception-based programs, teen pregnancy rates reached all-time highs in the 1990s. Whitehead reviews and critiques the comprehensive sexuality program "Learning about Family Life" specifically and the technocratic system of sex education in general.

In Reading 21, "What's Wrong with Abstinence-Only Sexuality Education Programs?," Debra Haffner establishes that SIECUS (Sexuality Information and Education Council of the United States) believes in and supports abstinence as a way of controlling sexually transmitted diseases (STDs) and unwanted pregnancy. SIECUS, however, believes that abstinence should be taught to young Americans as part of a comprehensive sex education program. According to Haffner, teaching abstinence to the exclusion of other types of contraception and STD prevention is inadequate and ineffective. She addresses each of the federal requirements for abstinence-based program grant applicants and provides arguments against each recommendation.

R E A D I N G 20

Issue 8: What type of sex education program is most effective in preventing pregnancies and sexually transmitted diseases?

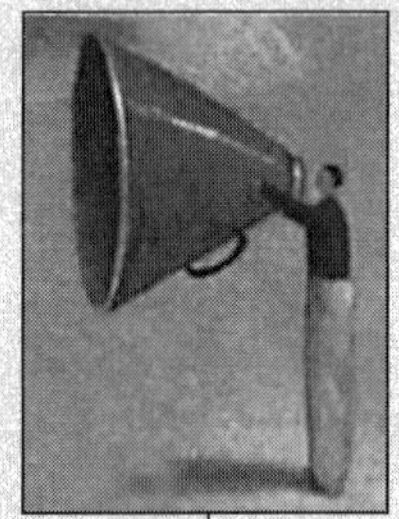

The Failure of Sex Education

"Comprehensive sex education," mandated in seventeen states, is the educational fad of the hour, yet there is little evidence that it "works"—prevents teenage pregnancy and stanches the spread of sexually transmitted disease. Defended by its professional-class originators as "getting real" about teenage sex, it fails to speak to the grim reality of what the author calls "the new sexual revolution" among the young.

Barbara Dafoe Whitehead

Amid rising concern about the hazards of teenage sex, health and school leaders are calling for an expanded effort to teach sex education in the schools. At the moment the favored approach is called comprehensive sex education. The nation's highest-ranking health officer, Surgeon General Joycelyn Elders, has endorsed this approach as the chief way to reduce unwed childbearing and sexually transmitted diseases (STDs) among teenagers. The pillars of the health and school establishments, including the National Association of School Psychologists, the American Medical Association, the National School Boards Association, and the Society for Adolescent medicine, support this approach. So do a growing number of state legislatures. Over the past decade seventeen states have adopted mandates to teach comprehensive sex education, and thirty more support it.

Sex education in the schools is not new, of course, but never before has it attempted to expose children to so much so soon. Comprehensive sex education includes much more than a movie about menstruation and a class or two in human reproduction. It begins in kindergarten and continues into high school. It sweeps across disciplines, taking up the biology of reproduction, the psychology of relationships, the sociology of the family, and the sexology of masturbation and massage. It seeks not simply to reduce health risks to teenagers, but also to build self-esteem, prevent sexual abuse, promote respect for all kinds of families, and make little boys more nurturant and little girls more assertive. As Dr. Elders explains, comprehensive sex education is not just about giving children a "plumbing lesson."

This approach is appealing for several reasons. First, it reaches the vast majority of American schoolchildren, through the public school system. Second, it is inexpensive. Principals have to do little more than buy a sex education curriculum and enroll the teacher or home-economics teacher in a training workshop, and their school has a sex-education program. Third, to panicky parents, worried about their ability to protect their children from AIDS and other STDs, comprehensive sex education offers a reassuring message: The schools will teach your children how to protect themselves.

Nonetheless, comprehensive sex education has provoked vigorous opposition, both at the grass roots and especially in the organized ranks of the religious right. Its critics argue that when it comes to teaching children about sex, the public schools should convey one message only: abstinence. In response, sex educators point to the statistics. Face facts, they say. A growing number of teenagers are engaging in sex and suffering its harmful consequences. It is foolish, if not irresponsible, to deny that reality. If more teenagers are sexually active, why deprive them of the information they need to avoid early pregnancy and disease? What's more, why insist on a standard of conduct for teenagers that adults themselves no longer honor or obey? As usual, the Surgeon General states the basic proposition memorably: "Everybody in the world is opposed to sex outside the marriage, and yet everybody does it. I'm saying, 'Get real.' "

This rhetoric is politically shrewd. It is smart to identify sex education with realism, honesty, and sexual freedom. (Its opponents are thereby unrealistic, hypocritical, and sexually unliberated.) Similarly, it is advantageous to link the sex-education campaign with the struggle against religious fundamentalism and, more generally, with opposition to religious argument in public life. When the issue is cast in Scopes-trial terms, it appears that an approach to sex education based in science will triumph over one rooted in blind faith.

But the sex educators' rhetoric is doubled-edged. As credentialed professionals, trained in the health and pedagogical sciences, advocates for a "reality-based" approach must at some point submit to reality tests. Their claims raise the inevitable question, How realistic is their approach to solving the problems associated with teenage sex? Or, to be more specific, What is the evidence that comprehensive sex education can achieve its stated goals? Does comprehensive sex education respond to the real-life circumstances of teenagers today? Does the new sex pedagogy take into account the realities of teenage sex in the 1990s?

The New Jersey Model

A few months ago I set out to answer these questions by venturing into a state with a long and strong commitment to comprehensive sex education. Few states have worked harder or longer than New Jersey to bring sexual enlightenment to schoolchildren. In 1980 the state adopted one of the nation's first mandates for comprehensive sex education—or family-life education, as it is called there—and it was the very first state to require sex education for children in the primary grades. Its pioneering efforts have earned New Jersey the equivalent of a three star rating from the Sex Information and Education Council of the U.S. (SIECUS), a national advocacy organization that promotes comprehensive sex education.

Virtually every public school student in New Jersey receives sex education (the average is twenty-four hours a year), and some schoolchildren, like those in the Irvington public schools, have an early and full immersion. Overall, teachers are trained and experienced, averaging close to ten years of teaching a family-life curriculum.

According to recent opinion polls, public support for sex education in New Jersey is strong. In one survey an overwhelming majority of adults said they favored teaching teenagers about sex in school, including controversial topics such as contraception, homosexuality, and "safer sex." Slightly more Catholics than Protestants surveyed favor sex education (88 percent to 84 percent), and support is nearly as high among parents as among nonparents. Parents tend to be more knowledgeable about the content of sex-education programs, and a majority say their school's offerings are excellent or good. Another survey, conducted by Rutgers University's Eagleton Institute, found that 61 percent of parents with school-age children say they would permit their child to get condoms from the schools.

Politically, therefore, sex education has been an all-but-unqualified success in New Jersey. Since 1980 popular support has steadily increased, and over that period the state mandate has held up against repeated legislative challenges, including a recent proposal to stress sexual abstinence.

The key to this success is a well-organized advocacy effort. A state mandate alone rarely achieves the goal of comprehensive sex education, because local school authorities often fail to act vigorously to observe the mandate. It takes a strong and sustained campaign to win over parents and teachers, beat back political opponents, and stiffen the spines of timid school administrators. In New Jersey two closely allied organizations advance the sex-education cause. Rutgers, the state university, administers grants and provides office space to the advocacy campaign. It is, though, the small but ubiquitous New Jersey Network for Family Life Education that conducts the daily business of winning support for sex education across the state.

The Philosophy of Sex Education

Susan Wilson runs the Network from her handsome gated home in Princeton. (The Network is officially headquartered at Rutgers.) Wilson, who has been an indefatigable crusader for comprehensive sex education for more than a decade, helped to write and pass the state mandate in the late 1970s, while she was a member of the State Board of Education. A few years later she took over as the head of the Network. With a budget of about $200,000 this year, mostly from foundations and the state government, Wilson and her small staff publish a newsletter, testify at hearings, train teachers, develop sex-education materials, fight efforts to overturn the mandate, and perform the scores of other duties required in their advocacy work. But Wilson's single most important task, which she clearly enjoys, is traveling up and down the state making the case for comprehensive sex education.

Because the case that she makes represents today's comprehensive-sex-education orthodoxy, it deserves close attention. It has several tenets. First, children are "sexual from birth." Like many sex educators, Wilson rejects the classic notion that a latency period occurs between the ages of about six and twelve, when children are sexually quiescent. "Ever since I've gotten into this field, the opponents have used that argument to frighten policymakers," she says. "But there is a body of developmental knowledge that says this is not true." And, according to Wilson, it is not simply that children are born sexual or that their sexuality is constantly unfolding. It is also that sexuality is much broader than most imagine: "You are not just being sexual by having intercourse. You are being sexual when you throw your arms around your grandpa and give him a hug."

Second, children are sexually miseducated. Unlike Europeans, who learn about sex as matter-of-factly as they learn about brushing their teeth, American children grow up sexually absurd—caught between opposing but equally distorted views of sex. One kind of distortion comes from patents. Instead of affirming the child's sexuality, parents convey the message that sex is harmful, shameful, or sinful. Or, out of a misguided protectiveness, they cling to the notion of childhood innocence and fail to provide timely or accurate information about sex. The second kind of distortion comes from those who would make sex into a commodity. While parents withhold information, the media and the marketplace spew sexual misinformation. It is this peculiar American combination of repressiveness and permissiveness that leads to sexual wrong thinking and poor sexual decision-making, and thus to high rates of teenage pregnancy and STDs.

Third, if miseducation is the problem, then sex education is the solution. Since parents are failing miserably at the task, it is time to turn the job over to the schools. Schools occupy a safe middle ground between Mom and MTV. They are places where "trusted adults" can teach children how to protect themselves against the hazards of sex and sexual abuse.

Moreover, unlike homes, schools do not burden children with moral strictures. As Wilson explains, schools can resolve the "conflict between morality and reality" by offering unbiased statements of fact. Here, for example, is how a teacher might handle the subject of masturbation in a factually accurate way: "Some people think it is okay to masturbate and some people think it is not okay to masturbate, but most people think that no harm comes to you if you masturbate." Consequently, when it comes to sex, schools rather than homes offer a haven in the heartless world.

A fourth and defining tenet is that sex education must begin in the earliest grades. Like math or reading, comprehensive sex education takes a "building blocks" approach that moves from basic facts to more sophisticated concepts, from simple skills to more complex competencies. Just as it would be unthinkable to withhold math education until the sixth grade, so, too, is it unwise to delay the introduction of sex education until the eighth grade.

In the beginning, before there is sex, there is sex literacy. Just as boys and girls learn their number facts in the first grade, they acquire the basic sex vocabulary, starting with the proper names for genitalia and progressing toward an understanding of masturbation, intercourse, and contraception. As they gain fluency and ease in talking about sexual matters, students become more comfortable with their own sexuality and more skillful in communicating their feelings and desires. Boys and girls can chat with one another about sex, and children can confide in adults without embarrassment.

Early sex education readies grade school children for the onslaught of puberty. By the time they reach adolescence, they are cognitively as well as biologically primed for sex. Moreover, with early sex training, teenagers are much more likely to engage in what Wilson and her colleagues consider responsible sexual conduct: abstinence, noncoital sex, or coitus with a condom. Since abstinence will not lead to pregnancy or STDs, and noncoital and protected sex are not likely to do so, comprehensive sex education will help to reduce the incidence of these problems among teenagers.

This is the philosophy of comprehensive sex education. But how to translate it into lessons for little children? Although the state mandate allowed school districts to shop around for a suitable curriculum, at first not much was available for primary schoolers. Most teachers had to improvise a curriculum or adapt higher-grade-level texts to the early grades. What was missing was a standard text: a Dick and Jane reader for the Michaels and Ashleys of the post-sexual-revolution generation.

Family Life

Rutgers University Press seized the opportunity. With a growing number of states adopting comprehensive-sex-education mandates, and with the 595 school districts of New Jersey seeking to meet their state mandate, the market for a sex primer looked promising. The press set out to fill that market niche. It assembled a small, sympathetic advisory panel, including Susan Wilson, and then hired Barbara Sprung, an independent consultant from New York City, to write its pathbreaking sex-education text.

A graduate of Sarah Lawrence and the Bank Street College of Education, Barbara Sprung spent eight years as an elementary school teacher before she embarked on a second career as a diversity-education specialist. During the 1970s and the 1980s, working first for a feminist organization and then for her own organization, Educational Equity Concepts. Sprung produced books, teachers' guides, and other materials based on a "nonsexist, multicultural, disability-sensitive, early childhood approach." The Rutgers project was her first venture into sex education.

With her advisers, she came up with *Learning About Family Life,* a "textbook package" described in the Rutgers University Press marketing brochure as a "pioneering" approach to family-life education for schoolchildren in kindergarten through third grade. The textbook also carries a pioneering price tag—$250 a package. As befits a fundamental text, the curriculum sets forth its guiding principles: "Sexuality is a part of daily living, as essential to normal functioning as mathematics and reading." And as befits a primer, it offers the sex basics. Here is a representative sampling:

> *On female genitalia:* "The vulva is the area enclosing three parts: a vagina, the opening you urinate from, and a clitoris. . . . Clitoris is a small sensitive part that only girls have, and it sometimes makes you feel good."
>
> *On sexual intercourse:* "To have sex, the man and woman lie very close to each other so that their bodies are touching. Usually it happens in bed, and they don't have any clothes on. Together the woman and man place the man's penis inside the woman's vagina, and while they are loving each other, many sperm come from the testicles into the man's penis. After a while, the sperm come through the little hole at the end of the man's penis, and they swim up the vagina and meet the egg in the fallopian tube."
>
> *On masturbation:* "Grown-ups sometimes forget to tell children that touching can also give people pleasure, especially when someone you love touches you. And you can give yourself pleasure, too, and that's okay. When you touch your own genitals, it's called masturbating."
>
> *On sex:* "When you are older, you can decide if you want to have sex. Most people do, because they like it and it's a very important way of showing that we love someone."

These sex facts are presented in a particularly captivating form. Unlike standard sex-education curricula, which are about as exciting to read as an IRS Form 1040, *Learning About Family Life* tells a story. The text follows a fictional class of primary school children and their teachers, Ms. Ruiz and Mr. Martin, as they experience a series of family events during the course of the school year. The teachers and children are characters in a continuing saga, full of drama and incident. Primary school teachers tell Sprung that children eagerly ask, "When are we going to talk about those kids in Class 203 again?" Little wonder. This is sex education packaged as *Sesame Street.*

Like *Sesame Street, Learning About Family Life* deals with the social and family issues of the day. During the year Classroom 203 encounters the following events: Ms. Ruiz's pregnancy and childbirth, the death of Mr. Martin's father, the drug arrest of Martine's cousin, the birth of a child to Joseph's teenage sister, the arrival of Natan's grandmother from Russia, Sarah's trip to see her divorced father, and the visit of Seth's HIV-infected uncle. These events and others, presented in forty-three vignettes, provide an occasion for straight talk about genitalia, sexual intercourse, pregnancy and childbirth, HIV and AIDS, masturbation, sexual abuse, physical disability, drug abuse, death, divorce, grandparents, and all kinds of families.

As they read about Classroom 203, children acquire a scientific sex vocabulary. "Adults in the children's families probably don't use accurate terms like anus and buttocks," the teachers' resource guide warns. "You, as the teacher, are the best role model for creating comfort." Indeed, the teacher is to insist on replacing even words that are perfectly apt for a six-year-old's vocabulary with more-scientific terms. In a lesson on pregnancy, Brian talks about how his mother's tummy felt when the baby was growing inside. Ms. Ruiz says, "I know we are used to saying *baby* and *tummy.* But *fetus* and *uterus* are more accurate words." And when it comes to a hot issue like masturbation, a teacher's cool command of the facts is crucial: "Masturbation is a topic that is viewed negatively in many families, based on long-standing cultural and religious teachings. Assure parents that your approach will be low keyed and will stress privacy, but also make it clear that you will not perpetuate myths that can mar children's healthy sexual development." Teachers must also debunk the myth that masturbation is only for boys. Girls must be granted equal time to ask masturbation questions.

There is something radically new about comprehensive sex education. As a philosophy and a pedagogy, it is rooted in a technocratic understanding of teenage sexuality. It envisions a regime of teenage sexual self-rule.

If girls need nudging in the sex department, boys need coaxing in the emotions department. Indeed, one of the strongest themes in the text is the problematic nature of boys. Boys are emotionally clogged, unable to cry or to express feelings. And little boys may enter grade school with the idea that such sex-related matters as pregnancy, child bearing, and baby care are only for girls. Therefore *Learning About Family Life* enlists boys in nurturing and "feelings" activities. These may be difficult for boys who come from macho backgrounds. But here again the school provides a cultural haven. If the lessons in nurturing conflict with a boy's family or cultural teachings, the teachers' manual advises, the teacher should say, "In school, talking about feelings is a part of learning."

In early sex education feelings talk and sex talk are closely related for good reason: little schoolchildren do not have the capacity to understand big adult issues directly. But many are now exposed to big adult issues at an early age, and so it is necessary to find routes to understanding. Early sex education thus turns to affective pathways and to a therapeutic pedagogy.

Stuff Happens

According to its publishers, *Learning About Family Life* provides a realistic slice of contemporary family life. Nonetheless, it is a highly selective slice. There is a vignette designed to expose children to an "amicable divorce." But there is no corresponding vignette to give children a picture of an amicable, much less a long-lasting, marriage. (Susan Wilson believes that you "can't beat kids all over the head" with marriage.) There is a story about sex as a way to show love, but no story about commitment as a way to show love. There is an effort to give children positive messages about expressing sexuality, but no effort to give children positive messages about the advantages of not expressing sexuality before they are grown. And this family world is only thinly populated by men. Ms. Ruiz is a well-defined character in the story: the male teacher, Mr. Martin, is more of a bit player, taking center stage in one story to talk about masturbation and in another to cry. There are grandmothers but no grandfathers. A brand-new father makes a cameo appearance to show off his nurturing skills, but the only other father is divorced and a plane ride away.

Here is the dilemma: *Learning About Family Life* is caught between two competing tendencies. On the one hand, it works hard to reflect the real-life family circumstances of many children. It deals with some hard-edged issues: sexual abuse, unwed teenage motherhood, drug dealing, and divorce. On the other hand, it takes a deeply sentimental view of these gritty realities. Consider, for example, the story "Joseph Is an Uncle":

Joseph's seventeen-year-old sister has a new baby. She is not married. The baby's father is gone. Joseph's parents are mad and sad at the same time. His sister is tired and out of sorts. Yet things work out. The family rallies round. An aunt takes care of the baby during the day. Joseph's sister returns to school. Joseph shows the photograph of his new nephew to his best friend, but he doesn't want anyone else to know about his sister's baby. His friend encourages him to show the photo to Mr. Martin and Ms. Ruiz.

Of all the sex tales, Joseph's story merits the closest attention. Early sex education, after all, purports to help children avoid the fate of Joseph's teenage sister. So what are we to make of this story? First, though illegitimacy is not treated cavalierly, it is depicted as a family crisis that is quickly resolved, because all the folks pitch in. Apparently there are no longer-term consequences for Joseph's sister or his little nephew—such as poverty, welfare dependency, or diminished school and job prospects. Second, in a curriculum designed to teach personal responsibility, the text misses an opportunity to do so. Unwed teenage parenthood is not an affliction visited on people like hurricanes or drought, yet that is the message of the story. Among the families in Classroom 203 stuff happens.

Finally, think about the baby's father. Joseph's sister's boyfriend has sex as an expression of love, exactly as the sex primer describes, but then he takes off. Though *Learning About Family Life* has stern messages for boys about caring and sharing, it ducks the basic question of male responsibility. A seven-year-old boy listening to this story might well conclude that illegitimacy is a girls' topic.

As it turns out, then, early sex education is not straight talk at all but a series of object lessons. And these are offered not so much with a nose for the facts as with an eye to the sex educators' philosophy. *Learning About Family Life* is no less didactic in its views on family life than Dick and Jane. To be sure, a truly fact-based approach would have to deal with some hard truths. For example, it would have to say that unwed teenage parenthood carries grave consequences for teenagers and their babies; that not all families are equally capable of caring for children; and that absent long-term commitment, responsibility, and sacrifice, love does not conquer all. Since some children grow up in broken or unwed teenage families, there is an understandable concern that children not feel stigmatized by such facts. Yet such tender concern raises a tough question: If the classroom is the source of unbiased factual information, how can the problems of illegitimacy and broken families be dealt with without touching on the key facts in the matter?

The Pedagogy of Sex Education

In the middle grades sex education takes a more technical turn. At eleven and twelve many young people are approaching the threshold of puberty while others are already in full pubertal flower. (Today the average age of menarche is twelve and a half.) Now, as hormones kick in, children are ready to express themselves sexually. Thus the focus of sex education shifts from sex literacy to building sexual skills. This is when students must acquire the knowledge and technical skills to manage their emerging sexuality.

Sex-education advocates agree that abstaining from sex is the best way to avoid STDs and early pregnancy. But they reject an approach that is limited to teaching abstinence. First, they say, abstinence-based teaching ignores the growing number of adolescents who are already sexually active at age twelve or thirteen. One Trenton schoolteacher said to me, "How can I teach abstinence when there are three pregnant girls sitting in my eighth-grade class?" Second, abstinence overlooks the fact that, as Susan Wilson explains, "it is developmentally appropriate for teenagers to learn to give and receive pleasure."

Consequently, the New Jersey sex-education advocates call for teaching middle-schoolers about condoms, abortion, and the advantages of "protected" sex. But given the risks to teenagers, they are not crazy about sexual intercourse either. Indeed, Wilson says, Americans are fixated on "this narrow little thing called intercourse." The alternative is a broad thing called noncoital sex or, in the argot of advocates, "sexual expression without risk."

Noncoital sex includes a range of behaviors, from deep kissing to masturbation to mutual masturbation to full body massage. Since none of these involves intercourse, sex educators see them as ways for teenagers to explore their sexuality without harm or penalty. And from a broader public-health perspective, risk-free sexual expression has great potential. According to the Rutgers education professor William Firestone, who conducted a study of sex-education teaching in New Jersey for the Network for Family Life Education, noncoital sex offers "real opportunities to reduce dangers to many teens who engage in sexual behavior, despite recommendations for abstinence." Yet as Firestone's survey research shows, many teachers shrink from this approach. Wilson says, "We hardly ever talk to teens about necking and petting and admiring your body and maybe massage."

As Wilson points out, noncoital sex is most practicable when teenagers can communicate with each other. "A lot of people think that once you start down the road to sex, you can't stop, and that's the problem. But I think that by talking about these things and by role playing, you give kids control and you give them the language to say, 'That's enough—I don't want any more. I don't want to have intercourse.' "

Since safe petting and good talking go together, middle school students need to continue to practice their communication skills. But in teaching these skills teachers cannot rely on old-fashioned didactic methods. Middle school students are still short-term thinkers, reckless in deed. Therefore sex education in middle school does not yet enter the realm of thinking and ideas but remains lodged instead of the realm of what one teacher calls "feelings and values."

"Hello, Vulva"

I attended a teacher-training conference sponsored by the Network for Family Life Education to get acquainted with the way sex is taught. In New Jersey, as in other states with mandates for comprehensive sex education, such one-day workshops are a mainstay of teacher training. For a small investment of time and money—a day out of the classroom and $35—teachers learn the latest in sex-education theory and practice. On the day I attended, the crowd was made up of physical-education, home-economics, and health teachers with a scattering of elementary school nurses as well. Almost all were women.

Deborah Roffman, an independent sex-education consultant from Maryland who teaches in several private middle and high schools, was the keynote speaker. (Like Roffman, most of the trainers at this conference came to it from the world of advocates, family planners, and private consultants. Only one teaches in the public schools.) She was an engaging speaker with the timing and phrasing of a good comedian. (*Teacher in audience:* "What do you say when a student asks you to define 'blow job'?" *Roffman:* "You say it is oral sex." Pause. *Roffman again:* "But what if the student's next question is 'Does that mean you talk while you screw?' ") To kick off the conference, Roffman gave a rousing talk, urging teachers to adopt bolder teaching methods. I was curious to see what she had in mind, so I attended her workshop.

She began the workshop sessions with these instructions: "Turn to the person next to you. Make eye contact. Say 'Hello, penis.' Shake hands and return the greeting: 'Hello, vulva.' " This warmup exercise underscores a central idea in sex pedagogy: for teachers no less than for students, talking about sex provokes anxiety and embarrassment. Such embarrassment stands in the way of good communication, and good communication is crucial to responsible sexual conduct.

So is emotional literacy. To become more emotionally articulate, middle-schoolers engage in a series of feelings exercises. The purpose is to help students "normalize" and share common growing-up experiences. Roffman handed out a list of sample questions: "What is the worst thing your parents could find out about a child of theirs who is your age?" "Have you ever experienced the death of someone close to you?" "What is a way in which your parents are 'overprotective'?" In the middle schools as in the elementary schools, there is a continuing effort to break down boys' emotional reserve. Encourage your students to sit boy-girl, Roffman suggests, and ask the biggest boy in the class the first feelings question.

The Consortium for Educational Equity, at Rutgers, offers a similar set of feelings-and-values exercises in a sex curriculum designed for seventh- and eighth-graders. Some are sentence-completion exercises. In one, seventh-graders are asked to complete the sentence "If someone loves me, they . . ." and then elsewhere to "compare their ideas [about love] to [Eric] Fromm's and [Leo] Buscaglia's material on love." In another, students are to "write a positive self-statement . . .— 'I am strong' . . . 'I am happy' . . ."—and then discuss the "impact of positive self-statements on feelings of self-esteem."

Other exercises draw on more therapeutic methods, such as role-playing and small-group work. There are gender-reversal exercises, in which girls and boys each play the role of the opposite sex. In small groups students may brainstorm about ways to deal with an unwanted pregnancy or come up with a list of their expectations of nonmarital sex.

Some of the gender-reversal exercises sound like birthday-party games. In one exercise, called the Fish-Bowl, girls are seated in a circle in which there is one empty chair. Boys form a circle around the girls. Girls talk about what they like and dislike about boys. If one of the boys wishes to speak, he sits in the empty chair in the girls' circle. After a time the boys repeat the exercise, with the girls in the outer circle.

Because of its intimate subject matter, the feelings-and-values classroom institutes a new code of classroom conduct. There are confidentiality rules. Roffman's middle school students are told that nothing said in sex-education class goes out of the class without students' express permission. In discussions middle-schoolers must protect the privacy of individuals who are not class members: except for classmates', no names may be used. Another rule is that any student who does not want to answer a question may pass. In some classes students agree to use only "I" statements, rather than "you" statements, in order to express their thoughts more positively.

In therapeutically oriented classrooms, moreover, the teacher assumes the role of confidant and peer. Like students, teachers are encouraged to share personal experiences. An idea book for New Jersey teachers, published by the Network, tells the inspirational story of a high school teacher who talks to his class about his vasectomy and how he feels about it. Yet although they are advised to share experiences, teachers are not to impose their opinions, even when it comes to arguably the most important question: "What is the right time to begin having sex?" The teacher is encouraged to turn the question back to the students: "How would you begin to make that decision?"

Sex educators defend this approach with the language of empowerment. Students, they say, must acquire the knowledge and skills to answer these questions for themselves. After all, grown-ups aren't around to supervise teenagers every minute of the day. Teachers can't follow students home, and working parents can't check up on teenagers who are home alone. Why not invest teenagers with the power to make wise choices on their own?

Reality Tests

On its face, this new therapeutic sex pedagogy does not seem all that therapeutic or all that new. Teenage girls have enjoyed self-inventory tests at least as long as *Seventeen* magazine has been around. And there's nothing particularly revolutionary about small-group discussions of feelings and values. This, after all, is why teenagers invented the slumber party.

But on second glance there is something radically new about comprehensive sex education. As both a philosophy and a pedagogy, it is rooted in a deeply technocratic understanding of teenage sexuality. It assumes that once teenagers acquire a formal body of sex knowledge and skills, along with the proper contraceptive technology, they will be able to govern their own sexual behavior responsibly. In brief, what comprehensive sex education envisions is a regime of teenage sexual self-rule.

The sex educators offer their technocratic approach as an alternative to what they see as a failed effort to regulate teenage sexuality through social norms and religious values. Face facts. In a climate of sexual freedom the old standard of sexual conduct for teenagers—a standard separate from adult sexual standards—is breaking down. Increasingly teenagers are playing by the same sexual rules as adults. Therefore, why withhold from adolescents the information and technologies that are available to adults?

To be sure, sex educators have a point. Traditional sexual morality, along with the old codes of social conduct, is demonstrably less effective today than it once was in governing teenage sexual conduct. But although moral standards can exist even in the midst of a breakdown of morality, a technocratic view cannot be sustained if the techniques fizzle. Thus comprehensive sex education stands or falls on the proven effectiveness of its techniques.

For a variety of reasons the body of research on sex-education programs is not as rich and robust as we might wish. However, the available evidence suggests that we must be skeptical of the technocratic approach. First, comprehensive sex education places its faith in the power of knowledge to change behavior. Yet the evidence overwhelmingly suggests that sexual knowledge is only weakly related to teenage sexual behavior. The researcher Douglas Kirby, of ETR Associates, a nonprofit health-education firm in Santa Cruz, California, has been studying sex-education programs for more than a decade. During the 1980s he conducted a major study of the effectiveness of sex-education programs for the Department of Health, Education and Welfare, and he has since completed a review for the Centers for Disease Control of all published research on school-based sex-education programs designed to reduce the risks of unprotected sex. His research shows that students who take sex education do know more about such matters as menstruation, intercourse, contraception, pregnancy, and sexually transmitted diseases than students who do not. (Thanks to federal funding for AIDS education in the schools, students tend to be very knowledgeable about the sources and prevention of HIV infection.)

But more accurate knowledge does not have a measurable impact on sexual behavior. As it is typically taught, sex education has little effect on teenagers' decisions to engage in or postpone sex. Nor, according to Kirby, do knowledge-based sex-education programs significantly reduce teenage pregnancy. And although teenagers who learn about contraception may be more likely to use it, their contraceptive practices tend to be irregular and therefore ultimately unreliable.

Comprehensive sex education assumes that knowledge acquired at earlier ages will influence behavior. Yet the empirical evidence suggests that younger teenagers, especially, are unlikely to act on what they know. An analysis of a Planned Parenthood survey concludes that a "knowledgeable thirteen-year-old is no more likely to use contraceptives than is an uninformed thirteen-year-old." As Kirby puts it, "Ignorance is not the solution, but knowledge is not enough."

If knowledge isn't enough, what about knowledge combined with communication skills? Sex education does appear to diminish teenagers' shyness about discussing sexual matters. One study shows that girls who have had sex education may be more likely to talk about sex with their parents than those who have not. Since talking with their mothers about sex may help some girls avoid pregnancy, this is a mildly positive effect. There does not seem to be a parallel effect for boys, however.

Overall, parent-child communication is far less important in influencing sexual behavior than parental discipline and supervision. One study, based on teenagers' own reports of levels of parental control, shows that teenagers with moderately strict parents had the lowest level of sexual activity, whereas teens with very strict parents had higher levels, and those with very permissive parents had the highest levels. Moreover, there is a strong empirical relationship between diminished parental supervision and early sexual activity.

In boy-girl communication, girls say that they want help in rejecting boys' sexual overtures. In a survey taken in the mid-1980s, 1,000 teenage girls aged sixteen and younger were asked to select from a list of more than twenty sex-related topics those areas where they would like more information and help. The girls were most likely to say they wanted more information on how to say no without hurting boys' feelings. This is especially noteworthy given that all the girls in the survey were sexually active, and some were mothers.

Beyond "no," better communication about sex does not seem to contribute to higher levels of sexual responsibility. To be sure, there has been little research into this aspect of teenage sexuality. But even absent research, there is good reason to be skeptical of the claim. If free and easy sex talk were a key determinant of sexual behavior, then we might expect the trends to look very different. It would be our tongue-tied grandparents who had high rates of illegitimacy and STDs, not today's franker and looser-lipped teenagers.

"You Are Not Ready for Sex"

Unsurprisingly, there is not a shred of evidence to support the claim that noncoital sex, with or without communication, will reduce the likelihood of coitus. William Firestone, of Rutgers, who wrote the study for the Network for Family Life Education, concedes that his enthusiasm is empirically unfounded. In fact, several studies show just the opposite. Outercourse is a precursor of intercourse. But do we need studies to tell us this? Is it not graven in our memory that getting to third base vastly increases the chances of scoring a run? In fact, it could be argued that teaching noncoital sex techniques as a way of reducing the risks of coitus comes close to educational malpractice.

And what about empowering students to make their own sexual decisions? Douglas Kirby's work shows that teaching decision-making skills is not effective, either, in influencing teenage sexual behavior. Similarly, there is little empirical support for the claim made by comprehensive sex education's advocates that responsible sexual behavior depends on long years of sexual schooling. In fact, the evidence points in the opposite direction. Math and reading do require instruction over a period of time, but sex education may be most effective at a key developmental moment. This is not in grade school but in middle school, when pre-teens are hormonally gearing up for sex but are still mainly uninitiated.

In pursuit of a more effective sex pedagogy, researchers have turned away from technocratic approaches and dusted off that old chestnut, norms. According to Kirby's research review, several new and promising sex-education programs focus on sending clear messages about what is desirable behavior. When middle-schoolers ask "What is the best time to begin having sex?" teachers in these programs have an answer. It is "Not yet. You are not ready for sex."

Evidently, too, sex education works best when it combines clear messages about behavior with strong moral and logistical support for the behavior sought. One of the most carefully designed and evaluated sex-education courses available is Postponing Sexual Involvement, a program developed by researchers at Grady Memorial Hospital, in Atlanta, Georgia, and originally targeted at minority eighth-graders who are at high risk for unwed motherhood and sexually transmitted diseases. Its goal is to help boys and girls resist pressures to engage in sex.

The Grady Hospital program offers more than a "Just say no" message. It reinforces the message by having young people practice the desired behavior. The classes are led by popular older teenagers who teach middle-schoolers how to reject sexual advances and refuse sexual intercourse. The eighth-graders perform skits in which they practice refusals. Some of them take the part of "angel on my shoulder," intervening with advice and support if the sexually beleaguered student runs out of ideas. Boys practice resisting pressure from other boys. According to the program evaluator, Marion Howard, a professor of gynecology and obstetrics at Emory University, the skits are not like conventional "role plays," in which students are allowed to come up with their own endings. All skits must end with a successful rebuff.

The program is short: five class periods. It is not comprehensive but is focused on a single goal. It is not therapeutic but normative. It establishes and reinforces a socially desirable behavior. And it has had encouraging results. By the end of ninth grade only 24 percent in the program group had had sexual intercourse, as compared with 39 percent in the nonprogram group. Studies of similar programs show similar results: abstinence messages can help students put off sex. It is noteworthy that although the purpose of the Grady Hospital program was to help students postpone sex, it also had an impact on the behavior of students who later engaged in sexual intercourse. Among those who had sex, half used contraception, whereas only a third did in a control group that had not taken the course.

As it is typically taught, sex education has little effect on teenagers' decisions to engage in or postpone sex. Nor do knowledge-based sex-education programs significantly reduce the incidence of teenage pregnancy.

Postponing Sexual Involvement and similarly designed sex-education programs offer this useful insight: formal sex education is perhaps most successful when it reinforces the behavior of abstinence among young adolescents who are practicing that behavior. Its effectiveness diminishes significantly when the goal is to influence the behavior of teenagers who are already engaging in sex. Thus teaching sexually active middle school students to engage in protected intercourse is likely to be more difficult and less successful than teaching abstinent students to continue refraining from sex. This seems to hold for older teens as well. In a 1991 study Kirby points to one curriculum for tenth-graders, Reducing the Risk, which has been successful in increasing the likelihood that abstinent students will continue to postpone sex over the eighteen months following the course. However, although the program emphasizes contraception as well as sexual postponement, it does not increase the likelihood that already sexually active tenth-graders will engage in protected sex. "Once patterns of sexual intercourse and contraceptive use are established," Kirby writes, "they may be difficult to change." For that reason the Grady Hospital researchers have developed a program for sixth-graders, since 44 percent of the boys taking their course in the eighth grade were already sexually experienced (this was true of just nine percent of the girls).

It does not follow, however, that this approach will work for younger children. The evidence strongly suggests that children who are sexualized at very early ages are likely to be victims of sexual abuse and other forms of traumatic sexualization. Teaching refusal skills to a "sexually active" nine- or ten-year-old is not the answer. Such children need far more intensive care and support than can be provided in the classroom.

In a sharp break with the Surgeon General's approach, President Clinton's welfare-reform proposal strongly endorses the Grady Hospital approach. Similarly, the President's recent bully-pulpit message to teenagers, counseling sexual postponement and marriage before parenthood, is strikingly at odds with the Surgeon General's message to "get real." Thus the Administration finds itself in the awkward position of advancing contradictory approaches to sex education and pregnancy prevention.

Judging by the available evidence, the President has the stronger case. None of the technocratic assumptions of comprehensive sex education hold up under scrutiny. Research does not support the idea that early sex education will lead to more responsible sexual behavior in adolescence. Nor is there reason to believe that franker communication will reduce the risks of early-teenage sex. Nor does instruction about feelings or decision-making seem to have any measurable impact on sexual conduct. Teaching teenagers to explore their sexuality through noncoital techniques has perverse effects, since it is likely to lead to coitus. Finally, although teenagers may be sexually miseducated, there is no reason to believe that miseducation is the principal source of sexual behavior. As we will see, the most important influences on teenage sexual behavior lie elsewhere.

Moreover, if comprehensive sex education has had a significant impact on teenage sexual behavior in New Jersey, there is little evidence to show it. The advocates cannot point to any evaluative studies of comprehensive sex education in the state. Absent such specific measures, one can only fall back on gross measures like the glum statistics on unwed teenage childbearing in the state. In 1980, 67.6 percent of teenage births were to unmarried mothers;

eleven years later the figure had increased to 84 percent. Arguably, the percentage might be even higher if comprehensive sex education did not exist. Nevertheless, it is hard for advocates to claim that the state with the nation's fourth highest percentage of unwed teenage births is a showcase for their approach.

The absence of empirical support for comprehensive sex education does not, however, discomfit or deter its advocates. Up and down the sex-education ranks, from the Surgeon General to local advocates, there has been little effort to make a reasoned case for comprehensive sex education. Challenged, the sex educators simply crank up their rhetoric: Criticize sex education, they say, and you contribute to the deaths of teenagers from AIDS.

Nor, for that matter, has there been much critical challenge from the research community. Perhaps this is because comprehensive sex education is a policy crafted outside the precincts of the academy. It is not rooted in a single discipline, or even a set of disciplines, but can best be described as a jumble of popular therapies and philosophies, including self-help therapies, self-esteem and assertiveness training, sexology, and certain strands of feminism.

The unifying core of comprehensive sex education is not intellectual but ideological. Its mission is to defend and extend the freedoms of the sexual revolution, and its architects are called forth from a variety of pursuits to advance this cause. At least in New Jersey, the sex-education leaders are not researchers or policy analysts or child-development experts but public-sector entrepreneurs: advocates, independent consultants, family planners, freelance curriculum writers, specialty publishers, and diversity educators. However dedicated and high-minded they may be, their principal task is not to serve the public or schoolchildren but to promote their ideology.

For better or worse, sex-education advocacy is largely women's work. And there is an unmistakably female bias in the advocate's idea of what is sexually nice. It favors what thousands of American women have told Ann Landers: in their sex lives women would like more talking, more hugging, more outercourse. At the teacher-training workshop I attended, a family planner explained a classroom exercise designed to show all the things we can do without sexual intercourse: we can have children; we can show love and affection; we can gain self-esteem; we can achieve success in life. Reaching her summation, she proclaimed, We can have orgasm without sexual intercourse. After a moment, in the back of the classroom, one of the few men attending cleared his throat and politely protested this ideal of intercourse-free sex.

Comprehensive sex education reflects not just a gender bias but also a generational bias. Despite its verbal swagger, it offers a misty-eyed view of early-teenage sexuality. It assumes that the principal obstacles to responsible sexual conduct are ignorance, guilt, and shame. Once properly schooled in sex and freed of these repressive feelings, boys and girls can engage in mutual sexual pleasuring. But there is a dated quality to this view. Indeed, many of the arguments for sex education are filled with anecdotes from the fifties: Susan Wilson, for one, urges middle-aged teachers to think back and remember how inadequate their own sex education was. Though the educators' notions may accurately reflect what it was like for eighteen-year-old females to come of age before the sexual revolution of the 1960s, they have little to do with what fifteen-year-olds face in the 1990s. The MTV generation may indeed have a distorted image of sex, but it has not been distorted by shame or repression.

Thus comprehensive sex education flunks the reality test not just once but twice. Indeed, much of the evidence suggests that less-comprehensive, more-targeted sex education would be far more effective in reducing early sexual involvement and its associated risks. But more important, comprehensive sex education is woefully out of touch with the realities of teenagers' sex lives. Surely any policy with claims to steely-eyed realism must begin with an appraisal of what the evidence tells us about the sexual lives of today's adolescents, especially teenage girls.

The New Sexual Revolution

There is a new sexual revolution in America. Unlike the old sexual revolution, which has been documented and celebrated ever since its boisterous beginnings, in the late 1960s, the new sexual revolution has arrived unheralded. Its vanguard is found not among confident, self-dramatizing students on college campuses, but among gawky adolescents in the crowded hallways of the junior high.

The children of the Baby Boom generation are beginning to have sex at earlier ages than their parents did. In 1970, five percent of fifteen-year-old girls and 32 percent of seventeen-year-old girls reported having had sex; by 1988 the figures had increased to 26 percent of fifteen-year-olds and 51 percent of seventeen-year-olds. By age nineteen nearly 80 percent of young women have had sexual intercourse. As a result of earlier sexual initiation among girls, the historical gender gap in first sexual experience is narrowing; according to the 1988 National Survey of Young Men, one third of teenage males have had sex by age fifteen, and 86 percent by age nineteen. With early initiation, today's adolescents are more sexually active. They have more partners: among never-married sexually experienced teenage girls in 1971, 38 percent had had two or more sexual partners; by 1988 the figure had increased to

59 percent. And they have sex more frequently: the 1988 National Survey of Family Growth reported that 45 percent of never-married sexually active girls had intercourse at least once a week, as compared with 40 percent when the survey was administered in 1982.

But these figures alone do not capture what may be the most striking feature of the new sexual revolution: the rise in the proportion of younger teenagers engaging in sex. The largest relative increase in sexual intercourse among teenage girls has occurred among those fifteen years of age, from 4.6 percent in 1970 to 25.6 percent in 1988. (Below the age of fifteen, the evidence strongly suggests, sexual initiation is involuntary for a large proportion of girls who report having had sexual intercourse.)

Within this overall pattern of earlier sexual initiation there are significant racial and ethnic differences. African-American males are more likely than white or Hispanic males to engage in early sex. At age fourteen, 35 percent of black males have had intercourse; the comparable percentages for white and Hispanic males are seven and six respectively. Apparently because they begin their sexual careers earlier, black males also report more partners than white or Hispanic males (those who are sexually active at age fifteen, for example, report 6.4, 3.5, and 1.9 respectively). Though data comparing teenage girls from all three groups are not available, the evidence points to similar differences between African-American and white females. African-American girls are more likely to have had premarital sex in the early teen years than their white counterparts. However, the differences become less pronounced among older teens. For example, at age sixteen, 24 percent of white girls, and 33 percent of black girls, report having experienced sexual intercourse: by age nineteen the percentages are nearly identical: 76 percent of white girls and 79 percent of black girls.

Family structure strongly influences early sexual activity as well. Daughters in single-parent families are more likely to engage in early sex than girls who grow up in two-parent families. Several factors may be involved: less supervision in the home, less exposure to adults' sexuality, and the lack of a father's steady affection and protection. Girls whose relationships with their fathers have been severely damaged by divorce or their parents' nonmarriage are more likely to engage in a frantic quest for male approval and to seek love through early sex than are girls from intact families. Both parents and teenagers in divorced families have more permissive attitudes toward sexual intercourse outside marriage. In fact, there is evidence of a kind of sexual trickle-down in families, not just from parent to child but also from older siblings to younger. Teenagers with sexually active siblings are likelier to begin having sex at an early age.

Religiously observant teens are likelier than others to refrain from early sex: the highest level of premarital intercourse occurs among teens with no religious affiliation. At the same time, the University of Michigan sociologist Arland Thornton reports, cause and effect can work in the other direction. Early sexual activity can dampen religious ardor.

In the midst of this sexual upheaval one trend is quite clear: the new sexual revolution has been a disaster for teenage girls. Even more now than in the past, girls bear the heavy burdens and penalties of nonconjugal sex. Early sexual initiation puts girls at increased risk for sexually transmitted diseases. This is partly because teenagers who are sexually active at an early age have more partners and partly because young teenage girls are likely to have older, sexually experienced partners. Some researchers also contend that teenage girls are at greater risk for STDs than adult women because their cervical lining is not yet fully mature and is therefore more vulnerable to pathogens. Whatever their causes, STDs can lead to serious, sometimes permanent, damage to the reproductive system, including infertility, chronic pelvic pain, ectopic pregnancy, and cervical cancer.

And despite reported high levels of contraceptive use among adolescents, teenage girls continue to get pregnant. A million teenage girls each year find themselves pregnant. About 37 percent of teenage pregnancies end in abortion and about 14 percent in miscarriage. Roughly half of all these pregnancies result in childbirth, and since less than 10 percent of teenagers today give their babies up for adoption, teenage childbearing commonly results in teenage motherhood—usually unwed motherhood.

This fact constitutes one of the more perplexing aspects of the new sexual revolution. Teenage girls have greater control over their fertility today than they had in the past, and yet the percentage of births to unwed mothers continues to rise, having already increased from 30 percent among teenagers in 1970 to nearly 70 percent in 1990. In some cities in America 85 or 90 percent of all teenage births are to unwed mothers. Twenty-five percent of all babies born to teenagers are not first children. And the earlier a teenager begins her maternal career, the more children she is likely to have.

Teenage childbearing on this scale has monumental social consequences, both for the mothers and for their young children. In fact, if one wanted to spawn a generation of vulnerable families, one would seek to increase the number of families headed by fifteen- and sixteen-year-old mothers. A single teenage mother is less likely to complete high school or to be employed than her peers, and her child is at greater risk than other children for a host of health and developmental problems, and also for physical and sexual abuse. Both mother and child are likely to experience poverty and its predictable social consequence, chronic welfare dependency. If these risk factors for poverty are present—teenage childbearing, failure to complete high school, and nonmarriage—then it is all but inevitable that the mother and her child will live in poverty: 79 percent of all children born to mothers with those three risk factors are poor.

Exploitative Sex

Beyond these statistical measures researchers are beginning to piece together a portrait of teenage sexuality in the 1990s. There is still much to learn, but recent research tells us two things: first, fifteen-year-old sex is riskier than eighteen-year-old sex; and second, early-teenage sex is often exploitative sex. This evidence indicates that few young teenagers are ready or able to engage in kinder, gentler sex. In fact, sexual encounters between fifteen-year-olds are likely to be nasty, brutish, and short.

To begin with, there are sharp polarities in the way male and female teenagers approach sex. Despite changes in teenage sexual behavior, boys and girls continue to view love and sex relationships in different ways. Girls look for security, and boys seek adventure. Boys are after variety, and girls want intimacy. The classic formulation still seems to hold true: girls give sex in order to get love, and boys give love in order to get sex. According to one study, more than 60 percent of sexually experienced girls were going steady with or engaged to their first sexual partner, whereas less than 40 percent of teenage boys had their first sex with a steady or a fiancee. Boys were more than twice as likely as girls to have had their first intercourse with someone they had only recently met. As Freya Sonenstein, of the Urban Institute, and her colleagues report, "A typical picture of an adolescent male's year would be separate relationships with two partners, lasting a few months each."

Such gender polarities are most pronounced in early adolescence. Boys and girls both experience physical changes during puberty, but these changes carry different psychological meanings. For boys, increases in body weight and size bring an enhanced sense of power and dominance, whereas similar changes frequently provoke ambivalence and anxiety among girls. In a culture obsessed with skeletal thinness as a standard of female beauty and achievement, weight gain can inspire feelings of "grossness" and self-disgust among teenage girls. Carol Gilligan and other researchers have noted a decline in young adolescent girls' feelings of competence and confidence at roughly the same time that adolescent boys are becoming more assertive and, well, cocky.

The younger a girl is when she begins to have sex, the more vulnerable she is to its risks. She is less likely than an older teenager to be in a steady relationship, to plan her first intercourse, or to use contraception. Thus girls who were fifteen or younger at first intercourse are almost twice as likely as eighteen-year-olds to experience pregnancy within the first six months of sexual activity. Nor can it be said that a fifteen-year-old girl really chooses to engage in sex, given the enormous gap between physical readiness on the one hand, and emotional and cognitive readiness on the other. On this point Laurie Schwab Zabin, a researcher at Johns Hopkins University, writes, "Whether or not to engage in coitus, whether or not to contracept, whether or not to bear a child when faced with an unintended conception—are all decisions. Unfortunately, they are often not true 'choices.' " David Ellwood, the assistant secretary of Health and Human Services, puts it even more plainly: "There seems to be ample evidence to support almost any model of teenage behavior except a model of pure rational choice."

Girls who are sexually active at early ages are likely to experience coercive sex. Teenager girls tend to have first sex with male partners who are three or more years older, whereas teenage boys are likely to have their first sexual encounter with girls who are less than a year older. Thus the balance of power is dramatically skewed. Surely one has to be skeptical of claims of "voluntary" sex between girls and much older partners. As one researcher put it, "Could one possibly call the pairings of eleven-year-old girls and twenty-five-year-old men 'dates'?"

Indeed, age disparities between girls and their sexual partners are often markers for sexual abuse. In one study of abused teenage mothers and mothers-to-be, only 18 percent of the girls reported abuse by men near their age, while 46 percent reported abuse by men ten or more years older. Sexual abuse is a significant factor in girls' early sexualization. Studies show that teenage girls who have been sexually abused are significantly more likely to engage in voluntary sexual intercourse and are likely to have intercourse at an earlier age, to be more sexually active, and to engage in a wider range of sexual activities than girls who have not been abused.

Girls' sexual conduct, unlike that of boys, is governed less by hormones than by social controls. But in a cultural climate of sexual freedom, girls have lost much of their authority in boy-girl relationships. Until quite recently girls organized, managed, and regulated the social pursuits of their peer groups, with the strong support of adults. In romantic relationships girls exercised their power by withholding sex, keeping boys in the role of craven sexual petitioners. At the same time, they moved their boyfriends in the direction of commitment and monogamy. "Going steady," the ultimate romantic achievement for teenage girls, offered a pseudo-marriage that might include parceling out some of the sexual favors of marriage. Of course, this system was seriously flawed. In the intimacy of a steady relationship, girls could lose control, "give in," and go all the way. Then they had to deal with the dire consequences of their sexual transgression—a guilty conscience, a ruined reputation, and sometimes an unwanted pregnancy.

The sexual revolution overturned this system of social controls by giving women technological control over their fertility. Its emblematic moment came when college health services began providing birth-control pills to eighteen- and nineteen-year-old women. Liberated from many of the penalties of premarital sex and the burdens of a sexual double standard, women were able to behave like men in their sexual pursuits. Yet although a single standard for men and women promised greater honesty and equity in relationships, it tilted away from women's goals of intimacy and commitment in the direction of what one sociologist has aptly called sexual "freedom with a male bias": no holds barred and no strings attached. (A nosy mother, I once asked my college-age daughter if there were any differences in the way young men and women conducted their sex lives on campus. "Only that girls wait for a phone call the next day," she said.)

In the 1980s, with the advent of AIDS, the condom, an all-purpose contraceptive, gained new favor. As an appurtenance of the sexual culture, the condom led to a second shift in the control of sexuality: it brought back protection with a male bias. Although pressure to engage in early sex did not diminish, teenage girls' ability to protect themselves did. One of the great ironies of the new sexual revolution is that having won the "right" and the freedom to engage in sex at an early age, girls must resort to some of the old wiles and cajolery to get their male partners to use protection. Although girls may carry Trojans in their purse, as the Surgeon General urges, they cannot wear them.

The Lure of Motherhood

Recent thinking about unwed teenage pregnancy has focused on the links between teenage motherhood and the economic incentives of the welfare system. Charles Murray and others argue that poor teenagers choose motherhood because it offers economic rewards such as health care, day care, and an apartment of one's own. Yet some of the most compelling research on unwed childbearing among poor teenagers suggests that the strongest incentives for early teenage motherhood may be psychological rather than economic. As Judith Musick argues in her book *Young, Poor and Pregnant,* early pregnancy and childbearing must be understood as a response to the developmental demands of adolescence.

According to Musick, whose research is based on her work as a developmental psychologist and her six years as the director of the Ounce of Prevention Fund, a public-private venture that runs pregnancy-prevention and teenage-parent programs in Illinois, many of the girls most at risk for unwed motherhood grow up without adequate nurturance and protection. Some experience early and traumatic sexualization in households where they are left in the care of their mothers' boyfriends or other "play daddies." Thus the emotional lives of many of the most vulnerable girls are defined by "repeated experiences of personal harm at the hands of those who should be their protectors."

As these girls become teenagers, they bring limited inner resources to the key developmental task of adolescence: the formation of a stable identity. Whereas a more resilient teenager is ready to face the classic questions of adolescence—Who am I? and What will I do with my life? and How will I be different from my mother?—the fragile girl may still be wrestling with questions associated with an earlier developmental stage: Who cares about me? and Whom can I depend on? and Where can I find safety and security?

Through pregnancy and early childbearing a young woman finds a way to reconcile her contradictory needs for autonomy and security. She may be able to draw closer to her mother and to place a claim on maternal affection, albeit indirectly, through a grandchild. And she may even gain the fleeting attention of a wayward boyfriend or a faraway father. Thus early sexual activity and maternity offer a way to retrieve childhood and enter adulthood simultaneously.

The absence of empirical support for comprehensive sex education does not discomfit its advocates. They simply crank up their rhetoric: criticize sex education, they say, and you contribute to the death of teenagers from AIDS.

Not to be ignored in this developmental drama are the universal satisfactions of motherhood itself. If most new mothers are thrilled with their infants, why would young girls not feel a surge of ecstatic fulfillment? And if mothers everywhere enjoy dressing and showing off their newborns, why would a teenage mother not derive maternal pleasures from such activities? For a disadvantaged girl with few outlets to express herself, exhibit her talents, or win recognition, becoming a mother is a way to be fussed over and admired.

Reinforcing the immediate benefits of maternity are the psychological costs of postponing sex and motherhood. Within the peer group as well as the family, going to school and doing homework can be far less appealing than showing off a baby, particularly if a girl's older sisters and friends have babies of their own. Moreover, as Judith Musick explains, pursuing a dream that does not include early motherhood involves a painful and radical kind of split from mothers and other influential women in a girl's life. So threatening is this separation that many teenage girls on the threshold of change—enrolling in high-school-equivalency classes, completing a job-training program, breaking off with a violent boyfriend—fall back into an abusive relationship, get pregnant a second time, or go back to an old drug habit.

Thus changes in economic incentives, however politically attractive, may not be enough to reduce unwed teenage childbearing. It may be necessary to alter the psychological-incentive structure as well, including "prettifying" the unglamorous business of going to school, doing homework, and earning respectable grades. The process may also include fostering strong relationships with adult women mentors who can exercise firm guidance and give direction as well as support. Finally, it may require some imaginative measures to "uglify" unwed teenage motherhood or even to re-establish some of the disincentives that worked in the past, including separation of the girl from her peer group. Perhaps teenage mothers should attend special high schools, as they do in some cities, rather than mixing with the general high school population. This contemporary version of being "sent away"—though it would not interrupt education—would segregate teenage mothers from nonpregnant teenagers and perhaps change a peer culture that views schoolgirl pregnancy as an unobjectional, even enviable, event.

The Retreat from Adolescence

Adolescence is a modern social invention, designed to deal with a modern problem: the lengthening period between biological and social maturity. Earlier in the nation's history girls entered puberty and left school at about the same time—around age fifteen or sixteen. Although most young women waited another five or six years before marrying, they continued to live at home; teenager marriages were not common until the 1950s. By the beginning of this century, however, the age of menarche was declining and the period of formal schooling was lengthening. At the same time, parents, churches, and schools were relaxing their close supervision of young women. Many young people were living in cities, where the seductive attractions of the street, the saloon, and the dance hall replaced the more wholesome pastimes of rural life. Under these new social conditions youthful risk-taking became perilous, its penalties more severe.

As a social invention, therefore, adolescence represented a clear effort to define, order, and regulate a life stage that was becoming socially chaotic. Among other things, adolescence provided institutional reinforcement for the moratorium on youthful sexual activity, giving young people the opportunity to acquire the competencies and credentials of adulthood before they took on the responsibilities of marriage and parenthood.

In the past decade or so, however, a new way of thinking about teenage sexuality has emerged. It, too, recognizes the gap between biological and social maturity, but responds with a different set of controls. The new approach contends that teenagers should be expected to express themselves sexually as part of their normal growing up, but should be able to do so protected from the risks of early sexual activity. The way to protect teenagers is to give them the interpersonal skills and the technical tools to manage their own sexuality.

These competing traditions assign radically different responsibilities to adults. In the classic model, adults are the custodians of the moratorium. They secure and maintain this special life stage by establishing familial and institutional controls over teenage sexuality. Indeed, this approach requires some measure of sexual restraint, or at least discretion, on the part of adults in order to set an example. In the contemporary model, adults have a more limited responsibility. Their job is to train teenagers in the management of their own sexuality and to provide access to contraceptives. In the new technocracy adults are called upon to staff teenagers in their sexual pursuits while teenagers themselves are left to decide whether or not to engage in sex. Refusing sex, no less than having sex, becomes a matter of following individual dictates rather than following socially instituted and culturally enforced norms.

One can, of course, imagine a creative synthesis of the two models: a little more freedom for the kids, a little less supervision from the busy grown-ups. But this is not what has happened. In the past decade the technocratic approach has gained ground while the classic approach has steadily lost it. This has brought about a corresponding shift in adult responsibility. Increasingly the litmus test of adult concern is one of access: will grown-ups give teenagers the skills and tools to manage their sex lives? Seen in the broader historical context, two seemingly opposing responses to teenage sex—handing out condoms and teaching refusal skills—reflect the same trend toward technocratic solutions and diminished adult responsibility.

There has been a similar shift in public concerns. For most of this century the debate over youthful well-being covered a broad social terrain. The deliberations of the decennial White House Conference on Children, which began in 1909 and ended in the early 1970s, ranged widely from improving health and schooling to building character and citizenship. Today public ambitions and public concern for adolescents' well-being are narrower. Attention has turned to the task of managing the collapse of the moratorium. As a consequence, the entire public debate on the nation's youth has come down to a few questions. How do we keep boys from killing? How do we keep girls from having babies? How do we limit the social havoc caused by adolescent acting out?

There has been, as well, a shift in the notion of responsibility among health and school professionals. As an idea, adolescence is closely identified with the work of the American psychologist G. Stanley Hall. But it was a liberal reform coalition of school, health, and social-work professionals that took the idea of adolescence and translated it into a set of new institutions designed to protect vulnerable city youth from the burdens and responsibilities of too-early adulthood. The juvenile justice system, the youth center, and child-labor laws are all part of that institutional legacy. This coalition also fought hard for sex education in the schools. But today a similar liberal coalition is turning its back on that larger legacy.

The health and school establishments did not create the problems associated with teenage sex. Thus it is impossible not to view their response to these problems with a measure of sympathy. On the front lines of the new sexual revolution, overwhelmed by the clinical evidence of breakdown—thirteen-year-olds with gonorrhea, sixteen-year-olds giving birth for the third time—the youth-serving professionals respond with the tools of the clinic. At the same time, they seem to have lost sight of the meaning and purpose of adolescence and of their own historical role in creating and sustaining it.

Despite its confident assertions, comprehensive sex education implicitly acknowledges a lifting of the moratorium and a return to a more Darwinian sexual environment. What sex educators are offering now is training in sexual survival. Once the kids have been equipped with refusal skills, a bottle of body oil, and some condoms, "reality-based" advocates send them into the world to fend for themselves. Perhaps that is the best protection that today's school and health leaders are able to offer from a harsh and predacious sexual environment. But it is not realism. It is retreat.

FRAME the DEBATE

Form at end of book

Issue 8: What type of sex education program is most effective in preventing pregnancies and sexually transmitted diseases?

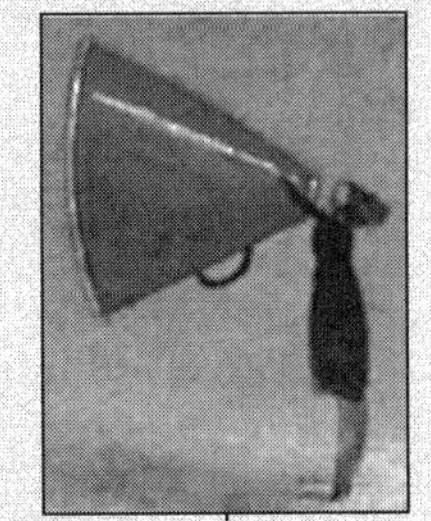

What's Wrong with Abstinence-Only Sexuality Education Programs?

Debra W. Haffner, M.P.H.

SIECUS President/CEO

SIECUS supports abstinence. I repeat, SIECUS supports abstinence. But SIECUS does not support teaching young people *only* about abstinence.

SIECUS's *Guidelines for Comprehensive Sexuality Education: Kindergarten—12th Grade* state that one of the four primary goals of comprehensive education is "to help young people exercise responsibility regarding sexual relationships, including addressing abstinence and [how] to resist pressures to become prematurely involved in sexual relationships."[1]

Abstinence is one of the 36 topics covered in the *Guidelines,* and messages about abstinence are included in age-appropriate sections. (See "What the SIECUS *Guidelines* Say about Sexual Abstinence" on page 114.)

SIECUS does ***not*** believe in abstinence-only approaches to sexuality education that have as "their exclusive purpose teaching the social, psychological, and health gains to be realized by abstaining from sexual activity."[2] (This is what the newly funded $50 million federal program will require grant recipients to teach American youth. See "Excerpts: *Draft Block Grant Guidance, Abstinence Education Provision of the 1996 Welfare Law,*" on page 8.*)

SIECUS does, however, support programs that are abstinence-based—such as *Proposing Sexual Involvement* and *Will Power, Won't Power*—that provide young people with clear messages about abstaining in the context of a broader, more comprehensive program. (See "Abstinence-Only Curricula *Without* the Fear" on page 22 for abstinence-based programs that are sound pedagogy for their target population.*)

*Does not appear in this publication.

Abstinence-only sexuality education is not effective. Proponents of such sexuality education make broad claims that sound exciting. They argue that if you tell young people to abstain from sexual intercourse, they will. These "just say no" programs promise to keep young people from developing "too serious" relationships, from being emotionally hurt, from experimenting with intimacy and sexual behaviors, and, of course, from getting pregnant and from contracting an STD or HIV.

There is no reason to believe that these claims are true. There are *no* published studies in the professional literature indicating that abstinence-only programs will result in young people delaying intercourse. In fact, a recent $5 million abstinence-only initiative in California not only did not increase the number of young people who abstained, but, in one school, actually resulted in more students having sexual intercourse after having participated in the course.[3] Proponents of abstinence-only fear-based programs often recite their own in-house evaluations as proof that these programs are effective. Yet, they have not published their evaluations in peer-reviewed literature and are not willing to make them available for review by outside researchers.

Comprehensive sexuality education is, on the other hand, an effective strategy for giving young people the skills to delay their involvement in sexual behaviors. Several reviews of published evaluations of sexuality education, HIV prevention, and teenage pregnancy prevention programs have consistently found that:

- sexuality education does not encourage teens to start having sexual intercourse or to increase their frequency of sexual intercourse.[4]
- programs must take place before young people begin experimenting with sexual behaviors if they are to result in a delay of sexual intercourse.[5]

What's Wrong with Abstinence-Only Sexuality Programs? Debra W. Haffner, SIECUS REPORT, April/May 1997. Reprinted by permission.

What the SIECUS Guidelines *Say about Sexual Abstinence*

Subconcept

Abstinence from sexual intercourse is the most effective method of preventing pregnancies and STD/HIV.

Developmental Messages

Level 2 (preadolescence, ages 9 through 12, later elementary schools)

- Intercourse is a pleasurable activity for most adults.
- Children are not ready for sexual intercourse.

Level 3 (early adolescence, ages 12 through 15; middle school/junior high school)

- Young teenagers are not mature enough for a sexual relationship that includes intercourse.
- Abstinence from sexual intercourse is the best method to prevent pregnancy and STD/HIV.
- Teenagers who date need to discuss sexual limits with their dating partner.
- People need to respect the sexual limits set by their partners.
- Teenagers in romantic relationships can express their feelings without engaging in sexual intercourse.
- There are many ways to give and receive sexual pleasure and not have intercourse.
- Teenagers considering sexual intercourse should talk to a parent or other trusted adult about their decisions, contraception, and disease prevention.
- Most adults believe school-age teenagers should not have sexual intercourse.
- Most religions teach that sexual intercourse should only occur in marriage.
- Abstinence from intercourse has benefits for teenagers.
- Teenagers who have had sexual intercourse can choose to be abstinent.

Level 4 (adolescence, ages 15 through 18; high school)

- Many American teenagers have had sexual intercourse and many have not.
- Sexual intercourse is not a way to achieve adulthood.
- Teenagers in romantic relationships can express their sexual feelings without engaging in sexual intercourse.
- Many adults experience periods of abstinence.

- teenagers who start having intercourse following a sexuality education program are more likely to use contraceptives than those who have not participated in a program.[6]
- HIV programs that use cognitive and behavioral skills training with adolescents demonstrate "consistently positive" results.[7]

Indeed, a recent World Health Organization review of 35 studies found that the programs most effective in changing young people's behavior are those that address abstinence, contraception, *and* STD prevention.[8] In addition, the National Institutes of Health's Consensus Panel on AIDS said in February 1997 that the abstinence-only approach to sexuality education "places policy in direct conflict with science and ignores overwhelming evidence that other programs [are] effective."[9]

Fear-based, abstinence-only programs also fail to address many of the antecedents of early first intercourse. Extensive research conducted during the past two decades has clearly delineated a portrait of a young person who begins intercourse prior to age 14.

Education programs cannot influence some of the factors such as early physical development, lower age of menarche or a higher testosterone level, older siblings, single-parent household environments, or mothers with lower educational attainment.

Sexuality education programs can, however, potentially address other factors such as young people's perception of their friends' and siblings' sexual behaviors, the timing of first dating, steady relationships, and beliefs about gender role stereotypes.

Other venues such as counseling and mentoring programs can address these other antecedents of early first intercourse: lower school performance, lower reading and writing skills, lack of parental support, lower church attendance, depression, and other problem behaviors, such as substance use (including alcohol and nicotine), and school delinquency.[10]

Federal Requirement #1:

The new welfare program requires that sexuality education classes in the United States teach that "abstinence from sexual activity outside marriage is the expected standard for all school-age children."

Although adults may very well want this as a standard, it is far from accurate in describing the reality of today's teenagers.

Almost all American adolescents engage in some type of sexual behavior. Although most policy debates about sexuality education have focused on sexual intercourse and its negative consequences, young people actually explore their sexuality from a much wider framework that includes dating, relationships, and intimacy.

The welfare reform legislation never even defines "sexual activity." Since the definition includes the word "activity" rather than "intercourse," one must assume that it is broader and includes a prohibition against other activities besides sexual intercourse. This is, however, never stated. For clarification, the Medical Institute for Sexual Health MISH defines *abstinence* as "avoiding sexual intercourse as well as any genital contact or genital stimulation."[11] Other fear-based curricula define it as any behaviors beyond hand holding and light kissing.[12]

The reality is that sexual behavior is almost universal among American adolescents. A majority of American teenagers date, over 85 percent have had a boyfriend or girlfriend and have kissed someone romantically, and nearly 80 percent have engaged in deep kissing.[13]

The majority of young people move from kissing to more intimate sexual behaviors during their teenage years. More than 50 percent engage in "petting behaviors." By the age of 14, more than 50 percent of all boys have touched a girl's breasts, and 25 percent have touched a girl's vulva. By the age of 18, more than 75 percent have engaged in heavy petting.[14] From 25 to 50 percent of teens report that they have experienced fellatio and/or cunnilingus.[15] A recent study found that of those teens who are virgins, nearly one third reported that they had engaged in heterosexual masturbation of or by a partner. One tenth of virgins had participated in oral sex, and one percent had participated in anal intercourse.[16]

More than half of American teenagers in schools have had sexual intercourse. The latest data from the Youth Risk Behavior Surveillance System of the U.S. Centers for Disease Control and Prevention found that 54 percent of high school students had sexual intercourse, a rate virtually unchanged since the study began in 1990.[17] By the time they reach the age of 20, 80 percent of boys and 76 percent of girls have had sexual intercourse.[18]

At each stage of adolescence, higher proportions of boys and girls have had sexual intercourse today than 20 years ago. The largest increase occurred between 1971 and 1979. The increase was modest in the 1980s. It appeared to level off in the 1990s.[19] It is important to note, however, that these trends started much earlier than the 1970s. In fact, the modal age for first intercourse was 17 for men and 18 for women in the 1950s and 1960s. It was 16 for men and nearly 17 for women in the 1970s and 1980s. This is a one-year change over a 40-year span.[20]

Federal Requirement #2:

The new federal program also requires that grantees teach that "abstinence from sexual activity is the only certain way to avoid out-of-wedlock pregnancy, sexually transmitted diseases, and other associated health problems."

On the surface, it is hard to argue with this statement. The SIECUS *Guidelines* themselves state that "abstinence from sexual intercourse is the most effective method of preventing pregnancies and STDS/HIV." Yet, after learning that abstinence is the "only certain way" to avoid pregnancy and STDS/HIV, young people may get the impression that contraception and condoms are not effective. In fact, many of the fear-based approaches to sexuality education discuss methods of contraception only in terms of their failure rates.[21] Indeed, professionals who work directly with adolescents in schools and clinics can attest that adolescents vows of abstinence fail far more than condoms do.

Messages that contraception and condoms are not effective could, unfortunately, reverse the significant strides that American youth have made toward having safer sex during the past two decades. Consider these statistics:

- In 1979, fewer than 50 percent of adolescents used a contraceptive at first intercourse.
- In 1988, more than 65 percent used them.
- By 1990, more than 70 percent used them.[22]

Teenagers who receive contraceptive education in the same year that they become sexually active are 70 to 80 percent more likely to use contraceptive methods (including condoms) and more than twice as likely to use the pill.[23]

It is vitally important that programs encourage young people who engage in intercourse to use contraception and condoms. According to the National Institutes of Health, "although sexual abstinence is a desirable objective, programs must include instruction in safe sex behavior, including condom use."[24]

Federal Requirement #3:

The new abstinence-only programs must also teach that "a mutually faithful monogamous relationship in the context of marriage is the expected standard of human sexual activity."

This "information" is clearly not true in American culture. The fact is that the vast majority of Americans begin having sexual relationships (including sexual intercourse) as teenagers. Fewer than 7 percent of men and 20 percent of women aged 18 to 59 were virgins when they were married.[25] Only 10 percent of adult men and 22 percent of adult women report that their first sexual experience was with their spouse, many of whom had their first intercourse when they were engaged prior to marriage.[26] Indeed, this "norm" was probably never true: a third of all Pilgrim brides were pregnant when they were married.[27]

There are currently more than 74 million American adults who are classified as single because they have delayed marriage, decided to remain single, are divorced, or have entered into a gay or lesbian partnership. More than three quarters of these men and two thirds of these women have had sex with a partner in the past 12 months.[28] Most of them would take offense at this new "standard of human behavior." Under this new program's definition, schools will teach young people that these adults must remain celibate throughout their lives.

The concept of chastity until marriage may have made more sense a hundred years ago when teenagers reached puberty in their middle teens. For them, marriage and other adult responsibilities closely followed. Today's young people are different: They reach puberty earlier, they have intercourse earlier, and they marry in their middle twenties. In fact, women and men marry several years later today than they did in the 1950s. The current mean age for first marriage is 26.7 years old for men and 24.5 years old for women.[29]

Federal Requirement #4:

The new federal programs must also teach that "sexual activity outside of marriage is likely to have harmful psychological and physical effects."

There is no sound public health data to support this statement. It is certainly true that sexual relations can lead to unplanned pregnancies, STDS, and HIV. It is also true that intimate relationships can be harmful for some people. But the reality is that the majority of people have had sexual relationships prior to marriage with no negative repercussions. For example, one study reports that when premarital sexual intercourse is satisfying, it has a positive effect on relationships for both males and females.[30] The largest study of adult sexual behavior found that more than 90 percent of men and more than 70 percent of women recall that they wanted their first intercourse to happen when it did; only 6.9 percent of men and 21 percent of women had first intercourse on their wedding night.[31]

Consensus Statement

The National Commission on Adolescent Sexual Health recognizes that adolescent sexuality is a highly charged emotional issue for many adults. It urges, however, that policymakers recognize that sexual development is an essential part of adolescence and that the majority of adolescents engage in sexual behaviors as part of their overall development.

More than 50 national organizations have endorsed the Commission's consensus statement that says "society should encourage adolescents to delay sexual behaviors until they are ready physically, cognitively, and emotionally for mature sexual relationships and their consequences."

These organizations urge, however, that "society must also recognize that a majority of adolescents will become involved in sexual relationships during their teenage years. Adolescents should receive support and education for developing the skills to evaluate their readiness for mature sexual relationships."[32]

The reality is that the majority of American adults believe that young people need to be told more than "just say no." Although 60 percent believe that premarital sexual relations for teenagers is always wrong,[33] more than three-quarters of adults also believe that teenagers need information and access to contraceptive services and STD prevention information.[34] Abstinence-only programs, which include misinformation about sexual behaviors and promote fear and shame, are unlikely to prove effective.

If Congress and the states are serious about helping young people delay sexual behaviors and grow into healthy, responsible adults, they will support a comprehensive approach to sexuality education that has a proven track record in accomplishing these goals.

References

1. National Guidelines Task Force, *Guidelines for Comprehensive Sexuality Education, Kindergarten—12th Grade* (New York: Sexuality Information and Education Council of the United States, 1991).
2. *Congressional Record*/U.S. Senate, Sept. 15, 1995, pp. 513647–9.
3. D. Kirby, M. Korpi, R. P. Barth, and H. H. Cagampang, *Evaluation of Education Now and Babies Later (ENABL): Final Report* (Berkeley, CA: University of California, School of Social Welfare, Family Welfare Research Group, 1995).
4. J. J. Frost and J. D. Forrest, "Understanding the Impact of Effective Teenage Pregnancy Prevention Programs," *Family Planning Perspectives,* 27:5 (1995): 188–96; D. Kirby et al., "School-based Programs to Reduce Sexual Risk Behaviors: A Review of Effectiveness," *Public Health Reports,* 190:3 (1997): 339–60; A. Grunseit and S. Kippax, *Effects of Sex Education on Young People's Sexual Behavior* (Geneva: World Health Organization, 1993).
5. D. Kirby et al., "School-Based Programs," 339–60.
6. A. Grunseit and S. Kippax, *Effects of Sex Education,* 339–60.
7. J. J. Frost and J. D. Forrest, "Understanding Prevention Programs."
8. A. Grunseit and S. Kippax, *Effects of Sex Education.*
9. National Institutes of Health, *Consensus Development Conference Statement,* Feb. 11–13, 1997.

10. K. A. Moore, B. C. Miller, D. Glei, and D. R. Morrison, *Adolescent Sex, Contraception, and Childbearing: A Review of Recent Research,* (Washington, DC, Child Trends, Inc., 1995).
11. *National Guidelines for Sexuality and Character Education* (Texas: Medical Institute for Sexual Health, 1996), p. 7.
12. L. Kantor, "Scared Chaste? Fear-based Educational Curricula," *SIECUS Report,* 21:2 (1992): 1–15.
13. R. Coles and F. Stokes, *Sex and the American Teenager* (New York: Harper and Row, 1985) and Roper Starch Worldwide, *Teens Talk About Sex: Adolescent Sexuality in the 90s* (New York: Sexuality Information and Education Council of the United States, 1994).
14. Ibid.
15. S. Newcomer and J. Udry, "Oral Sex in An Adolescent Population," *Archives of Sexual Behavior,* 14 (1985): 41–6.
16. M. A. Schuster, R. M. Bell, D. E. Kanouse, "The Sexual Practices of Adolescent Virgins: Genital Sexual Activities of High School Students Who Have Never Had Vaginal Intercourse," *American Journal of Public Health* (November 1996) 86:11, 1570–76.
17. *Morbidity and Mortality Weekly Report,* Sept. 27, 1996, 45: SS–4; YRBS, 1990.
18. Alan Guttmacher Institute, *Sex and America's Teenagers* (New York: The Alan Guttmacher Institute, 1994).
19. Ibid.
20. E. Laumann et al., *The Social Organization of Sexuality—Sexual Practices in the United States* (Chicago: The University of Chicago Press, 1994).
21. L. Kantor, "Scared Chaste? Fear-Based Educational Curricula."
22. D. Haffner, editor, *Facing Facts: Sexual Health for America's Adolescents* (New York: Sexuality Information and Education Council of the United States, 1994).
23. J. Mauldon and K. Luker, "The Effects of Contraceptive Education on Method Use at First Intercourse," *Family Planning Perspectives,* 28:1 (1996): 19.
24. National Institutes of Health, *Consensus Development Conference Statement,* Feb. 11–13, 1997.
25. E. Laumann et al., *The Social Organization of Sexuality.*
26. Ibid.
27. J. D'Emilio and E. Freedman, *Intimate Matters: A History of Sexuality in America* (New York: Harper and Row, 1988).
28. E. Laumann et al., *The Social Organization of Sexuality.*
29. U.S. Census Bureau, *Marital Status and Living Arrangements,* March 1994.
30. Rodney M. Cate, Edgar Long, Jeffrey J. Angera, and Kristen Draper, "Sexual Intercourse and Relationship Development," *Family Relations,* April 1993, p. 162.
31. E. Laumann et al., *The Social Organization of Sexuality.*
32. D. Haffner, editor, *Facing Facts.*
33. E. Laumann et al., *The Social Organization of Sexuality.*
34. Gallup Poll, "Attitudes Toward Contraceptives," March 1985.

FRAME the DEBATE

Form at end of book

WiseGuide Wrap-Up

Today's teens face AIDS/HIV, chlamydia, herpes, syphilis, gonorrhea, human papillomavirus, and a variety of other sexually transmitted diseases. In addition, the rates of unplanned and unwanted pregnancies have escalated to all-time highs. While no one wishes to see children subjected to these risks and problems, gaining consensus on how to best approach prevention and sex education is perhaps the single greatest hurdle for health educators to overcome.

Sex education programs are most often categorized as abstinence-based programs or comprehensive contraception-based programs. Both include aspects of risk reduction, behavior modification, and choice making. They differ in their primary message and core values. While contraception-based programs strive to be relatively value-free, abstinence-based programs are generally centered on a strong core of values or dogmas. Measuring the outcomes of these differing types of programs has two serious problems. The first problem is lack of agreement as to what constitutes an abstinence- or contraception-based program. The second problem involves what constitutes "success"—pregnancy rates, sexually transmitted disease rates, or self-report data regarding behavioral choices such as remaining celibate or monogamous.

R.E.A.L. Sites

This list provides a print preview of typical **Coursewise** R.E.A.L. sites. (There are over 100 such sites at the **Courselinks**™ site.) The danger in printing URLs is that web sites can change overnight. As we went to press, these sites were functional using the URLs provided. If you come across one that isn't, please let us know via email to: webmaster@coursewise.com. Use your Passport to access the most current list of R.E.A.L. sites at the **Courselinks** site.

Site name: SIECUS Believes

URL: http://www.siecus.org/about/abou0002.html

Why is it R.E.A.L.? This site offers a variety of information regarding human sexuality and sexuality education. Members of SIECUS are generally in favor of comprehensive informational programs and the right of the individual to make choices concerning their sexuality. SIECUS states, "All people have the right to comprehensive sexuality education that addresses the biological, sociocultural, psychological, and spiritual dimensions of sexuality from the cognitive domain (information), the affective domain (feelings, values, and attitudes), and the behavioral domain (communication and decision-making skills)."

Key topics: sex, sex education, abstinence, contraception

Try this: Read the "SIECUS Believes" page of policy statements regarding human sexuality and education. Select one policy statement described by SIECUS (for example, on sex education, school-based sex education, sexuality and religion, sexuality and the media, sexual orientation, etc.). Find an opposing viewpoint from another web site. Compare both policy statements, and organize a list of points and counterpoints for each side. Compare how well SIECUS and your selected site support their position statements with factual information, provable statements, ethical standards, emotional appeals, and spiritual beliefs.

Site name: The Sinclair Intimacy Institute's Online Encyclopedia of Sex

URL: http://www.sexualitydata.com

Why is it R.E.A.L.? This site is an electronic encyclopedia of sexuality-related information. It represents an effort to provide easily accessed and comprehensive sexual information.

Key topics: sexuality, sex education

Try this: Visit this site with several sexuality questions in mind. After reading the responses to your queries, evaluate the site in terms of the accuracy of information and biases. What impact does this type of site have on adolescent sex education? Can the free distribution of the sexually related information found at this site help or harm efforts to control the rising rates of adolescent sexually transmitted diseases and unwanted pregnancies?

Site name: A Case for Abstinence Education

URL: http://www.family.org/cforum/hotissues/A0000990.html

Why is it R.E.A.L.? This site is owned and operated by conservative columnist and radio host, Dr. James Dobson. This particular page ("A Case for Abstinence Education") features an article that criticizes SIECUS and Planned Parenthood for their efforts to have comprehensive sex education programs widely accepted in schools. The author, Peter Brandt, states, "In the final analysis, the primary driving force of the safe-sex ideology is sexual freedom for teens, not adolescent health." Links to other pages describe Focus on the Family's positions on the effectiveness of abstinence-based programs.

Key topics: abstinence, contraception, SIECUS, sex, sex education

Try this: Read "A Case for Abstinence Education," and visit the links: "Title V: The Most Outrageous List" and "Frequently Asked Questions about Title V." How well do the authors of these papers support their positions? What persuasion techniques (emotional appeals, moral high ground, factual information and statistics, etc.) do they use most often? How do you feel this site contrasts with the SIECUS site in terms of persuading individuals to make positive health decisions regarding their sexuality? Identify and describe three points on which you base your opinion.

Section 4 Summary

In the field of health education, no other topical area is surrounded by as much controversy as sex education. The topics of reproduction, sex, and human sexuality are laden with values and cultural dogma. Sex education may well be the one arena in which the importance of a multidimensional approach to health becomes paramount. Sex education requires the educator and the learner to examine their core values, their spiritual beliefs, the influences of family and community, and the influence of perceived and real cultural norms. Sexuality challenges the health educator to take a multidimensional approach to complex health content.

STAND! section 5

Drugs and Alcohol

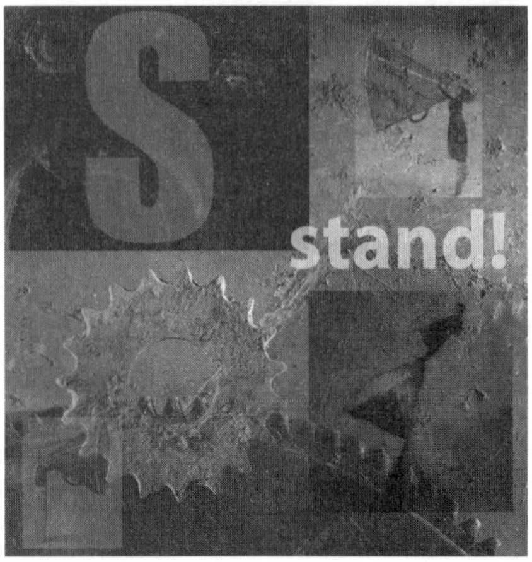

Learning Objectives

- Separate fact from hyperbole regarding the healthfulness of caffeine consumption.
- Examine the limits of the law in preventing drug-related birth defects and alcohol-related automobile accidents.
- Challenge contemporary knowledge regarding the nature of addiction.

Introduction

It often seems that substance abuse is as much a defining element of American culture as baseball, apple pie, and the family car. We are led to believe that drinking the right brand of beer can bring us untold happiness, romance, and sports aptitudes, that smoking the right brand of cigarettes can provide women with slim figures and sophistication, and men with masculinity and an unmatched freedom of spirit. Health, we are told, results from swallowing the right mixture of food supplement tablets and taking the right prescriptions for every human ailment. We like to think that every illness and ailment—whether physical or psychological, from cancer to depression—can be cured by taking licit or illicit drugs. For some Americans, drug taking is a part of their everyday life; for others, drug taking controls their lives.

At least 76 million Americans come from families where alcoholism is present, according to the U.S. Department of Health and Human Services. Despite all the health warnings, more than 61 million Americans still smoke cigarettes, 10 million smoke marijuana, and 7 million use smokeless tobacco. Drunk driving accounts for over 41,907 deaths every year. Clearly, we are a drug-taking culture, and drug abuse and alcoholism are major national health concerns.

The readings in this section examine and question contemporary knowledge regarding drug-taking behaviors most likely to affect Americans.

Caffeine: Harmless Drug or Serious Health Concern?

ISSUE 9

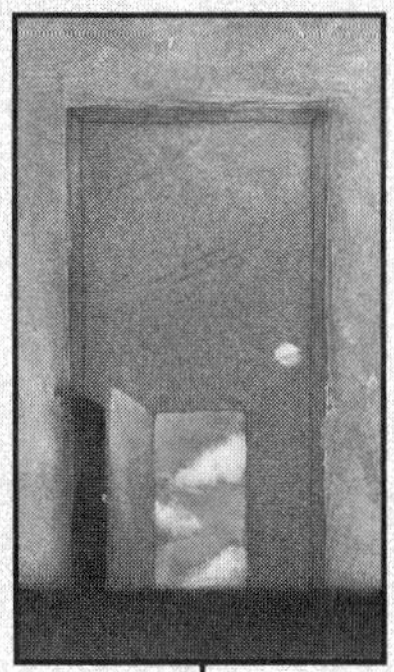

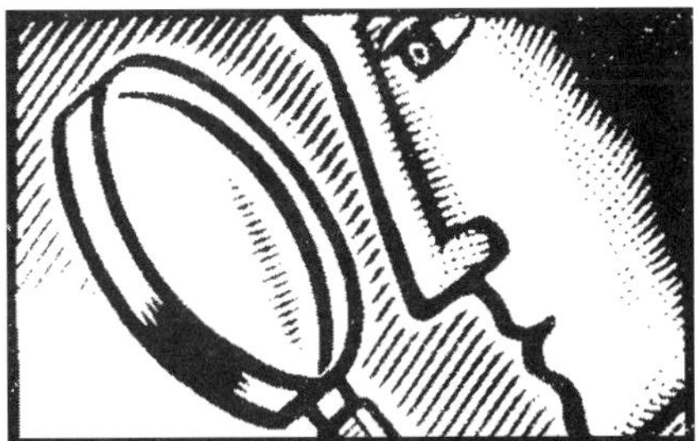

Take a Closer Look

1. In what way is caffeine purportedly related to osteoporosis?
2. What did the University of California 1994 study of women and osteoporosis find regarding caffeine consumption?
3. What did the research at Johns Hopkins University reveal regarding caffeine vs. placebo testing on mental alertness?
4. List at least three side effects of caffeine consumption identified in Reading 23.
5. What are at least four specific health risks that Reading 23 associates with caffeine consumption?
6. What is the mechanism by which caffeine exerts its mental stimulatory effects?
7. What does the *Nutrition Action Health Letter* suggest to lessen the calcium loss from consuming caffeine?
8. What was the primary finding of the Harvard School of Public Health with regard to caffeine consumption?
9. What other nondiet-related recommendations does Michael Lasalandra make in Reading 25 regarding colon cancer reduction?

WiseGuide Intro

Caffeine is likely the world's most popular stimulant. Nearly all adult Americans and many children regularly consume beverages containing caffeine. Coffee is the most popular caffeinated beverage, followed by colas and teas. In the past decade, espresso drinks, coffee houses, and espresso stands have emerged in nearly every community, particularly college towns.

Caffeine belongs to a group of natural stimulants called xanthines. The main effects of caffeine are central nervous system stimulation, elevation of the heart rate and blood pressure, cerebral vasoconstriction, and mild analgesia. In small doses, caffeine increases alertness and concentration; in large doses, however, it may cause heart palpitations, insomnia, depression, nervousness, stress symptoms, and reduced concentration. Caffeine is addictive. Tolerance develops with repeated use, and measurable withdrawal symptoms mark cessation of use. Although caffeine is usually benign and its stimulant properties mild, health-conscious people are becoming increasingly concerned about their caffeine consumption and its possible link to a variety of health detriments.

Reading 22, "Caffeine: Not So Bad for Your Bones after All," primarily reviews the research conducted at Penn State University on the effects of caffeine on bone density and calcium loss in women who drank coffee. The conclusions are discussed and contrasted with findings of researchers from Tufts University and the University of California.

Reading 23, "What Caffeine Can Do for You—and to You," reviews several of the main effects of caffeine consumption, confirms caffeine's addictive nature, and warns about the potential consequences of overconsumption of caffeine and its interaction with other drugs. The reading also examines the health risks of hypertension, heart palpitations, abnormal pregnancy, osteoporosis, and gastrointestinal problems associated with overconsumption of caffeine and offers some final advice regarding moderation.

Reading 24, "Caffeine: The Inside Scoop," briefly outlines the main effects of caffeine consumption and addresses some of the common health concerns regarding overconsumption of caffeine.

In recent years, coffee has been blamed for a variety of health detriments, including cancer. In Reading 25, "Study Finds Coffee May Help Battle Colon Cancer," Michael Lasalandra reviews the recent research out of the Harvard School of Public Health, which indicates a 24 percent drop in colorectal cancer rates among subjects who drank four or more cups of coffee per day. Lasalandra also lists several other health behaviors that may lower colorectal cancer risk and provides specific dietary advice.

READING 22

Issue 9: Is caffeine a harmless drug or a serious health concern?

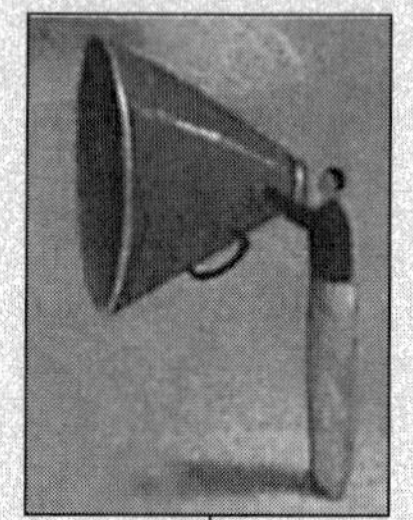

Caffeine:
Not So Bad for Your Bones after All

Although some studies have suggested that quaffing too many caffeinated beverages may weaken your bones, scientists at Pennsylvania State University now say it isn't so. The theory has been that since caffeine causes a small amount of calcium to be excreted in the urine, bone density might suffer from a long-term drain caused by several daily cups of java. Some research has suggested not just a connection between caffeine consumption and lower bone density but also an increased risk of fractures in older women. But it's difficult to tell whether those differences were due to caffeine per se or to other factors, such as smoking, body weight, lack of exercise and calcium intake.

In an attempt to clear up the confusion, the researchers at Penn State divided some 140 women ages 55 to 70 according to their caffeine consumption: low (up to two 6-ounce cups of coffee a day); medium (three to four cups); or high (five or more cups). They even measured the exact amounts of caffeine in each woman's coffee cup, sending samples off to a lab for analysis. But when age, weight, exercise, and estrogen replacement were factored in, the researchers couldn't find any change in bone density measurements related to caffeine intake.

Is this study the last word? Susan Harris, DSc, a researcher at Tufts who, has studied caffeine and bone loss, cautions that the researchers at Penn State studied *current* caffeine intake as it relates to *current* bone density. "It's better to look at caffeine intake over a period of years and compare that to changes in bone mass over the same period."

That's closer to what scientists at the University of California did back in 1994, when they linked lifetime coffee drinking with weaker spine and hip bones after questioning nearly 1,000 post-menopausal women. But the researchers also found that those women who drank a cup of milk every day throughout their adult lives—regardless of how much coffee they drank—had denser bones.

In fact, if you're meeting the current recommendations to consumer 1,000 to 1,500 milligrams of calcium a day, it looks as if coffee drinking is a moot point. Says Dr. Harris, "Any effect of caffeine is minor when compared to other risk factors for osteoporosis, like smoking, but caffeine becomes even less important if calcium intake is high enough."

FRAME the DEBATE

Form at end of book

Issue 9: Is caffeine a harmless drug or a serious health concern?

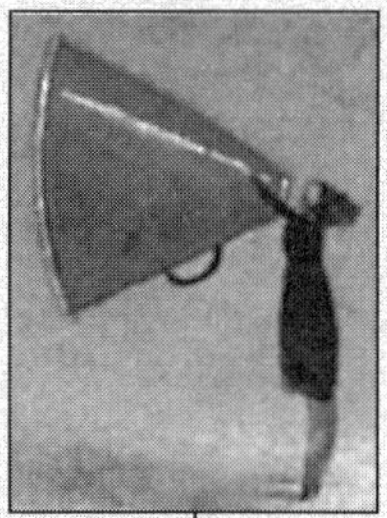

What Caffeine Can Do for You—and to You

It's America's favorite drug. Should you just say no?

Surge. Jolt. Aqua Buzz. Krank$_2$0. XTC. They sound like nicknames for underground drugs. Actually, they're brand names for soda, bottled water, and juice laced with caffeine. And the names aren't just hype: Caffeine is a mild stimulant that can fight fatigue, improve mood, and boost mental and physical performance.

Like any drug, caffeine has its drawbacks. For one thing, it's a potentially addictive drug, as the makers of caffeine-spiked drinks undoubtedly know. Miss your daily fix—whether it's from the "natural" caffeine in coffee and tea or the added caffeine in various foods, drinks, and drugs—and you may experience withdrawal symptoms. Consume *more* caffeine than you're used to, on the other hand, and you may experience "caffeine intoxication," marked by jittery nerves and insomnia. And the drug can cause or worsen various physical or emotional problems in certain individuals.

For most people, however, caffeine is relatively harmless—and can even be beneficial. Here's a rundown on the benefits and risks of caffeine.

A Stimulating Brew

Caffeine stimulates the central nervous system. That can lead to a variety of changes, many of them positive.

Mood

Coffee "quickeneth the spirits" and "maketh the heart lightsom," according to a seventeenth-century pitch for the brew—and modern science is confirming those claims. In one study, for example, researchers at Johns Hopkins University gave nine coffee drinkers a pill containing either caffeine or a placebo on each of 40 consecutive days. The volunteers, who didn't know which pill they were receiving on which day, reported feeling more awake, energetic, eager to work, confident, and friendly when they got the caffeine rather than the dummy pill. (That difference was not attributable to withdrawal symptoms on the placebo days.)

Mental Performance

Caffeine fights drowsiness, fatigue, and boredom. Studies have shown that as little as 32 mg of caffeine—the amount in one-third of a cup of brewed coffee—helps people pay attention to a long, repetitious series of tones or images and detect subtle, infrequent changes in the pattern. So caffeine can boost performance on monotonous tasks like typing, filing, or simple bookkeeping, and can help you stay alert during prolonged tasks like driving. If you're tired, caffeine can also sharpen moderately complex mental skills, such as recognizing words and manipulating numbers.

Physical Performance

Caffeine fights muscular fatigue, possibly by making the muscles' long-term fuel stores last longer. That effect can prolong the ability to exercise or perform lengthy physical tasks such as gardening or house cleaning. Some evidence suggests that caffeine may also speed the use of the muscles' short-term fuel stores, intensify muscle contractions, and mask the discomfort of vigorous exertion. Whatever the reason, the drug does boost performance of brief, intense activities like sprinting. (But see the warning below under "Health Risks" for people with hypertension.)

Caffeine Overload

While caffeine in moderation can clearly improve mood and performance, excessive doses can overstimulate the nerves, making the user feel restless, anxious, and irritable, making the hands tremble, and making it difficult to sleep. Too much caffeine can also cause facial flushing, diarrhea, and copious urination. The amount needed to trigger those effects depends on how sensitive you are to the drug as well as how much you regularly consume. Some individuals who rarely use caffeine experience symptoms after a single cup of coffee; even habitual users can become jumpy if they consume more than usual.

Giving up cigarettes can also cause caffeine overload, because certain compounds in the smoke speed up the body's disposal of caffeine. When a person stops smoking, blood levels of caffeine can increase up to 50 percent. So coffee drinkers who are trying to quit smoking may want to cut down on their coffee consumption before they stop smoking.

Caffeine Dependency

It doesn't take much to develop a dependency on the drug. In one study, fully half of the volunteers who ordinarily drank just one to three cups of coffee a day developed headaches, the main symptom of caffeine withdrawal, when they temporarily quit the brew. About 10 percent became depressed, anxious, or fatigued, and some complained of flu-like symptoms, nausea, and even vomiting; some felt sick enough to call their physician.

In general, the symptoms appear 12 to 24 hours after the last dose of the drug, peak on the second day, and persist for as long as a week (unless you take another dose of caffeine to stop the symptoms). That means that some people apparently experience early withdrawal symptoms every morning, before their first cup of coffee—and may experience full-blown symptoms if they miss that cup. Some people may also develop symptoms on weekends, simply because they sleep late or drink less coffee when they're not on their weekday work schedule.

Coffee is not the only substance that can leave you vulnerable to caffeine withdrawal. Two to four cans of caffeinated soda or two to four cups of tea can provide as much caffeine as a cup or two of regular coffee—enough to provoke symptoms if you skip the beverage for as little as half a day. Taking a caffeine-containing medication for more than a few days could also create dependency, triggering a reaction when you eventually go off the drug. (The American Medical Association and the Center for Science in the Public Interest have urged the U.S. Food and Drug Administration to require manufacturers to list the amount of caffeine in all foods and beverages. Meanwhile, see the table for the caffeine content of various foods and drinks, and the table on page 125 for caffeine in medications.)

Drug Interactions

Various drugs—including birth-control pills, the heart drug verapamil (*Calan, Verelan*), and the ulcer or heartburn drug cimetidine (*Tagamet*)—can hamper the body's ability to dispose of caffeine. So in people who take those drugs, even low doses of caffeine may trigger insomnia, irritability, or palpitations. Medications that stimulate the nervous system—including certain appetite suppressants, asthma drugs, thyroid hormones, and oral decongestants—also add to caffeine's jolt, with the same effects.

Similarly, caffeine decreases the sedative effect of benzodiazepine tranquilizers such as diazepam (*Valium*). And it can cause severe hypertension or abnormal heart rhythms in people taking an antidepressant monoamine oxidase (MAO) inhibitor, such as *Marplan, Nardil,* or *Parnate.* (For more on caffeine and drug interactions, see our December 1996 issue.)*

Health Risks—for Some

Over the past few decades, isolated studies have suggested that caffeine might increase the risk of cancer, coronary heart disease, fibrocystic breast disease, and other disorders. But more recent research has refuted most of those possibilities and demonstrated that caffeine actually poses significant health risks only in certain susceptible people. Here are the possible dangers:

- **Hypertension.** An unaccustomed dose of caffeine can raise blood-pressure levels temporarily; but while that might skew the results of a single blood-pressure reading, it wouldn't affect your health, even if you have hypertension. However, ingesting even normal doses of the drug before exercise or during stressful periods can accentuate the usual blood-pressure response to those occasions, and that could be dangerous in people with hypertension.
- **Abnormal heart rhythms.** People who consume caffeine in moderation generally do not run an increased risk of abnormal heart rhythms. Still, people who experience palpitations—a racing, pounding, or irregular heart beat—should try avoiding caffeine to see whether that helps.
- **Birth and pregnancy problems.** Some research suggests that women who regularly consume more than 300 mg of caffeine a day, the amount in roughly three cups of coffee, may reduce their chances of becoming pregnant and increase their chances of having a miscarriage or delivering an underweight baby. In addition, heavy caffeine consumption during pregnancy can overstimulate the fetus, causing abnormal heart rhythms before birth or jittery behavior right after birth. Heavy consumption may also push enough caffeine into the breast milk to make some breast-fed babies jittery. To be on the safe side, women who are either pregnant, trying to get pregnant, or breast feeding should restrict their caffeine or avoid the drug altogether.

*Refers to the December 1996 issue of *Consumer Reports on Health.*

Caffeine in Drinks and Chocolate

Food Item	Caffeine (mg)
Beverages	
Coffee	
Espresso, 2 oz	120
Regular, brewed, 6 oz	103
Instant, 6 oz	57
Instant, decaf. 6 oz	2
Tea	
Black, 6 oz[1]	53
Oolong, 6 oz[1]	36
Green, 6 oz[1]	32
Iced tea, instant, 12 oz	46
Soft drinks, 12 oz[2]	
Jolt Cola	72
Nehi Maxxvm Cola	70
Sundrop	63
Kick	58
Mountain Dew	55
Mello Yello, Surge	53
Coca-Cola Classic	47
Royal Crown Cola	43
Mr. PiBB, Dr. Pepper, Sunkist Sparkling Lemonade	41
Sunkist Orange	40
Squirt Ruby Red	39
Pepsi	37
A&W Cream Soda	28
Barq's	23
Slice Cola	11
Water, caffeine enhanced, 12 oz	
Java Water	71
Krank$_2$O	70
Water Joe	46
Aqua Java	43
Juice drinks, caffeine enhanced, 12 oz	
Java Juice	90
XTC	70
Chocolate	
Baking chocolate, unsweetened, 1 oz	58
Hershey Special Dark chocolate bar, 1.45 oz	31
Other milk chocolate candy bars, average, 1.55 oz	11

[1]Brewed in bag for three minutes.

[2]Diet sodas have roughly the same caffeine content as regular versions.

Caffeine in Medications[1]

Drug Class	Caffeine (mg)
Analgesics	
Actamin Super, Aspirin-Free Excedrin, Excedrin Extra Strength	65
Goody's Headache Powders, Supac, Vanquish	33
Anacin, Anacin Maximum Strength, Buffets II, Cope, Gelpirin, Gensan, P-A-C Revised Formula, Rid-A-Pain Compound	32
Cold Combinations	
Kolephrin, Kolephrin/DM	65
Fendol	32
Histosal	30
Stimulants	
Caffedrine, Keep Alert, NoDoz Maximum Strength, Ultra Pep-Back, Vivarin	200
Quick Pep	150
NoDoz, Pep-Back	100
Enerjets	75
Analgesics	
Cafergot, Ercaf, Ergo-Caff, Gotamine, Wigraine	100
Amaphen, Femcet, Fioricet, Fiorinal with Codeine No. 3, Idenal with Codeine, Medigesic, Pharmagesic, Two-Dyne	40
Synalgos-DC	30
Cold Combinations	
Citra Forte, Hycomine Compound	30
Muscle Relaxants	
Norgesic Forte, Norphadrine Forte, N3 Gesic Forte, Orphenagesic Forte	60
Norgesic, Norphadrine, N3 Gesic, Orphenagesic	30

[1]Table includes only those medications that contain 30 mg of caffeine or more per tablet. All drugs except the stimulants contain active ingredients in addition to caffeine.

- **Osteoporosis.** While caffeine tends to leach small amounts of calcium from the bones, that effect generally does not cause significant bone loss in people who consume adequate amounts of calcium. But the caffeine in as little as two cups of coffee a day may indeed cause noticeable bone loss in postmenopausal women who have a low intake of calcium—less than 800 mg per day, roughly half the recommended daily amount of 1500 mg; and those women are already at increased risk for developing osteoporosis, or fragile bones. Even if they do get enough calcium, postmenopausal women who have other risk factors for osteoporosis—such as a family history of the disease, early menopause, cigarette smoking, and being thin or inactive—may want to play it safe and avoid large doses of caffeine.
- **Ulcers and heartburn.** Consuming coffee or soda—even varieties that contain no caffeine—tends to stimulate the secretion of gastric acid, which can trigger heartburn in some people and aggravate an existing stomach ulcer. Caffeinated versions of those beverages may increase gastric-acid secretion somewhat more.
- **Anxiety and panic attacks.** Some evidence suggests that people who suffer from anxiety problems tend to feel better when they avoid caffeine. Large doses of the drug can trigger panic attacks in some people.

Finally, caffeine may worsen several other, typically less-serious problems: insomnia and incontinence, and possibly hot flashes during menopause, emotional distress before menstruation, and tinnitus, or ringing in the ears.

Summing Up

Caffeine can sharpen thinking (when you're tired), boost alertness, and improve physical speed and endurance. But caffeine can also cause overstimulation, interact with other drugs, and, if you abruptly stop taking it, trigger withdrawal symptoms. Most people can easily avoid all those pitfalls and consume caffeine safely. Only certain individuals may need to avoid the drug.

- To avoid both the jitters and possible withdrawal symptoms, keep your caffeine intake fairly steady—unless you're trying to quit.
- If you do want to quit, lower your intake gradually, over the course of a week or so. (That may be particularly important near the end of that week, since going from, say, five cups down to four reduces caffeine intake by 20 percent, while going from two cups to one would cut consumption by 50 percent—possibly enough to spark withdrawal symptoms.)
- Restrict caffeine or avoid it entirely if you face any of the health risks discussed above.
- Check to make sure it's safe to take caffeine together with your medications by asking your doctor or pharmacist or by consulting drug labels, our December 1996 report,* or a drug reference book such as *The Complete Drug Reference,* available in libraries or from Consumer Reports Books.

*Refers to the December 1996 issue of *Consumer Reports on Health.*

FRAME the DEBATE

Form at end of book

Issue 9: Is caffeine a harmless drug or a serious health concern?

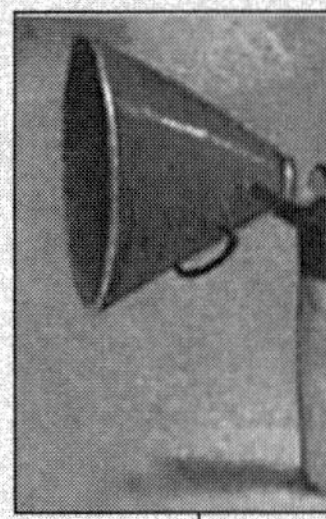

Caffeine: The Inside Scoop

D. Schardt and S. Schmidt

Caffeine is the world's most popular stimulant—four out of five Americans take it each day. However, scientists can't seem to agree on whether it has any real effect on our health. That is because we rarely consume caffeine by itself; we put milk and sugar in our coffee, combine it with sugars and other ingredients in our sodas, and generally complicate the research problem. Even the way coffee and tea are prepared can't make a difference. Caffeine "gives us a lift" because it lessens the effects of adenosine (a chemical that slows brain action) in our brains and temporarily makes it easier to concentrate and dampens fatigue. The effects peak within 30 to 60 minutes and take four to six hours to fully disappear. Typically, we consume about 200 mg/day (apprx. amount in two mugs instant coffee or four mugs of tea or two reg. NoDoz or 1 1/2 Excedrin). A chart of caffeine consumed from ordinary brand name products is provided.* Linking specific health conditions to what we eat is especially complicated with caffeine. Nevertheless, several conditions have consistently been linked to caffeine consumption. Here is what latest research shows on them:

1. **Osteoporosis.** Bones need calcium. About 5 mg of calcium are drained from the body for each cup of coffee or two cans of cola. Two tablespoons of milk added to the coffee make up that loss.
2. **Birth defects and miscarriages.** It's still uncertain whether caffeine at ordinary consumption levels has a direct effect. However, pregnant women consuming 250–300 mg/day have twice the risk of delivering underweight babies, who are then physically and developmentally at risk.
3. **Heart disease.** As long as you drink instant coffee or filtered drip coffee, recent studies see no higher risk.
4. **Cancer.** Caffeine is no longer implicated in pancreatic cancer, nor is there evidence that coffee has a role in the development of bladder, breast, colon, lung or prostate cancers.
5. **Infertility.** Recent studies show that caffeine impairs fertility, but usually only at three or more cups of regular coffee per day.

The bottom line is: if you are pregnant, or want to be, skip or limit caffeine-bearing beverages and products. To not deplete the calcium your body must have, drink as much milk as coffee/tea—or, add at least two tablespoons to each cup.

FRAME the DEBATE

Form at end of book

*Chart not included.

Issue 9: Is caffeine a harmless drug or a serious health concern?

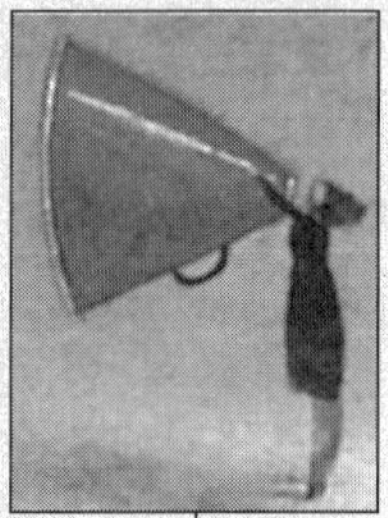

Study Finds Coffee May Help Battle Colon Cancer

Michael Lasalandra

Maybe you should skip the bran muffin and have an extra cup of coffee instead.

Now that it has been shown that eating a high-fiber diet does not protect against colon cancer, some are looking to java as a way to prevent the deadly disease.

Dr. Edward Giovannucci of the Harvard School of Public Health published a study last year suggesting that the risk of colorectal cancer drops 24 percent among those who drink four or more cups of coffee a day.

But before you go out and invest in a Starbucks franchise, take note. Giovannucci says the study is far from conclusive.

"I wouldn't tell people to go out and start drinking coffee, although there isn't much harm in it," he said.

Experts say the best ways to prevent colorectal cancer are still taking vitamins, staying in shape, taking an aspirin a day, avoiding red meat and getting regular screenings after age 50.

Giovannucci's paper, which reviewed all the literature on the subject of coffee and colorectal cancer, appeared in the *American Journal of Epidemiology.* But he downplayed its importance.

"I'm not sure the 24 percent reduction in risk is a cause and effect association," he said.

"It would be important if it is real, but it is hard to say in an epidemiological study that there isn't a bias or other factor that is accounting for this."

Giovannucci said the results were interesting enough to warrant further study, which is what Vanderbilt University in Nashville is planning to do. Vanderbilt is scheduled to open its Institute for Coffee Studies within the next six months, thanks to $6 million in funding from trade groups in leading coffee-producing nations.

"We're going to help people get over the idea that coffee is caffeine," said Vanderbilt's peter Martin. "Caffeine actually is a very small component of coffee. There are many other components that aren't well understood."

Some studies have suggested coffee can help relieve depression, treat alcoholism and prevent colorectal cancer. The institute's mission is to understand why.

Although it may not reduce the risk of colon cancer, eating lots of fruits, vegetables and cereals has been shown to help prevent diverticulitis, high blood pressure and heart disease. But preventing colorectal cancer may require more technology-oriented strategies.

Dr. Francis Farraye, a gastroenterologist at Harvard Vanguard Medical Associates, says those over 50 should discuss colorectal screening with their doctors.

There are several methods, including an annual stool test; a test in which a scope is inserted into the lower third of the colon, once every five years; a barium enema, done every five to 10 years; or a more invasive test in which a scope is inserted into the entire colon, usually once every decade.

FRAME the DEBATE

Form at end of book

WiseGuide Wrap-Up

Since the early nineteenth century, Americans have enjoyed coffee as a part of their daily existence, but recently, coffee and caffeine-containing beverages have become something of a raging fad. Diet colas, which are high in caffeine, have replaced coffee and tea as America's number one beverage, yet in the 1990s we have seen a national surge in the proliferation of espresso stands, lattes, and caffeine addicts.

Out of this modern caffeine craze have arisen concerns about the relative safety of caffeine. Caffeine may be linked to hypertension, arrhythmia, osteoporosis, and fibrocystic breast diseases. Controlled research, however, does not necessarily support the conclusion that caffeine is as harmful as some might fear. At the same time, however, caffeine should not be regarded as merely a benign substance that provides a cost-free lift. Caffeine addiction is very real, as are the withdrawal effects of headaches, restlessness, and anxiety upon cessation of caffeine consumption.

As with so many health behaviors, the solution to the caffeine controversy may lie in moderation.

R.E.A.L. Sites

This list provides a print preview of typical **Coursewise** R.E.A.L. sites. (There are over 100 such sites at the **Courselinks**™ site.) The danger in printing URLs is that web sites can change overnight. As we went to press, these sites were functional using the URLs provided. If you come across one that isn't, please let us know via email to: webmaster@coursewise.com. Use your Passport to access the most current list of R.E.A.L. sites at the **Courselinks** site.

Site name: Coffee Science Source: The Online Source for Coffee, Caffeine, and Health Information

URL: http://www.coffeescience.org/

Why is it R.E.A.L.? This site offers a variety of articles on coffee and caffeine. The articles are fairly well supported with research and reputable sources.

Key topics: caffeine, coffee, drugs, herbals, stimulants

Try this: Explore the site. Click on "Other Questions about Coffee and Health." Does this additional information cause you to reconsider your viewpoints on caffeine? How might your behavior change now that you have become more informed about the health aspects of caffeine consumption?

Site name: Naturopathic Medicine: Caffeine, Sugar and Bone Loss

URL: http://www.healthy.net/library/articles/naturopathic/art.CaffeineBone.np.htm

Why is it R.E.A.L.? This site offers alternative medical health advice and information. This particular article explores the effects of caffeine and sugar on bone loss .

Key topics: bone loss, caffeine, coffee, drugs, herbals, stimulants

Try this: Read the article and compare it to the recommendations of conventional (allopathic) medicine. Consider the evidence that caffeine may cause bone loss in children. How does this compare to conventional views of caffeine and osteoporosis? Are the concerns raised and the advice provided well grounded?

Addicted Pregnant Women: Are They Victims or Criminals?

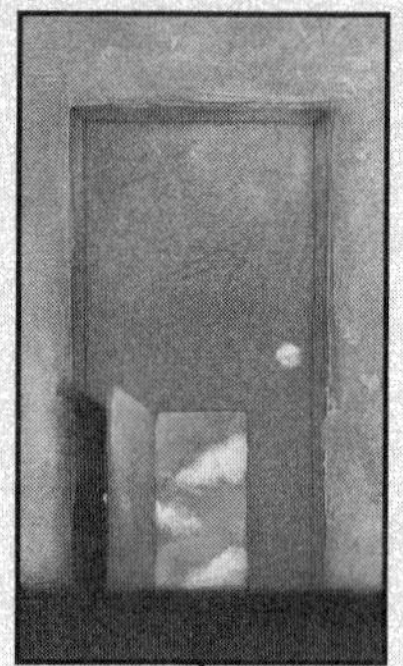

ISSUE 10

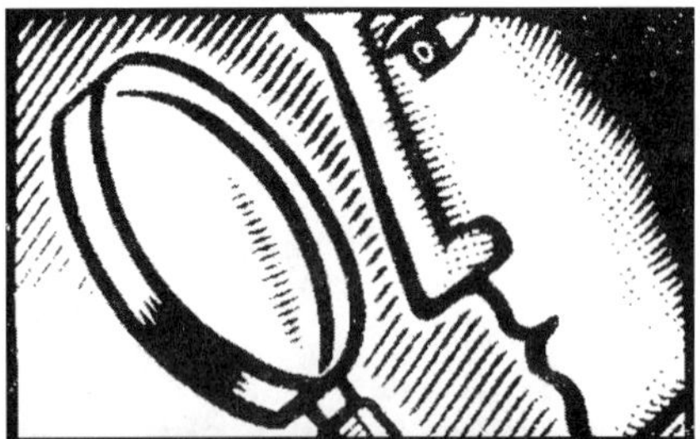

Take a Closer Look

1. What drug was found in Cornelia Whitner's system?
2. What charges did the State of North Carolina bring against Whitner?
3. Reading 27 posits five reasons why the Supreme Court should rule against mandatory treatment of pregnant chemically addicted women. Select two reasons, state the main thesis for each, and then write a paragraph rebuttal to each.

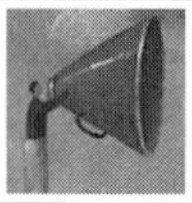

WiseGuide Intro

Fetal alcohol syndrome (FAS) is a collection of mental, physical, and behavioral symptoms in newborns that result from the mother consuming alcohol during the pregnancy. Fetal alcohol effects (FAE) is the name given to similar but less pronounced symptoms with the same etiology. FAS is considered the single most preventable cause of mental retardation.

Nationally, around 5,000 babies are born annually with FAS, and approximately 36,000 are born with FAE. Between 30 and 40 percent of heavily drinking pregnant mothers will give birth to babies with some degree of FAS or FAE. Although FAS and FAE can result from even moderate social drinking, they are most often associated with chronic alcohol consumption and high blood alcohol levels. The most critical time period for developing FAS is during the first trimester of pregnancy, when the fetus's brain and central nervous system develop.

Despite public education and product labeling, some women continue to drink throughout their pregnancies and therefore risk having a baby with either FAS or FAE. Some substance abuse organizations, politicians, and citizen groups want to adopt laws that restrict women's drinking while pregnant in an effort to reduce the prevalence of these preventable disorders. Opponents to legal sanctions against pregnant women who drink have denounced the laws as unconstitutional, ineffective, and an infringement on the rights of individual women to decide and to absorb the consequences of their behaviors.

In Reading 26, "Abuse Laws Cover Fetus, a High Court Rules," Tamar Lewin reviews a recent ruling of the Supreme Court of South Carolina that allows for prosecution of pregnant women who abuse drugs (but not specifically alcohol). The ruling upholds the argument that an unborn fetus is a "person" and therefore is protected by current child abuse laws. Lewin discusses the particular case and compares it to similar earlier cases in South Carolina. Feminists and health groups argue that fear of prosecution may deter pregnant addicts from seeking drug treatment and prenatal care.

Reading 27, " Why the Supreme Court Should Rule against Mandatory Treatment: Five Good Reasons," is an essay in response to a 1997 Canadian Supreme Court ruling that a woman and her fetus are one and that making laws to protect the fetus impinges on the rights of the mother. The authors of this reading oppose any laws that restrict the freedom of pregnant women to drink or abuse drugs during pregnancy. They feel that the laws would likely be enacted unfairly with regard to race and socioeconomic status. In addition, the authors address concerns about the effectiveness of forced treatment in lieu of volunteer treatment and about child protection services having too much power.

Issue 10: Are addicted pregnant women victims or criminals?

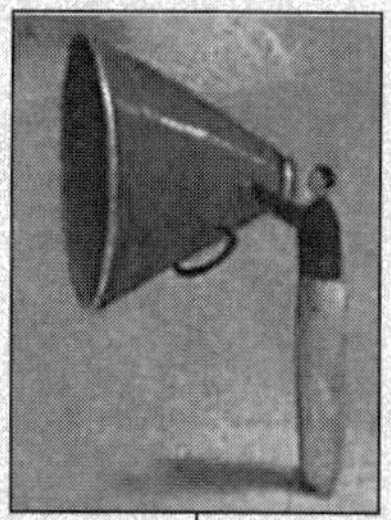

Abuse Laws Cover Fetus, a High Court Rules

Tamar Lewin

In a ruling that runs contrary to every other state supreme court that has addressed the issue, South Carolina's highest court this week upheld the criminal prosecution of pregnant women who used drugs, finding that a viable fetus is a "person" covered by the state's child-abuse laws.

The ruling came in the case of Cornelia Whitner, who in 1992 pleaded guilty to child neglect after her baby was born with traces of cocaine in its system. Ms. Whitner, 33, of Central, S.C., a tiny town in the northwest corner of the state, was sentenced to eight years in prison.

"The abuse or neglect of a child at any time during childhood can exact a profound toll on the child herself as well as on society as a whole," the state's high court said in its ruling on Monday. "However, the consequences of abuse or neglect which takes place after birth often pale in comparison to those resulting from abuse suffered by the viable fetus before birth. This policy of prevention supports a reading of the word 'person' to include viable fetuses." Ms. Whitner was released in 1994 after serving 16 months, when a lower court agreed to her request for a review of her case based on her claim of inadequate legal representation and the argument that the fetus had not been a person. Her baby is living with relatives.

Lawyers for Ms. Whitner, who plan to appeal the case to the United States Supreme Court, say that giving a fetus the same legal status as a child will have dire consequences: If women who use drugs during pregnancy can be prosecuted for child abuse, they say, what about women who drink or smoke while pregnant, or fail to get prenatal care?

"If fetus is a person, everything a pregnant woman does is potentially child abuse, abortion is murder, and women lose the right to make medical decisions on their own behalf during pregnancy," said Lynn Paltrow, a reproductive-rights lawyer from New York who represented Ms. Whitner, "The effect of declaring fetal personhood is to declare the pregnant woman's non-personhood." The question of whether a fetus is a person has arisen frequently over the last decade, both as a response to the growing number of babies being born with crack cocaine in their systems, and as an offshoot of abortion politics, a marker of the tensions between women's autonomy and fetal welfare.

Since 1990, prosecutors in at least 30 states have used a variety of criminal laws to bring charges against pregnant women who abuse drugs or alcohol. Some, as in South Carolina, have used child-endangerment statutes, while others turned to the drug laws, charging that women were delivering drugs through the umbilical cord. So far, only South Carolina has upheld such charges. State Supreme Courts in Florida, Kentucky, Nevada, Ohio and Wisconsin, and many lower courts, have struck them down, usually ruling narrowly that a fetus was not a person under the particular criminal law and avoiding broader constitutional issues.

In South Carolina, the high court ruled 3 to 2 against Ms. Whitner, with the chief justice one of the dissenters. The majority opinion said that a viable fetus was a person, unambiguously, under the plain meaning of the child abuse law.

Ms. Whitner's lawyers disagreed: "They heard the case in May '95," said C. Rauch Wise, of Greenwood, S.C. "When it takes five judges 29 months to decide what 'child' means, that's not plain or unambiguous." The court also rejected the argument that the prosecution had violated Ms. Whitner's constitutional right of privacy, saying, "It strains beliefs for Whitner to argue that using crack cocaine during pregnancy is encompassed within the constitutionally recognized right of privacy."

Courts in South Carolina, as in most other states, have long treated a viable fetus as a person in certain legal contexts: in 1960, for example, the South Carolina Supreme Court ruled that a wrongful death suit could be brought on behalf of an infant who died four hours after her birth as a result of injuries she received prenatally. More recently, the same court upheld murder charges against a man who stabbed his pregnant wife and in the process killed the fetus in her womb. So, the majority in the Whitner case said, consistency requires that a viable fetus be treated as a person under the child-abuse laws.

Many other states that treat a fetus as a person under the wrongful-death laws, however, refuse to do so under the child-abuse laws.

Many feminists and health groups argue that although prosecutors say they hope the threat of criminal charges will encourage pregnant drug-users to get treatment, the actual effect is to frighten such women away from the medical system.

Ms. Paltrow said the ruling would "hurt babies" by deterring pregnant women from seeking drug treatment and prenatal care for fear that their drug use might be discovered.

FRAME the DEBATE

Form at end of book

Issue 10: Are addicted pregnant women victims or criminals?

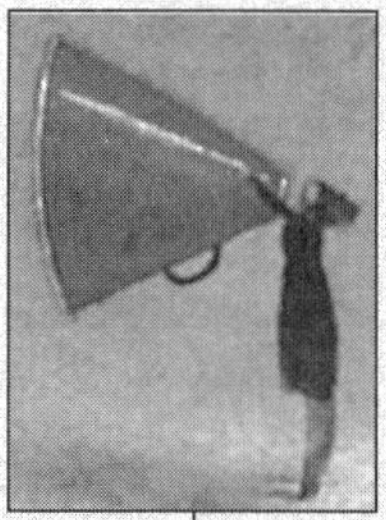

Why the Supreme Court Should Rule against Mandatory Treatment:
Five Good Reasons

For many of us, knowing that an expectant woman is using substances that could harm her fetus is very upsetting, maybe even enraging. It's hard not to focus on the defenseless fetus whose life may be affected by actions she or he has no control over.

From this perspective, it might seem like a good idea to use the law to pressure women who persist in using alcohol, drugs or solvents throughout their pregnancies into treatment. After all, it's for their own good—and the good of their unborn children—and the good of the rest of society, isn't it?

But is it really?

"It is easier to punish one pregnant woman than to alleviate the lethal conditions of many," notes Dr. Michelle Harrison. In her view, society's frustration with the problem of drug addiction and pregnancy, and our urge to protect the fetus from harm, drives us toward solutions that identify the pregnant woman as the cause.

"In our haste," she notes, "we may find ourselves responding to the need to 'do something,' relying on questionable data, and turning to solutions that defeat the ultimate purpose of caring for the woman and protecting the fetus."

Taking drastic action against individual women only deludes us into believing that we are dealing with the problem, and allows us to continue to do nothing about the root causes of substance use for women.

Aboriginal Women of Montreal is one of the many women's groups in Canada that advocate a more holistic understanding of the problem. They say: "Too much emphasis has been placed on the behaviour of "G" and not enough on other factors such as poverty, isolation, and an overtaxed social welfare system. "G"'s situation represents a much larger problem that cannot be solved by granting government agencies the ability to incarcerate these women. It would represent yet another failure of the social system to effectively deal with complex "human" problems which, in this case, requires valuing not only the unborn, but also valuing the pregnant woman who society has failed at every turn."

So before adopting a punitive position, we owe it to ourselves to take a closer look at the dangers of such a simplistic and individualistic approach—if we truly care about the health of women and children. Here are five good reasons why the Supreme Court should rule against mandatory addictions treatment for pregnant women.

1. Forced Treatment Just Doesn't Work

If the ultimate purpose of forced-treatment laws is to help pregnant women overcome their addictions and protect their unborn children from damage, they are a dismal failure. In fact, evidence from Britain and the United States shows they actually do more harm than good.

Rather than helping the pregnant women most at risk to get the services and support they desperately need, these laws just drive them underground. In the American states that have these laws, many women steer clear of health and social services for fear that they will be locked up or have their babies taken away. Obviously, this does nothing to improve the health and security of women and their future children.

2. Laws Like This Probably Won't Be Applied Equally to All Women

As with child welfare laws, forced-treatment laws have the potential to be applied very unfairly. Studies from other countries show that the majority of women confined against their will are poor or members of racial minorities.

This article is reprinted with permission from "Network," the publication of the Canadian Women's Health Network, Suite 203, 419 Graham Avenue, Winnipeg MB R3C 0MC.

The fact that "G" is Aboriginal and on social assistance suggests that such a pattern may occur in Canada as well.

3. A Law and Order Response Is a Quick Fix—It Doesn't Deal with the Systemic and Social Causes of Substance Use

Violence, sexual abuse, poverty, poor self esteem and lack of control over their lives are the reasons many women start down the path of addictions. Racism and other forms of discrimination only worsen this situation for women from marginalized groups, such as Aboriginal women.

Orphaned as a little girl, "G" went through a series of foster homes and ended up on the street at 16. Solvent-sniffing provided a cheap way out of a desperate and painful reality. "G" tried three times to get treatment for her addiction, each time when she was pregnant. But there were no spaces, or she didn't qualify, or she was put on a waiting list.

For example, "G" was admitted into a hospital through emergency, where she went through withdrawal and made a voluntary application to receive treatment. Instead of being given help, she was placed on a waiting list and discharged. Due to a bureaucratic bungle, her application failed to mention that she was receiving CFS services, which would have given her priority. She was left alone over a weekend. When the CFS worker visited her at home a few days later, she was sniffing glue once again. It was at this point that the agency sought a mandatory treatment order.

Those who work in the area of women and addictions have repeatedly called for more treatment programs for women who use substances and more resources to address the underlying causes. Yet few such programs are available, and government cutbacks continue to threaten these and other attempts to combat violence and poverty.

As the Women's Health Rights Coalition said in their presentation before the Supreme Court, resorting to "legal orders of confinement against women is totally unacceptable when innovative and voluntary treatment approaches have barely been tried, let alone exhausted."

4. This Could Be the Start of a "Slippery Slope" for Pregnant Women or All Women of Childbearing Age

Enshrining such a coercive regime in law would endanger, not just the most vulnerable, but all women in Canada today. If we grant fetuses the legal right to care, where would the line be drawn? There are many substances and activities that can affect the well-being of mother and child. Do we want the court to have the power to order interventions against women who smoke, who don't eat well, who work in dangerous or high-stress environments or who engage in risky sports?

And how would we deal with the fact that many substances are most harmful in the very first days and weeks of pregnancy, often before a woman knows she is pregnant? Are we prepared to institute controls over the behaviour of all women of child-bearing age?

Mandatory treatment isn't the only threat facing substance-using expectant women. Dr. Gideon Koren of the Toronto Hospital for Sick Children advocates strong measures to keep them from getting pregnant in the first place. He goes as far as to suggest using food vouchers as incentives to get women to accept Norplant, a long-acting contraceptive implant.

5. Child Welfare Agencies Should Not Be Given This Power

The child and family service system has been criticized by many over the years. Professionals and families have expressed concern about the conflicting mandates of these agencies. Having legal responsibility for supervising and apprehending children at risk as well as trying to do prevention work with families can create competing priorities.

All too frequently, women involved with the child welfare system try to hide their pregnancies because they fear their babies will be apprehended at birth. This is particularly problematic for Aboriginal peoples, says Kathy Mallet of the Original Women's Network.

According to her, the child welfare system has been detrimental to Aboriginal families for a long time. "They've been apprehending our children for years," she says. "They haven't been that friendly to our communities. Child welfare has always been our enemy, not our friend—this will just give them more power. Now the agency will be seen, not as a place to get help, but as a place that will put women into treatment and take away their kids. It will just make things worse, not better."

The brutal funding cutbacks faced by child welfare agencies today compound the problem. Exhausted and burned-out staff struggle to meet the ever-increasing needs of communities, with ever-diminishing resources. High levels of unemployment are taking a profound toll on individuals and families, creating and intensifying problems with violence and addictions. The ultimate solution lies, not in punishing society's victims further, but in redressing societal inequities and strengthening our system of social supports.

FRAME the DEBATE

Form at end of book

WiseGuide Wrap-Up

The issues of restricting the freedoms of pregnant addicts or of punishing them begin with concern about preventing birth defects such as fetal alcohol syndrome and crack baby syndrome. However, they extend into the legal issues of women's rights, the existence of fetal rights, and freedom from government intrusion and public intervention into one's personal health choices.

The readings in this section reviewed the issues surrounding the convictions of two addicted mothers by the Canadian court system and the South Carolina Supreme Court. The facts surrounding the mothers' addictions, their drug use, and the possible teratogenic effects of their drug use are not in dispute. What is at issue, however, is the question: At what point does benevolent law end and unnecessary and unreasonable intrusion begin?

R.E.A.L. Sites

This list provides a print preview of typical **Coursewise** R.E.A.L. sites. (There are over 100 such sites at the **Courselinks**™ site.) The danger in printing URLs is that web sites can change overnight. As we went to press, these sites were functional using the URLs provided. If you come across one that isn't, please let us know via email to: webmaster@coursewise.com. Use your Passport to access the most current list of R.E.A.L. sites at the **Courselinks** site.

Site name: Social Drinking during Pregnancy Risks Infant Health

URL: http://www.pslgroup.com/dg/404de.htm

Why is it R.E.A.L.? This site offers medical advice and research summaries for a variety of medical conditions.

Key topics: alcohol, alcoholism, fetal alcohol effects

Try this: Read the article, "Social Drinking during Pregnancy Risks Infant Health." Given the facts in this article, consider the following question: Does society have the right to restrict the rights of women who choose to drink during pregnancy? Defend your position with at least three of the facts presented in this article.

Site name: Fetal Alcohol Syndrome—Why Caution Makes Sense

URL: http://www.mayohealth.org/mayo/9810/htm/fetal.htm

Why is it R.E.A.L.? This site offers health advice on a variety of medical topics. This particular page gives an overview of the risks of alcohol consumption during pregnancy.

Key topics: alcohol, alcoholism, fetal alcohol effects

Try this: Read the article "Social Drinking during Pregnancy Risks Infant Health." Given these facts, consider the following questions: Does society have the right to restrict the rights of women who choose to drink during pregnancy? Defend your position by using at least three of the facts presented in this article.

Should the Legal Limit for Blood Alcohol Concentration for Drunk Driving Be Lowered?

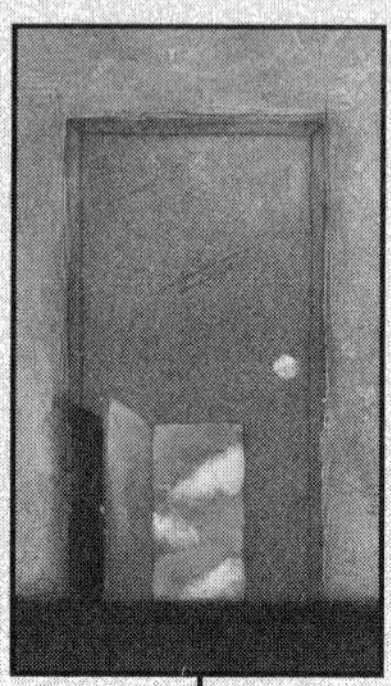

ISSUE 11

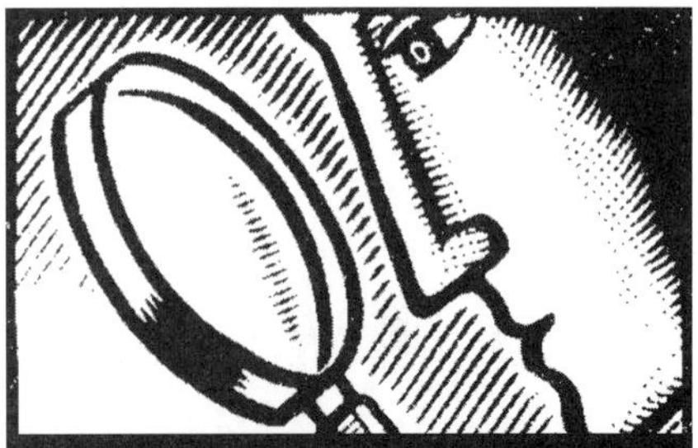

Take a Closer Look

1. According to the National Highway Traffic Safety Administration, how many drinks would the average 170-pound male need to consume in one hour to reach .08% BAC?
2. According to the National Highway Traffic Safety Administration, how many drinks would the average 137-pound female need to consume in one hour to reach .08% BAC?
3. What lobby does MADD feel is the primary opponent to .08 legislation?
4. What is the main argument that the opposition to .08 BAC legislation cites?
5. According to the American Beverage Institute, who causes most alcohol-related accidents?
6. What blood alcohol concentration is found among most drunk drivers killed in motor vehicle crashes?
7. What did the researchers from Data Nexus Inc. do with Ralph Hingson's data to find his conclusions spurious and flawed?

WiseGuide Intro

In 1997, drunk driving resulted in 16,520 fatalities, according to the National Highway Traffic Safety Commission. This accounts for nearly one death every 30 seconds. A multitude of approaches have been proposed for controlling this deadly drunk-driving problem. Currently, all fifty states have laws against drunk driving and impose legal sanctions against convicted drunk drivers that may include financial penalties, mandatory jail time, loss of driving privileges, and in some cases, retribution for damage to property and person.

The debate in this section deals with the legal definition of what blood alcohol concentration (BAC) constitutes drunk driving. In the U.S. House of Representatives, two bills have been proposed to lower the legal limit nationwide from a BAC of .10 percent to .08 percent. Advocacy groups such as Mothers Against Drunk Driving (MADD) say that this lower level will save hundreds of lives annually, while alcoholic beverage promotional groups, such as the American Beverage Institute and the Empire State Restaurant and Tavern Association (ESRTA), argue that the lower limit will only penalize social drinkers.

In Reading 28, "Reducing the Definition of Drunk Driving to .08% BAC," ESRTA outlines its opposition to the proposed revision of the drunk-driving BAC level from .10 percent to .08 percent. ESRTA uses research evidence from the National Highway Traffic Safety Administration and the Insurance Institute for Highway Safety to bolster its argument that the proposed lowered BAC level law would not likely save any more lives than the current regulations. According to ESRTA, a small group of chronic alcohol abusers who regularly reach high blood alcohol concentrations cause most drunk-driving fatalities, and social drinkers would thus be chastised unfairly by the proposed law.

In Reading 29, "House Rules Committee, under Influence of Alcohol and 'Hospitality' Industries, Strikes Down .08 BAC Drunk-Driving Amendment," MADD expresses its disappointment with the U.S. House Rules Committee for failing to support the Lowey-Canady-Moran-Castle-Gilman Amendment, which called for the nationwide reduction of the legal BAC for drunk driving to .08 percent from .10 percent. MADD accuses House representatives of buckling under pressure from the beverage industry, which opposes such regulation revision. According to MADD, adoption of the lower BAC limit would save 500 to 600 lives each year and would not penalize social drinkers. President Clinton supports the regulation revision, and the bill has strong supporters among the Senate.

In Reading 30, "The .08% BAC Debate: Social Drinking vs. Drunk Driving," the American Beverage Institute (ABI) argues that the new .08 percent BAC laws will only criminalize responsible social drinking. The ABI points out that chronic alcohol abusers with much higher BAC levels—not drivers with .08 percent BAC levels—cause most accidents. The ABI feels that federal .08 percent BAC legislation also circumvents states' rights to set their own laws. Obviously, their concern is the loss of business that such legislation will likely cause.

READING 28

Issue 11: Should the legal limit for blood alcohol concentration for drunk driving be lowered?

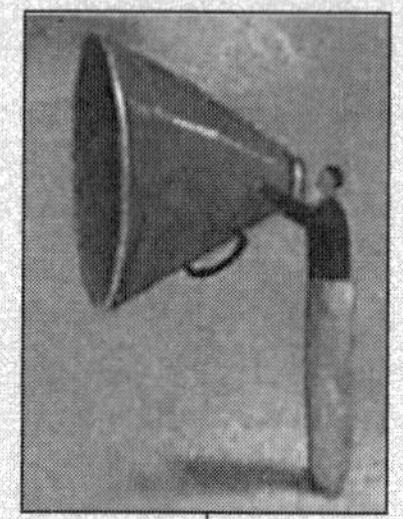

Reducing the Definition of Drunk Driving to .08% BAC

Despite a great deal of progress, drunk driving remains a serious problem. There are numerous bills under consideration by the State Legislature to make further improvements in the state's effort to combat this behavior, but legislation that lowers the definition of drunk driving from .10% BAC to .08% BAC causes us concern. This proposal is off target and distracts attention away from the people who are responsible for the great majority of alcohol related crashes and fatalities.

On the surface the legislation might appear to address the problem of drunk driving. Presented by its advocates as "the most important action that can be taken to deter drunk driving", a closer examination of this proposal reveals that heavy drinkers with high BAC levels cause most drunk driving fatalities:

- According to data from the National Highway Traffic Safety Administration (NHTSA), the average BAC level among fatally injured drinking drivers is .18 percent.
- Government studies conducted over the past 20 years show that 70–75 percent of those convicted of drunk driving have BAC levels of .15% or higher.
- A study completed for the Insurance Institute for Highway Safety found that 86% of the fatally injured drivers on weekend nights who have been drinking have BAC s in excess of .10 percent.
- The National Conference of State Legislators reports that in fatal accidents involving alcohol, only 5 percent of the drivers had a BAC level of .08 to .099% while 83 percent had levels of. 10% or higher.

While advocates of lowering the definition of drunk driving are quick to point out that many European nations have a lower BAC standard than the United States, they fail to mention that the nations cited have alcohol related traffic fatality rates higher than that of the U.S., some of them considerably higher.

There is no hard evidence that lowering the definition of drunk driving to .08% BAC improves traffic safety. Numerous studies undertaken to show that lower BACs reduce alcohol related fatalities have been inconclusive at best. In some cases, these studies have documented an increase in drunk driving after lowering the BAC level.

This information demonstrates that the people doing most of the damage drink far in excess of the current legal limits. They are not social or moderate drinkers. They drink irresponsibly and tend to have other identifiable symptoms of being problem drinkers. Lowering the definition of drunk driving to .08% BAC will have little effect on these individuals. In fact, efforts to lower the BAC could actually hurt highway safety efforts by diverting scarce law enforcement resources away from the real problem.

The main target of this proposal are drivers who currently drive within the legal limit. Establishing .08% BAC as the definition of drunk driving obviously will not have a positive impact on traffic safety. It is merely a symbolic gesture, especially since it is already illegal to drive with a BAC level of .05% or higher.

A more effective approach is to adopt measures which deter drunk driving among drivers with high BAC levels and to continue public education efforts. This combination of strategies is much more likely to make our roads safer—for everyone's benefit.

FRAME the DEBATE

Form at end of book

Reducing the Definition of Drunk Driving to .08% BAC. Empire State Restaurant and Tavern Association. Reprinted by permission.

Issue 11: Should the legal limit for blood alcohol concentration for drunk driving be lowered?

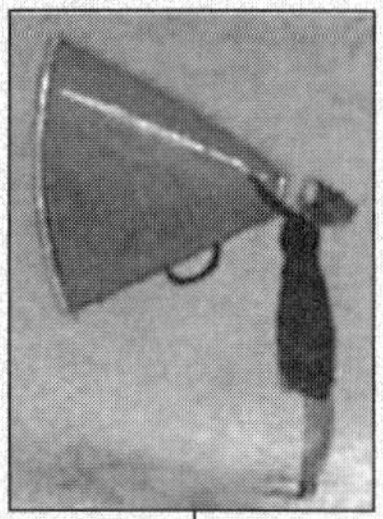

House Rules Committee, under Influence of Alcohol and "Hospitality" Industries, Strikes Down .08 BAC Drunk-Driving Amendment

MADD blasts committee's special interest cave-in, vowing: "The fight for .08 BAC is far from over, America's voice will be heard."

Washington, D.C. (March 31, 1998)—Following a hard-fought battle by Mothers Against Drunk Driving (MADD) and other safety advocates to lower the nationwide drunk driving standard to .08 percent blood alcohol content (BAC)—a measure that would save an estimated 500 to 600 lives every year—the U.S. House Rules Committee today squashed the legislation, under intense pressure from the opposing alcohol and "hospitality" industry lobby.

The Lowey-Canady-Moran-Castle-Gilman Amendment was expected to be offered to BESTEA when the $271 billion transportation bill is brought to the House floor tomorrow. The committee's decision kills any possibility the .08 BAC amendment will get a vote on the House floor. The .08 BAC amendment is supported by the Clinton Administration and is identical to the amendment passed in the Senate by an overwhelming 62–32 vote in early March.

"We are outraged at the obvious special interest cave-in by the Rules Committee," said MADD National President Karolyn Nunnallee. ".08 is a lifesaving law that the public has supported in every scientific poll on this issue. It is unconscionable that the committee would not let this bill go to a vote, especially with the strong Senate support. The American public wants a .08 BAC level, and the Rules Committee has ensured that no elected official from the House of Representative will be allowed to speak for their constituents by approving .08."

During the past two years, .08 legislation has been killed in more than two dozen states as lawmakers buckled under from alcohol and hospitality industry lobbyists who disseminated misinformation about .08 laws. MADD says the alcohol and "hospitality" industries defeated the federal .08 amendment with influence peddling and by spreading the myth that .08 would criminalize social drinking and reduce alcohol sales, and by hiding behind the states' rights argument. Supporters of .08 say these points are far from the truth.

"This law just makes sense," said Nunnallee. "At a .08 BAC level, everyone's critical driving skills are impaired and drivers with a .08 BAC are 11 times more likely to be involved in a fatal alcohol-related crash. The risk literally doubles at the .10 BAC limit, which is the current law in 34 states."

According to studies conducted by the National Highway Traffic Safety Administration (NHTSA), the

House Rules Committee, under Influence of Alcohol and "Hospitality" Industries, Strikes Down .08 BAC Drunk-Driving Amendment. MADD News 3/31/98. Reprinted by permission of Mothers Against Drunk Driving.

average 170-pound male would have to consume four drinks in one hour on an empty stomach before reaching .08 BAC. A 137-pound woman would have to consume three drinks in an hour under the same conditions to reach that level.

"The danger imposed by drunk drivers does not end at state lines and neither should the standards that define drunk driving," added Nunnallee. "The states' rights argument touted by opponents of .08 legislation is a smoke screen that hides what is really going on behind the scenes—alcohol and hospitality interests peddling big money to prevent lifesaving public policy."

Today, 34 states and the District of Columbia still define intoxicated driving as .10 BAC—the most lenient definition of drunk driving in the industrialized world. Currently, only 16 states have enacted .08 BAC laws. Washington State became the latest state to pass .08 when Governor Locke signed legislation yesterday.

"Today's irresponsible action by the House Rules Committee is only a small setback in the process of enacting a national uniform drunk driving standard of .08 BAC," said Nunnallee. "Strong support from the Senate and President Clinton ensures that .08 BAC stands a good chance of passage in the final version of the highway bill. MADD vows to continue fighting for.08 BAC. We are just terribly disappointed to find out that money—not safety—talks in the House of Representatives."

Nunnallee added, "The softer 'incentive grant' approach to .08 that was passed by the House transportation committee last week will not make it through state legislatures with the influence peddling of the alcohol and hospitality industries. The Rules Committee ignored the voices of America and refused to follow the lead of the Senate and the support of President Clinton and make .08 the law of the land."

FRAME the DEBATE

Form at end of book

Issue 11: Should the legal limit for blood alcohol concentration for drunk driving be lowered?

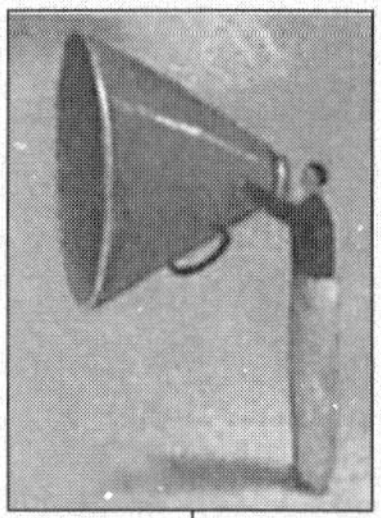

The .08% BAC Debate:
Social Drinking vs. Drunk Driving

.08% Debate Overview

Legislators and special interest groups are trying to tie provisions to the reauthorization of the Intermodal Surface Transportation Efficiency Act (ISTEA) that would equate social drinking with drunk driving—making it illegal for a 120-pound woman to drive after consuming just two glasses of wine in two hours!*

Under the plan, the federal government would reduce the funding of highway programs in any state that refused to lower its legal threshold for drunk driving from a .10% BAC (blood, alcohol concentration) level to a .08% BAC level.

But the .08% legislation misses the mark. Consider the following facts:

.08% Laws Criminalize Responsible Social Drinking

According to the National Highway Traffic Safety Administration (NHTSA), a 120-pound woman with average metabolism will reach the .08% BAC threshold if she drinks two six-ounce glasses of wine over a two-hour period. This woman is hardly what most people think of as a dangerous drunk driver. Yet under the proposed .08% legislation, she would face arrest, fines, jail, loss of license and much higher insurance rates.

Some advocates of the .08% legislation proclaim that the average-sized man must have four or five drinks in an hour to reach a .08% BAC. While this is a hypothetical possibility, it is an "example" designed to enrage rather than enlighten. In reality, few people drink four or five drinks in one hour, and then voluntarily quit. Rather, this pattern of a drink every 12 to 15 minutes is typical of product abusers who drink to high BAC levels over several hours.

.08% BAC Laws Do Not Save Lives

No unbiased, authoritive research has ever been able to show that lowering the BAC limit to .08% saves lives. Data from NHTSA show that the average BAC level among fatally injured drunk drivers is .18%—more than twice the proposed .08% limit—with more than 80% of these drivers having BAC levels of at least .14%. Lowering the legal BAC limit will have no effect on drivers who already ignore the current law.

Advocates of lowering the BAC limit frequently cite a study which claimed that California reduced alcohol-related fatalities by 12% by lowering the state BAC level to .08%. However, when the data were run by the state Division of Motor Vehicles using a more accurate measure, it was shown that there were "no statistically significant effects associated with . . . [California's] .08% law." In fact, the reduction in alcohol-related fatalities in California was smaller than the drop in the rest of the country, where BAC limits were generally set at .10%.

Eight out of the top 10 states ranked in 1996 for percentage of alcohol-related fatalities had .10% arrest levels. If .08% laws were proven to work, why weren't all ten .08% states?

.08% BAC Laws Ignore the Real Problem

According to a December 15, 1996 story in *The New York Times,* even the president of Mothers Against Drunk Driving (MADD) believes that the "problem may be down to a hard core of alcoholics who do not respond to public appeal." Government data reveal that no more alcohol-related fatalities occur between the .08% and .09% levels than do between the .01% and .03% levels—virtually negligible amounts of alcohol.

*"[T]he National Highway Traffic Safety Administration says a 120-pound woman who drives after drinking two six-ounce glasses of wine over a two-hour period could be driving 'drunk.' "—CBS Evening News, May 24, 1997

Lowering the BAC limit to .08% is like lowering the speed limit on the Interstate to 45 mph—the only people it will affect are those who obey the law and the police who have to enforce it. "Most professionals agree that lowering the presumptive level to .08% would simply exacerbate the [overloaded court system] problem," says the president of the Washington State Patrol Troopers Association. Chronic drunk drivers—like chronic speeders—will continue to flaunt the law and risk the lives of those who share the roads with them. The real way to reduce drunk driving is to target the real problem—high BAC drivers.

.08% BAC Laws Impose on States' Rights

In 1996, all 11 states that considered lowering their legal BAC limit decided against the policy change. Over the last ten years, the .08% proposal has been rejected more than 100 times by state legislators. By threatening to revoke highway funds, the proposed .08% federal legislation would force these states to implement policy changes already turned down by their own legislatures.

.08% BAC Laws Will Not Save 500–600 Lives a Year

Advocates of lowering the BAC limit claim to have research that proves that .08% BAC laws will save 500 to 600 lives per year. However, the research they refer to—a 4-page study, conducted by MADD board member Ralph Hingson—contains overt biases and fatal flaws that render it useless.

To study the effect of .08% BAC laws, Hingson paired .08% states with what he termed "nearby" .10% BAC states. Inexplicably, one of these "nearby" pairs consisted of California (a .08% state) and Texas (a .10% state). When researchers from Data Nexus, Inc. switched the comparison state from Texas to Arizona (leaving everything else the same), the study's conclusion was negated—.08 was shown to have no effect.

Even when the researchers replaced Texas with a combination of three states (MI, OH and PA) specifically determined to reflect California's population and geographic size, the results were still the same. In short, Hingson's method is flawed, the results do not replicate, and there is no evidence to suggest that .08% laws have had any effect.

FRAME the DEBATE

Form at end of book

WiseGuide Wrap-Up

According to the National Institute on Drug Abuse and the National Institute on Alcohol Abuse and Alcoholism, "Total costs attributed to alcohol-related motor vehicle crashes were estimated to be $24.7 billion [in 1992]. This included $11.1 billion from premature mortality and $13.6 billion from automobile and other property destruction."*

Nonetheless, the campaign to curb drunk driving in America is one of the greatest health promotion success stories of our time. The involvement of the public in terms of awareness and voluntary behavior change began in earnest in the 1980s and continues today, largely because of the leadership of citizen groups such as Mothers Against Drunk Driving (MADD) and voter support of the passage and enforcement of state and federal laws against drunk driving.

Few people would ever argue *for* drunk driving, but the issue now raised by the Empire State Restaurant and Tavern Association and the American Beverage Institute is: Are we going too far in our efforts to legislate against this problem?

Review the arguments for and against lowering the BAC level to .08 percent. Then weigh the relative benefits of stricter laws against the losses of individual health behavior freedom.

*From the "Executive Summary of the Economic Costs of Alcohol and Drug Abuse in the United States, 1992," http://www.health.org/pubs/qdocs/alcohol/economic.htm

R.E.A.L. Sites

This list provides a print preview of typical **Coursewise** R.E.A.L. sites. (There are over 100 such sites at the **Courselinks**™ site.) The danger in printing URLs is that web sites can change overnight. As we went to press, these sites were functional using the URLs provided. If you come across one that isn't, please let us know via email to: webmaster@coursewise.com. Use your Passport to access the most current list of R.E.A.L. sites at the **Courselinks** site.

Site name: Recent Liquor Industry Statistics

URL: http://www.health.org/pressrel/jan97/6.htm

Why is it R.E.A.L.? This site includes links to several alcohol-related informational pages.

Key topics: alcohol, alcoholism

Try this: Review the statistics on alcohol sales and advertising. Could these statistics bolster the argument that the beverage industry's efforts to subvert .08 BAC legislation are less than altruistic and more self-serving? Prepare a counter-argument to Reading 30 using these statistics and one other informational article from this site.

Site name: Impaired Driving Division

URL: http://www.nhtsa.dot.gov/people/injury/alcohol/

Why is it R.E.A.L.? This site has informational reports on traffic fatalities, drunk-driving laws, and scientific studies of the effects of alcohol on driving.

Key topics: alcohol, auto safety, drunk driving

Try this: At this site, read the articles ".08 Limit" and "Alcohol: Traffic Safety Facts for 1997." Use at least three factual statements from these articles to formulate two strong arguments either for or against a nationwide .08 BAC limit law.

Is It Time to Reexamine Our Approach to Addictions?

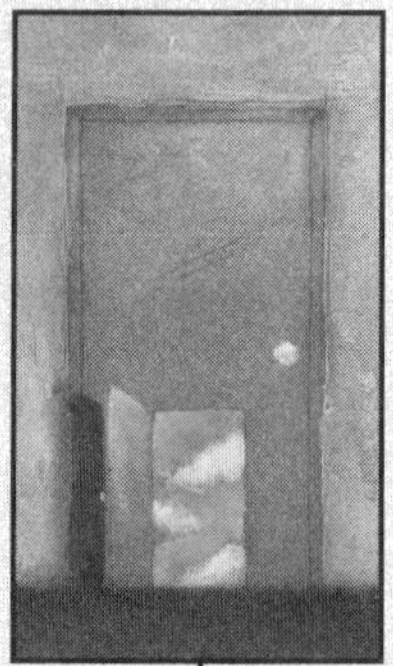

ISSUE 12

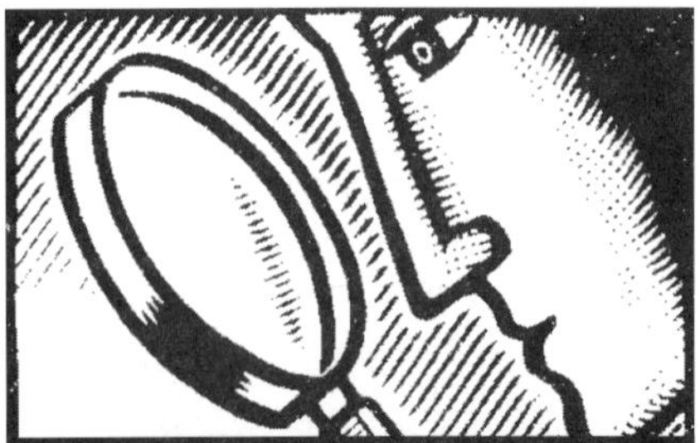

Take a Closer Look

1. In Reading 31, what therapies does Holder combine in his treatment of addictions?
2. How does the alignment of the spine influence addiction, according to Holder's theory in Reading 31?
3. What is auriculotherapy?
4. What are the guidelines for moderate drinking set forth by Moderation Management in Reading 32?
5. According to Drink/Link in Reading 32, what is the primary guideline for responsible drinking?
6. About how many participants are still drinking moderately a year after beginning a moderation program?
7. In Reading 33, Grinspoon and Bakalar suggest a simple self-test for alcoholism. Describe the self-test.
8. Regarding the possibility of a genetic cause of alcoholism, what do studies of twin sons of alcoholic fathers show?
9. In Reading 33, Fingarette identifies several points argued by critics of the disease model. List at least three.

WiseGuide Intro

The prevalence of alcoholism and addiction-related problems in the United States is staggering. Few single causes cost Americans as much in terms of loss of life and loss of quality of life. The National Council on Alcoholism and Drug Dependence (NCADD) reports that alcohol contributes to 100,000 deaths annually, making it the third leading cause of preventable mortality in the United States. According to NCADD:

> In 1992, more than 7 percent of the population ages 18 years and older—nearly 13.8 million Americans—had problems with drinking, including 8.1 million people who are alcoholic. Almost three times as many men (9.8 million) as women (3.9 million) were problem drinkers, and prevalence was highest for both sexes in the 18- to 29-years-old age group. (*Alcohol Health & Research World,* Vol. 18, No. 3, 1994, pp. 243, 245)

Most private and government agencies agree that alcoholism strikes about one in ten U.S. drinkers and that alcoholism has negatively affected four times as many. According to the National Center for Health Statistics,

> About 43 percent of U.S. adults—76 million people—have been exposed to alcoholism in the family: they grew up with or married an alcoholic or a problem drinker or had a blood relative who was ever an alcoholic or problem drinker." (*Advance Data,* USDHHS, No. 205, September 30, 1991, p. 1)

Effective, lasting treatment for chemical dependency is needed in America, but the approach to treatment is currently being reexamined, as is conventional understanding of addiction. For the past four decades, the "disease concept" has prevailed in alcohol and addiction treatment centers. The disease theory of addiction states that, because of its predictability and common symptoms, progressive nature, and the tendency for addicts to go through withdrawal and to relapse, addiction qualifies as an illness of mind, body, and spirit.

A great deal of research evidence on the physical causes and indicators of alcoholism is emerging. Viewing alcoholism and addiction as diseases rather than as character flaws relieves the addict of social stigmas, guilt, and self-loathing for lack of will power, fortitude, or character. Thus, proponents feel that the disease concept of alcoholism may also facilitate entry into treatment, as one might voluntarily enter into treatment for diabetes or other genetically linked diseases.

The disease theory of alcoholism may have gotten its start in the 1930s with Bill Wilson, founder of Alcoholics Anonymous. In 1960, Dr. E. M. Jellinek published his book, *The Disease Concept of Alcoholism,* which further promoted the concept that addictions are neither sins nor personality defects, but illnesses over which the afflicted has no control. In 1965 and 1966, the American Psychiatric Association and the American Medical Association (AMA) published statements that classified alcoholism as a disease, and in 1987, the AMA declared all chemical dependencies to be diseases.

Since the 1960s, the disease concept has prevailed, but in the past decade, new theories regarding addiction have emerged. The new theories reject the notions that "once an alcoholic, always an alcoholic" and that the only viable treatment for the alcoholic or substance abuser is complete and total lifelong abstinence. Critics of the disease concept argue that, while some individuals have severe obsessive compulsive disorders that involve alcohol or drugs, most individuals can consume alcohol in moderation if trained to do so. This is especially true in the case of individuals, such as college students, who have a personal history of episodic alcohol abuse. They should be called "heavy drinkers" instead of being mislabeled as alcoholics or hopeless addicts. They should not be forced to abstain from drinking for life but, rather, should be taught to drink responsibly. Critics of the disease concept of alcoholism also argue that the disease concept relieves alcoholics of all responsibility for their behavior. Responsibility and relearning of drinking habits are the cornerstones of most moderation programs.

In Reading 31, "The End to Addictions: A Startling New Treatment for Reversing *All* Addictions," Richard Leviton reviews the controversial work of chiropractor and physician Jay M. Holder. Holder, the director of a 300-bed Exodus Addiction Treatment Center in Miami Beach, Florida, is using a combination of chiropractic spinal adjustments and food supplement therapy to treat alcoholism and other addictions in an unconventional manner. Leviton presents a case study of a young alcoholic addict who underwent Holder's five-point treatment battery, consisting of spinal adjustments and amino acid supplements. Holder's theory is that every addicted individual has at least one spinal vertebrae out of place, which creates a condition that chiropractors call "subluxation." According to Holder, addiction and spinal vertebrae misalignment may be linked to the dorsal horn of the spinal cord, which extends the length of the cord and links the limbic portions of the midbrain.

The spinal adjustments at Dr. Holder's treatment centers are accompanied by large oral doses of four specific amino acids: L-phenylalinine, D-phenylalinine, L-glutamine, and L-tyrosine. The spinal adjustments are intended to ". . . remove the interference to the natural flow of brain chemicals," while the amino acids are intended to " . . . restore the brain reward cascade." In addition, the case study involved regular attendance at Narcotics Anonymous meetings and addiction counseling at least once per week. Dr. Holder's use of nonconventional acupuncture of the ear may also be added to the addiction recovery regimen.

Leviton states that the national retention rate for conventional addiction programs is around 72 percent, whereas with Dr. Holder's nontraditional treatment, the retention rate is 96 percent. The cost of the treatment ($870 to $1,030) is far cheaper than conventional addiction costs of $16,000 per month (seen in the case study presented in the article). Leviton implies that Holder's unconventional therapy may have uses in the treatment of attention deficit disorder and crack babies, as well as of adult drug and alcohol addicts.

Since the 1940s, the alcohol treatment field has embraced the theory that abstinence is the only viable treatment option for alcoholics and heavy drinkers. In Reading 32, "Half Steps vs. 12 Steps," Michel Marriott presents a brief overview of an alternative treatment approach to alcoholism promoted by a self-help group called Moderation Management (MM). Moderation Management enthusiasts believe that, contrary to the total abstinence advocated by Alcoholics Anonymous (AA), heavy drinkers can return to moderate, controlled drinking.

Like AA, the moderation programs usually require a drying-out period of sobriety, and all have a set of rules to follow, such as not drinking every day and specific drink limits for males and females. Research from Canada seems to support the controlled moderation theory, with 50 percent of moderation program enrollees maintaining their moderate drinking behaviors one year after beginning their programs. A supporting statement from a 1994 National Institute on Alcohol Abuse and Alcoholism document is quoted in the article. The president of the National Council on Alcoholism and Drug Addiction, however, is skeptical of moderation programs and believes they could be a dangerous delusion.

In Reading 33, "Alcohol Abuse and Dependence," Lester Grinspoon and James B. Bakalar examine the treatment of alcoholism. The Harvard Medical School authors take a traditional disease concept approach to this review. They begin with the first step of getting alcoholics to admit and recognize their problem, followed by a period of detoxification. A prescriptive battery of medications is suggested to ease withdrawal symptoms. Psychotherapy and the development of inner controls are suggested. Grinspoon and Bakalar briefly review behavior therapy aimed at modifying conditioned responses, as well as the self-help support group, Alcoholics Anonymous (AA). They also focus on the relative benefits of moderation- and abstinence-based treatments, spontaneous recovery, and alcoholism prevention.

Reading 33 also presents a debate between Herbert Fingarette, Ph.D., and George E. Vaillant, M.D. Fingarette argues for the rejection of the disease concept of alcoholism. A great deal of disease theory is derived from the early works of Jellinek, who identified the common symptoms and the progressive and often fatal nature of alcoholism. Fingarette, however, points out that Jellinek's work was based solely on AA members and a sample size of fewer than 100 self-selected respondents. Fingarette then provides evidence that the search for biological or "genetic" markers may also be methodologically flawed. He states that it is implausible that any biological or psychological markers could override a sober person's voluntary inclination to stay sober. Alcoholics, he points out, can and do, in fact, control their drinking voluntarily in certain situations. Thus, according to Fingarette, the conclusion that alcoholism is a disease marked by lack of control is false. Lastly, Fingarette argues that the disease concept of alcoholism is scientifically flawed and may serve only to precipitate alcohol abuse.

Vaillant argues for the retention of the disease concept of alcoholism. Vaillant begins his thesis by first attacking Fingarette's lack of personal experience in working with alcoholics. Vaillant makes immediate use of the "straw man" tactic, as he points out five major arguments often posited by his opposition (those who reject the disease concept of alcoholism). Then, one by one, he knocks down the arguments with counterpoints. He systematically poses counterarguments to the following points: (1) the unknown root cause of alcoholism, (2) the prevalence of diagnostic problems between heavy drinkers and true alcoholics, (3) the tendency for alcoholics to drink in reaction to situational and psychological factors, (4) the labeling and disparagement of free will, and (5) the classification of alcoholism as a maladaptive behavioral disorder and not as a potentially life-threatening state of physical illness. Vaillant concludes by pointing out that labeling alcoholism as a disease may actually increase the number of alcoholics who enter treatment. Alcoholism, he concludes, is best viewed through social and learning models, but best treated through medical intervention.

Issue 12: Is it time to reexamine our approach to addictions?

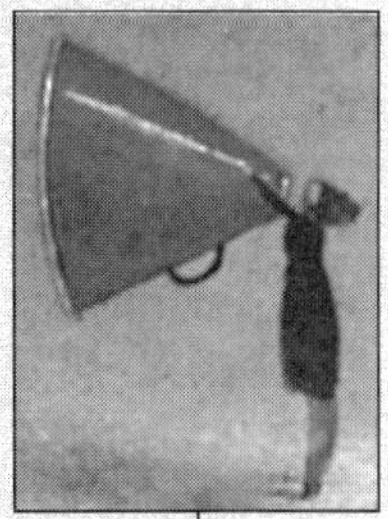

The End to Addictions: A Startling New Treatment for Reversing *All* Addictions

Dr. Jay M. Holder shows why chiropractic, acupuncture, and amino acids may be the groundbreaking answer to the leading cause of death in America. His bold new multifactorial approach has a high success rate and is cost effective. It could spell the end to addictions—to alcohol, cocaine, heroin, nicotine, gambling, attention deficit disorders in adults and children—in a generation.

Richard Leviton

In the first days of its second century, chiropractic may have a bold, effective, and inexpensive solution to the alarming problem of addictions. An estimated 20% of the U.S. population suffers from some form of addiction and over 80% of all crime is traceable to addictions or substance abuse. Even more shocking, evidence supports the conclusion that addiction, which most physicians now regard as a disease, is the leading cause of death in America, accounting for 69% of drownings, 68% of manslaughters, 49% of murders, 50% of all traffic fatalities, and 35% of all suicides. Add to this, deaths from drug overdose and related substance abuse complications, and you have a health problem of staggering proportions.

Emerging in the face of these grim statistics is the completely surprising revelation that the solution to this proliferation of addictions may be in our own therapeutic backyard. According to Jay M. Holder, D.C., M.D., Ph.D., a Miami chiropractor-physician and one of the prime movers in the 50,000 member-strong chiropractic profession, this 100-year-old primary health care profession may hold the answer to addictions literally in its hands. Chiropractic, after all, means "done with the hands," and if the rest of the profession grabs hold of Dr. Holder's theories and innovations, chiropractic may start to make a profound difference in turning around our most serious health problem in ways that nobody ever thought it could.

Dr. Holder is no ordinary chiropractor. In 1991, he was the first American physician to receive the Albert Schweitzer Prize in Medicine, the profession's most prestigious award, to the acclaim of doctors from 70 nations. That year he also was named Chiropractor of the Year by the Florida Chiropractic Association. Dr. Holder received Florida's first state grant to study the use of acupuncture to treat chemical dependency. In 1992, the State of Florida House of Representatives awarded Dr. Holder an Official Commendation for his medical excellence in addiction treatment.

In practice for 20 years, Dr. Holder directs two chiropractic clinics, in Miami and Miami Beach, Florida, including the 300-bed Exodus Addiction Treatment Center. He directs the Holder Research Institute which invents medical devices, formulas, and educational programs; he runs the American College of Addictionology and Compulsive Disorders which trains and board certifies professionals to work as addictionologists; and he travels, lectures, and teaches constantly.

"Our program integrates five modalities—chiropractic, amino acids, ear acupuncture, counseling, Alcoholics Anonymous—but I emphasize that of all these, the one that offers the greatest benefit for the dollar invested is chiropractic."

Not only is he phenomenally busy, but Dr. Holder is getting unheard-of clinical results in treating addictions. In 1993, the U.S. Senate, reviewing Dr. Holder's success rates, said: "In the realm of addictionology, these figures compare with Michael Jordan's performance in basketball."

So if a physician with this caliber of credentials says chiropractic, as the leading component of a 5 part addiction treatment program, can help addictions, we're well advised to give him an ear—both ears. Here is a typical case that shows how Holder reverses addictions.

The End to Addictions: A Startling New Treatment for Reversing *All* Addictions, Richard Leviton, ALTERNATIVE MEDICINE DIGEST, issue 7. Reprinted with permission by ALTERNATIVE MEDICINE MAGAZINE, tel. 888–333–HEAL.

Johnny, age 26, came to Dr. Holder depressed, very sick, displaying psychotic behavior, and strung out on alcohol and cocaine. He'd already seen four psychiatrists who had given him different mood-altering drugs, but they only made him worse. He'd started two addiction treatment programs, but finished neither. Johnny had attended Alcoholics Anonymous meetings but quit, finding them boring. He'd go off drugs for a few weeks, maybe several months, then relapse, and slip back into the habit.

Johnny's future didn't look promising. His parents refused to pay for any more treatment programs, which were running $16,000 a month. The insurance companies had written him off as hopeless, and if Johnny had gone to see any other physician besides Dr. Jay Holder, chances are they'd have recommended he attend more AA meetings and wished him well.

The trouble is, this is most often the guarantee of a dead end, which is why an estimated 35 out of 36 addicts never make it to treatment, fare very poorly, and often die. The 1 out of 36 is lucky enough to enter an addiction treatment program. A chronic addict, Johnny was down and out, and likely to stay permanently down. Of course, that's not the way Dr. Holder saw things.

After taking his case history, Holder began examining Johnny on the treatment table. Using a unique diagnostic and chiropractic treatment system called Torque Release Technique which Holder co-developed with chiropractor Marvin A. Talsky, D.C., Holder was able to tell which vertebrae in Johnny's spinal column were out of alignment. Chiropractors call this condition a *subluxation;* here any one of your spine's 33 vertebrae is partially dislocated. But the concept has a deeper meaning for Dr. Holder. "To us, a subluxation means a separation from wholeness that interferes with your body's ability to function in a whole way."

Every addicted person will have a subluxated spine with at least one or more vertebrae out of alignment, Holder says. Using a handheld spinal adjustment instrument he invented himself, called the Integrator™, Holder makes a few adjustments (never more than 3 in one visit) on Johnny's spine, using a minimum of force and pressure.

In addition to correcting Johnny's subluxations, Dr. Holder will start him on a series of 4 amino acids (precursors to or building blocks for proteins, normally found in foods) taken daily as oral supplements. These include L-phenylalanine (750 mg daily), D-phenylalanine (750 mg daily), L-glutamine (300 mg), and L-tyrosine (900 mg daily).

If this were anywhere else than the U.S., Dr. Holder would also give Johnny 400 mg of the amino acid L-tryptophan. Unfortunately, although the substance's efficacy has been proven, the FDA forbids its use in this country. Dr. Holder will keep Johnny on this amino acid combination for at least a year.

The idea is that the chiropractic adjustment will remove the interference to the natural flow of brain chemicals but you still need to shore up the body's supplies of these substances, vital for addiction recovery, for a fair amount of time. The amino acids will help Johnny make important changes in his behavior, which are crucial to the success of his treatment program and will help to guarantee that he stays off drugs for good in the future. Specifically, the amino acids, especially phenylalanine, the "addiction-treatment king," will help "restore the brain reward cascade" and its bodywide sense of well-being; it will greatly reduce stress and lift depression as well.

In addition, Johnny is attending Narcotics Anonymous meetings every day and receiving expert addiction counselling at least once a week, both of which are provided in Dr. Holder's clinic. He may also receive some acupuncture treatment on his ears. "We integrate all 5 modalities for the best results," Holder explains, "but I emphasize that of all the modalities, the one that offers the greatest benefit for the dollar invested is chiropractic."

The next day, Dr. Holder adjusts Johnny again, and makes sure he takes his amino acid capsules. On the third day, Johnny comes in with his family. They can't believe the changes in his condition and want to know what kind of miracle Dr. Holder has performed on their son.

"He doesn't yell or mope anymore," says Johnny's mother. "He has more attention, smiles frequently, even goes to work on time," says his father. And Johnny says: "I don't cry at night any more and I no longer dream about my drug. My appetite is completely gone. I feel no nagging to go back and take some more cocaine."

Holder isn't surprised. He's seen results like this often with many other chronically addicted people. "Under chiropractic care, they show a remarkable difference compared to any other addiction treatment program. They become open, relaxed, and compliant as their anxiety and depression lift. Their heads clear, their thinking improves, they get in touch with their feelings, and they open up to group therapy and the treatment program with a surprising intensity." A couple of years later Johnny pays Dr. Holder a visit. He's still off drugs and is getting married—and he's never relapsed.

There is, technically, no cure for addictions because, as the saying goes, "once a pickle, never a cucumber." Addiction treatment experts, including Dr. Holder, speak in terms of recovery and the ability to stay off drugs more or less permanently. So there is the possibility of successful and long-lasting intervention and recovery and Dr. Holder has put together the 5 elements that produce these previously unheard-of results. In case you're wondering if this is too good to be true, Dr. Holder has the statistics to prove chiropractic can get results like this.

The key factor in addiction studies is how long an addicted person will stay in the treatment program which typically runs 28 days. Experts call this the retention rate. The national retention average is 72%, which means out of 100 people in treatment, 28 will quit. Those who finish the program stand an 85% chance of staying drugfree 5 years later. So if you can get more people to finish the program, you basically come as close as possible to "curing" them—Dr. Holder calls it "securing an on going recovery"—of their addictions. Dr. Holder knew he could improve the odds and he did, by a great deal.

Holder was getting highly impressive results with his new developments in ear acupuncture, but then he found something even better—chiropractic. In a special trial with 100 addicts, when Holder gave them 20 chiropractic adjustments over a 30 day period, he got the retention rate up to 100%.

First, using acupuncture to treat six specific points on the ears, Holder got the retention rate up to 96%. But even here, Dr. Holder made an important contribution to the field of auriculotherapy, or treating acupuncture points on the ear. Classical Chinese medicine describes 5 ear points which can produce beneficial results in treating all addictions.

Then Dr. Holder, working with new information about the energetics of the ear, identified 3 completely new treatment points, again for all addictions. That new information has to do with the fact that there are 4 cranial nerves that have nerve endings throughout the ear and these are the points treated with needles.

Before Dr. Holder refined his understanding of the contribution subluxation-based chiropractic could make in addiction treatment, he had been using ear acupuncture 100% of the time; now he uses it with about 20% of his patients, when they need an extra energy boost to lift their depression and cut drug appetite.

Ear acupuncture is excellent for helping to relax the patient, which in turn allows addicted persons to be more compliant and open to the complete therapy program. It also enables them to feel less apathetic and more motivated to stay off drugs; further, it cuts down on drug craving and reduces their sense of physical and emotional withdrawal.

What's innovative about Holder's use of auriculotherapy is that he no longer uses the traditional needles. Instead he uses a Stim-Flex 400, which is a small handheld probe that delivers between 2.5–160 Hz in microcurrent to specific ear points for 8–16 seconds per point, maximum. This is in comparison to needle-delivered ear acupuncture which can require anywhere from 45–60 minutes. The microcurrent problem approach is thus far more efficient and specific, and helps release the pleasure-producing brain chemicals called endorphins much more quickly and more thoroughly than needle treatment.

So Holder was getting highly impressive results with his new developments in ear acupuncture, but then he found something even better: chiropractic. In a special trial with 100 addicts, when Holder gave them 20 chiropractic adjustments over a 30 day period. he got the retention rate up to 100%. "That is unheard of; it's never happened before in addiction treatment," Holder says. Bear in mind that at a national average of only $30 per chiropractic adjustment, this astounding success rate cost only about $600 per addicted person per month. Add to this $30 for a one month's supply of amino acids and $240–$400 a month for 4 addiction counselling sessions, and you have a total addiction treatment program cost of about $870–$1030. Johnny's unsuccessful treatment by comparison, had been costing his family $16,000 per month.

Johnny's parents saw the results but, naturally, they couldn't understand how chiropractic could have achieved it. The answer is almost as startling as the treatment's success.

But you first have to define a few basic terms, says Holder, such as what is addiction? "Simply put, addiction is compulsive use in spite of negative consequences." You keep using a substance even though you know it's bad for you. There are 5 types of addictions, including work, food, sex, drugs-chemicals, and gambling, and each one has many factors. "But these 5 categories are all symptoms of one disease—addiction."

According to research Holder has collected and thought about deeply, there are two key factors at play in causing addictions. First, according to Holder's colleague, Kenneth Blum, Ph.D. of the University of Texas Health Science Center at San Antonio, there is a genetic cause. Dr. Blum discovered the same specific genetic flaw (called "the A_1 allele of the D_2 dopamine receptor") in 69% of severe alcoholics compared to only 20% of non-alcoholic people.

It was Dr. Blum who developed the unique amino acid treatment plan for addictions, as the result of 30 years of painstaking research. "Because the brain reward cascade is a linear sequence of brain chemicals, Dr. Blum determined that certain intervention approaches could help to balance this important function and produce beneficial *restorative* effects," Dr. Holder explains. The amino acids, in other words, are necessary precursors, or building blocks, for the brain reward cascade chemicals (called neurotransmitters) which are chronically deficient in the addicted person.

Second, according to Holder's research, an estimated 90% of babies born through forcep or suction-cup assisted deliveries, arrive in this world with a subluxation. If the infant has the genetic defect associated with addiction and gets its spine dangerously stretched and misaligned at birth, then the chances of becoming an addicted adult are very high, Holder claims.

What's the connection between a subluxated spine and addictions? It has to do with a precise sequence of chemical changes in your brain called brain reward cascade. If this cascade goes well with no interferences, you feel good, full of well-being and pleasure: if the sequence is interfered with, you may start looking to mood-altering substances or activities to fill the gap. These brain chemicals are called neurotransmitters and they must be released in the right sequence (like falling dominoes) for you to feel good.

The biochemical bottom line here at the end of this cascade is called dopamine, and, for those born with the genetic defect, their dopamine will never work right. If your brain releases it, you feel good. The dopamine reward may be the biochemical secret to understanding addictions.

When your spine is out of alignment, or subluxated, says Holder, it interrupts this important biochemical sequence in your brain. You start experiencing disturbing emotions and crave substances to change, relieve, or suppress your feelings. But how does a subluxation somewhere in your back interfere with the flow of chemicals in your brain? This is where Holder's theory gets *very* interesting. Your brain is not just in your head, but in your spine as well.

Brain scientists explain that your emotions take place in the midbrain (also called the *limbic* system). Your sense of well-being, biochemically speaking, is seated in the limbic system. The brain reward cascade takes place here. Now, the limbic system has outposts throughout the spinal cord in little anatomical features called the "dorsal horn," according to groundbreaking research by the renowned scientist Dr. Candace Pert who discovered this in 1988. In other words, your limbic system is represented throughout the entire spinal cord.

This means if your spine is subluxated anywhere along its length, this condition interferes with your limbic system and the flow of feel-good chemicals in your head. If you are a person with the specific genetic flaw associated with addictions, you will probably never have that same feeling of self-contentment, pleasure, and total well-being available to the rest of the nonaddicted population. You may take up addictive substances or activities to compensate.

There is yet another intriguing link. It turns out that children who have Attention Deficit Hyperactivity Disorder (ADHD) or Tourette's Syndrome, also have this identical genetic defect. In other words, Holder explains, compulsive disorders affecting children is our nation's number one pediatric complaint. They affect 5–8% of boys and 2–19% of girls, and are highly similar in cause to addictions. This also means that what successfully treats adult addictions can be highly useful with hyperactive children. Holder proved this by reversing abnormal brain waves in ADHD patients using his Torque Release Technique.

The good news and the beauty of the approach is that when you remove the addict's subluxation, as Dr. Holder did with Johnny, you allow the brain reward cascade of feel-good biochemicals to run properly again, perhaps for the first time in the person's life. This in turn enables you to feel good and no longer seek outside substances to produce a sense of well-being.

There are about 50,000 chiropractors practicing in America today. This means that any addicted person or child with hyperactivity who goes to a chiropractor who treats subluxations can probably expect some immediate relief from their addicted or compulsive behavior, Holder says. You might say that chiropractic gets the dopamine flowing again, balancing the brain reward cascade. While a chiropractor who removes subluxations will most likely help an addicted person to start feeling better, you get even better results by far if your chiropractor is trained in all the protocols of addictionology.

If you go to a chiropractor trained in Dr. Holder's Torque Release Technique (TRT) or to one who has graduated from Dr. Holder's Certified Addiction Professional (CAP) program, you're likely to get the best results. "Because addiction is a multifactorial disease, you need a multifactorial approach to get the best results. We consider TRT the 'faster car' for addiction treatment," Holder says. Through his American College of Addictionology, Dr. Holder is training health professionals all over the U.S. in a 120-hour Certified Addiction Professional program; he's also teaching TRT to as many chiropractors as he can manage.

The result is that chiropractic is poised to make a dramatic leap forward in what they can offer the public as the nation's second largest primary health care profession. As a leading modality in alternative medicine, Holder says, chiropractic offers the public something that conventional medicine cannot: a *drugfree* addiction treatment program. Johnny never got better with the drugs his psychiatrists prescribed because they were mood-altering substances; they simply reinforced his addiction, making him dependent on yet other chemical substances to feel better.

This is the big news. We now have a bold new approach to treating addictions that has a very high success rate and is highly cost-effective. It works so well because it removes the interference (the subluxation) to the brain reward cascade and allows you to feel good about yourself," Holder says.

Dr. Holder is getting astonishing results in places where previously no one dared to tread. This is the area of pregnant cocaine addicts. Normally women in this condition find no sympathy in America's 8000 addiction treatment programs on account of the staggering insurance liabilities. Even worse, the local governments tend to regard them as criminal child abusers and arrest them, severing them from their children, and thus creating families that are even more broken and dysfunctional.

The statistics are grim, says Dr. Holder, but there are some communities in the U.S. today where 15% of all babies born are drug babies, born to mothers who were addicted while carrying the fetuses. In contrast, 15 years ago, this situation was unheard of, which means the incidence of drug babies has been growing by 1% a year. If this continues for another two generations, we could be looking at a situation in which there are no normal babies born at all, Dr. Holder says. This is why his was one of ten addiction treatment programs that made a bold proposal to the federal government a few years ago to take a new approach.

A colleague of Dr. Holder, Matthew Gissen, executive director of Village Treatment Center, came up with an innovative concept in treatment program design. The solution was what Drs. Holder and Gissen call, affectionately, the "pregnant mommie house." This is a refitted 7-story building in Miami where addicted pregnant women come for treatment. They have their babies and continue the treatment program for up to 2 years—without the fear of arrest, reprisal, or punishment for so-called child abuse. The approach worked so well, says Dr. Holder, that today there are about 50 similar programs scattered around the U.S.

One day Dr. Holder walked into the pregnant mommie house. A young woman grabbed his arm with a happy gleam in her eye. She brought him into her room where she proudly displayed her healthy newborn baby, barely a week old. She asked Dr. Holder to cradle her son and share the moment, as this was truly a special, rare moment, in which all the work of doctor and patient came to a happy resolution.

"If you could just see the look in that mother's eyes, her pride and self-esteem that she had experienced the miracle of recovery, that she had accomplished something truly important for her son," says Dr. Holder. There she was, a drugfree mother with her drugfree newborn. The drug addiction would not be passed on to the next generation, not with this mother. "She was actually realizing *in that moment* that she had conquered a life-threatening disease and would not pass it on to her child—you couldn't leave that room with a dry eye," Dr. Holder adds.

All of this leaves chiropractic looking pretty good on its 100th anniversary. Acupuncturists get excellent results in treating addictions but there are only 7000 of them for a population of 256 million. Conventional doctors can't successfully treat addictions because there is no addiction training in medical school and doctors prescribe mood-altering drugs that can keep the addicts addicted to substances and at risk to relapse.

Chiropractors are thus the logical primary intervention resource to deal with the nation's number one cause of death," says Holder. How this daring claim plays out in the profession's next 100 years remains to be seen, but nobody expects recovered addicts like Johnny to argue the point.

FRAME the DEBATE

Form at end of book

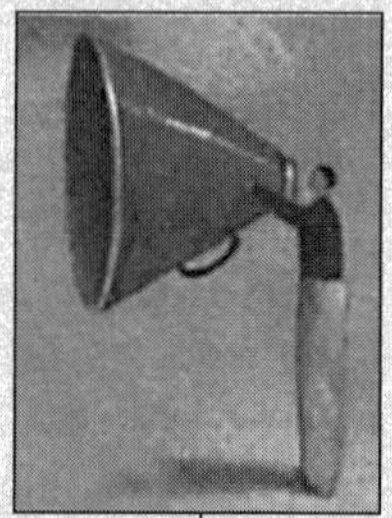

Issue 12: Is it time to reexamine our approach to addictions?

Half Steps vs. 12 Steps

Health: Can moderation help problem drinkers?

Michel Marriott

With Myron Stokes in Detroit, Patricia King in San Francisco and Bob French in Seattle.

On every Tuesday evening a modest room in a church annex in Ann Arbor, Mich., stirs with the business of repairing broken lives. Alcohol has licked each of the eight or so people gathered here more than once. So they have turned to each other in this circle of chairs and affection to try a program of reform. But this is not a meeting of Alcoholics Anonymous. In fact, few in this support group, who, like AA members, wish to remain anonymous, call themselves alcoholics. This is Moderation Management, or MM. Instead of hearing alcoholics support each other's vows to never drink again, MM members listen to "Ralph," who for decades eased his daily commute from the suburbs with booze. Now, he wants not to abstain completely, but just to drink less. "Betty," a housewife, says she used to drink a bottle of wine nightly. "Now I drink a fraction of that." The gathering nods.

For roughly 60 years, Alcoholics Anonymous and similar programs have dominated therapeutic thinking, treating alcoholism not as a behavior but as a disease—insisting on abstinence. But a growing number of moderation programs across the country are challenging that model. Moderation advocates distinguish between "chronic drinkers," who are "severely dependent on alcohol," and who have long histories of substance abuse, and "problem drinkers," whose bouts with alcohol have lasted five years or less and do not suffer physical withdrawal when they abstain. Proponents of moderation contend that problem-drinkers can still maintain careers and families—and they can learn to manage their drinking without eliminating it entirely. Moderation supporters acknowledge that their approach isn't for everyone. But they also cite studies, including one by the American Society of Addictive Medicine, indicating that problem drinkers outnumber hard-core alcoholics four to one.

New Rules for Sobriety

Like Alcoholic Anonymous with its 12 steps, Moderation Management has steps, guidelines and limits.

MM Limits

- *Do not drink every day:* MM suggests that you do not drink more than three or four days per week.
- *For women:* Do not drink more than three drinks on any day, and no more than nine drinks per week.
- *For men:* Do not drink more than four drinks on any day, and no more than 14 drinks per week.

Source: Moderate Drinking by Audrey Kishline

Most moderation programs have codes of conduct much like AA's 12 steps—but without spiritual references. Drink/Link, a seven-year-old program in Northern California, teaches people not to drink more than one drink an hour. MM suggests abstinence for three or four days a week. Practically all of the programs insist that problem drinkers begin with alcohol-free periods of 30 to 90 days. At the University of Washington in Seattle, researchers are preaching "harm reduction." Using a mock bar and nonalcoholic beer, students are taught that some of drinking's effects, like slurred speech, can be psychosomatic—you expect to feel drunk, and you do. So, students are told, they don't need to drink that much to have a good time.

Some problems drinkers, especially those who fail at cutting back, use moderation as a road to abstinence. Albuquerque, N.M., psychologist Reid Hester says this slower process of kicking the habit is called "warm turkey." Success rates for moderation programs are hard to determine. Research in Canada showed that after a year about 50 percent of those using moderation were drinking within its guidelines, but critics ask whether these programs will be effective over the long haul. Many participants say they now live normal lives without being stigmatized. "The monkey fell off my back when I realized that I wasn't an alcoholic, that I wasn't out of control," says Audrey Kishline, who founded Moderation Management and wrote a new book, *Moderate Drinking: The New Option for Problem Drinkers.* Kishline says that many European countries widely use moderation. In the United States evidence mounts that one treatment model may not fit all. A 1994 publication of the National Institute on Alcohol Abuse and Alcoholism says that "moderate drinking may be an acceptable goal" for some drinkers with a "relatively mild" problem.

The stakes are high in this emotional clash of philosophies: there are some 15 million alcoholics and problem drinkers in the United States. To Kevin, a recovering alcoholic from Chicago, all the moderation talk is a "kind of rationalization to keep drunks drinking. If I could drink like that, I wouldn't have the problem." Many who treat alcoholics are equally skeptical of what they see as a dangerous delusion. Paul Wood, president of the National Council on Alcoholism and Drug Dependence, worries that alcoholics might get wind of the moderation message and tumble off the wagon. "Every alcoholic's great dream," he says, "is to be a moderate drinker again." For most experts, AA's "one day at a time" still beats moderation's one drink at a time.

FRAME the DEBATE

Form at end of book

R E A D I N G 3 3

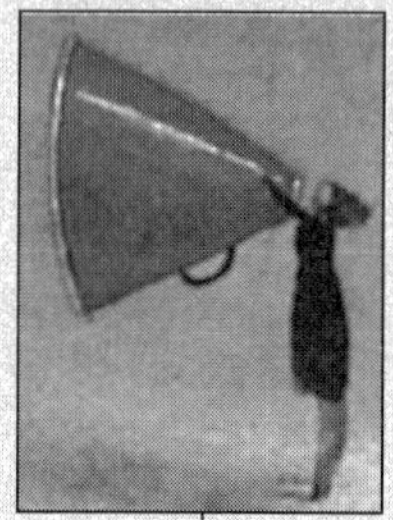

Issue 12: Is it time to reexamine our approach to addictions?

Alcohol Abuse and Dependence

Lester Grinspoon, M.D.
and James B. Bakalar, J.D.

With contributions from Paul S. Appelbaum, M.D., Herbert Fingarette, Ph.D., Marc A. Schuckit, M.D., and George E. Vaillant, M.D.

Treatment of Alcoholism

Alcohol abuse is not only the world's most common drug problem but one of the hardest to treat. The best approach is uncertain at every stage, from diagnosis to precarious recovery. No two cases respond to the same handling. But the situation is far from hopeless; even some of the most severely ill alcoholics recover with or without formal treatment, and health care professionals can help to create conditions for recovery.

The first step is to identify and acknowledge the disorder. Alcohol abusers, feeling ashamed and guilty, often refuse to admit the problem to themselves and try to conceal it from their families, friends, and physicians, who in turn may avoid acknowledging it for fear of being intrusive or having to take responsibility. Probably more than half of the alcoholics seen by doctors are not diagnosed correctly, even though the problem that brings them to the doctor's office is often related directly or indirectly to drinking.

Denial and obliviousness are not the only sources of misunderstanding. In a society that has so many heavy drinkers, it is not always easy to decide when a drinking problem has become so serious that special help is needed. Professionals are often as doubtful and confused about these issues as the lay public. Drinkers are not neatly divided into the healthy and the diseased, or the many who have no problems and the few who have many. Alcoholism can be hard to observe day by day, even if it's easily recognizable over a period of years.

Even when the signs of alcoholism are unmistakable, our society has not decided how to assign the task of coping with the problem or treating the disorder. Medical and mental health professionals often take it on reluctantly, doubtful whether they can help. Alcohol abusers themselves must often assume the burden, either as individuals or in groups like Alcoholics Anonymous. The alcoholic's family may be asked to deal with it, or society as a whole may be expected to take responsibility for preventing the disorder by proper transmission of drinking customs and regulation of alcohol sales.

Detoxification

Although a few experimental drugs offer promise, there is no established sobering agent—nothing that counteracts the effects of alcohol or speeds its breakdown and passage out of the body. Stimulants reverse some of alcohol's effects on thinking and motor coordination, but they are unreliable and have dangers of their own. Opiate antagonists do not affect alcohol intoxication or alcohol withdrawal.

Many alcoholics can withdraw on their own, but some are so severely dependent that they have to be detoxified—supervised as they go through a gradual withdrawal. The most common withdrawal symptoms are tremors, nausea, dry mouth, sweating, weakness, and depression. These symptoms begin six to eight hours after sudden withdrawal, reach their greatest intensity after ten to thirty hours, and subside in a few days. In especially severe cases (about 5 percent), the high fever, accelerated heart rate, agitation and hallucinations of withdrawal delirium (delirium tremens) began about two days after withdrawal. Many alcoholics are withdrawn in a clinic or hospital, either for the sake of their health and safety or simply to avoid temptation.

Withdrawal can be eased by substituting another central nervous system depressant—usually a benzodiazepine such as diazepam (Valium®) or chlordiazepoxide (Librium®)—and gradually reducing the dose to zero over a period of a week. The drug atenolol, which suppresses the sympathetic nervous system, reduces tremors and lessens the danger of cardiovascular symptoms by lowering heart rate, blood pressure, and body temperature in withdrawing alcoholics. It affects anxiety, agitation, and hallucinations less, but there is some evidence that it may speed up withdrawal by a day or two and reduce the need for benzodiazepines. Antipsychotic drugs are used only for delirious hallucinations.

Detoxification is relatively easy; the most complicated and frustrating part of treatment is preventing relapse. The most important principle is to deal with alcoholism itself immediately and directly. It is usually useless to try to solve some other psychological or social problem first and hope that drinking will then stop. Whatever the original cause of drinking, it eventually comes to dominate the alcoholic's life, and continuing uncontrolled alcohol use makes any kind of therapy impossible. The family, in particular, should not be blamed. Wives, husbands, and children need help in dealing with the problem, not treatment for themselves. That kind of help is supplied by family counseling and by mutual aid groups like Alanon and Alateen.

Psychotherapy has a limited effect on alcoholics. It can hardly help them while they continue to drink, because alcohol abuse prevents real (as opposed to merely verbal) insight. Even for a temporarily sober alcoholic, psychotherapy alone is not enough. Patients who formally acknowledge their drinking problems may still harbor the conviction that they are basically different from other alcoholics. Therapy aimed at individual insight runs the danger of encouraging that belief and thus distracting attention from alcohol itself.

Nevertheless, psychotherapy can be helpful as part of the treatment. Emotional problems that result from drinking do not necessarily disappear immediately when the drinking stops; and some patient's have problems unrelated to their drinking that hinder recovery from alcoholism. A psychotherapist must begin by helping the patient recognize that alcohol abuse is the main problem. Patients need to be educated about the role alcohol has played in their lives. The therapist must not hesitate to give direct advice. Alcoholics must be confronted with the consequences of their actions and at the same time supported as they try to cope with the world in a sober state and create a new life for themselves. Keeping track of alcohol consumption is important to guard against a serious relapse.

Alcoholics must learn to develop internal controls, and they must be encouraged not to avoid difficulties and challenges because of fear that they might get drunk. They have to be helped to find substitutes for drinking as a way to spend leisure time. Psychotherapists also work with the family and encourage the patient to meet with other recovering and recovered alcoholics. Insight therapy is effective only when the patient attains stable sobriety, which usually takes a year or more. Before that, it may create anxiety and cause a relapse. Patients must understand that they should call the therapist instead of taking a drink, not after taking a drink.

Drug Treatments

Drugs are generally not very useful for sober alcoholics, and some drugs create a serious danger of dependence. A few alcoholics suffering from severe depression will be helped by antidepressants, but more often the depression results from alcohol abuse and clears up a week or two after withdrawal. Recent experiments suggest that lithium sometimes blocks the euphoria produced by alcohol and reduces the desire to drink. Although lithium is usually prescribed for mood disorders, it helps alcoholics who are not depressed as much as those who are.

The only drug now commonly given to recovering alcoholics is disulfiram (Antabuse®), which prevents the body from breaking down and excreting alcohol normally. Acetaldehyde, a toxic metabolite of alcohol, accumulates and causes nausea whenever the patient drinks. Disulfiram is not so much a treatment as one way to make treatment possible. Patients who take the drug every morning are likely to avoid drinking because they know the consequences are unpleasant. Instead of constantly having to choose whether to drink, they face the choice only once a day. The main problem is compliance. Disulfiram will not work unless the patient is committed to long-term change and needs protection only against momentary lapses. A common side effect is inflammation of nerve tissue (neuritis) causing numbness, pain, or paralysis in an affected area. Great care is necessary, because alcohol can be lethal to a patient taking disulfiram.

Behavior Therapy

Behavior therapists assume that alcohol abuse is a learned habit that can be unlearned by altering contingencies—the factors in a given situation that determine whether or not a person takes a drink. Early behavior therapists thought that alcoholics had become conditioned to use drinking as a way to relieve anxiety. To break this supposed conditioning, they experimented with such techniques as chemical and electrical aversion—giving electric shocks or injecting a nauseating drug while the alcoholic drank. These treatments have not been very successful, and most experts now think that conditioned anxiety is not the main cause of alcohol abuse.

More recently behavior therapists have emphasized cognitive behavioral therapy. Alcoholics are encouraged to identify and record the situations and feelings that cause them to drink. Then they are trained to avoid these situations and feelings and to substitute other responses. They may be taught how refuse drinks politely and how to monitor the level of alcohol in their blood by paying close attention to physical sensations. The therapist also encourages better diet and exercise. The aim is to learn a skill, the social skill of controlled drinking. Abstinence is not regarded as the ultimate goal but as one way, which may or may not be the best, to exercise self-control.

Alcoholics Anonymous

Group therapy allows alcoholics to rebuild the personal relationships they have lost through drinking. The results are new hope, new skills, and a new sense of community or family. Patients gain a sense of social effectiveness and power over their circumstances by finding a place in the group and helping others while helping themselves. Some varieties are couples therapy, psychodrama, and group therapy with a professional leader.

By far the most popular form of group treatment is Alcoholics Anonymous, one of the oldest and most respected mutual aid organizations. Founded in the 1930s by Bill Wilson, a recovered alcoholic, AA now sponsors 60,000 groups in 112 countries. In the United States it reaches 650,000 alcoholics a year; only half as many are treated by alcoholism clinics and physicians combined. The organization is decentralized and local chapters are largely autonomous. Rules are flexible and there is no hierarchy: Alcoholics Anonymous is sustained only by its members; contributions are not accepted from outsiders, and the name and image of AA are not used for any purpose except its main mission. Anonymity permits confidentiality and promotes humility. It allows principles to be placed before personalities and prevents the development of a leadership cult. Mental health and medical professionals may make referrals and serve as consultants, but they do not direct policy.

The Twelve Steps

The basic strategy of AA is known as the Twelve Steps. Recovering alcoholics must admit their powerlessness over alcohol and seek help from a higher power, which can be understood in any way an individual member chooses. Members are urged to pray or meditate to get in touch with that power. They are asked to make a 'moral inventory,' confess the wrongs they have done, beg forgiveness, make amends, and carry the message to other alcoholics. Alcoholics Anonymous takes the position that anyone who has once been an alcoholic is always an alcoholic; the disease can be arrested but vulnerability is permanent. The most famous AA slogans are "It's the first drink that gets you drunk," which states the goal of abstinence, and "One day at a time," which places present action before long-term planning and dreaming.

Members of AA are told that alcohol is the source of their problems but that they nevertheless must assume responsibility for their own recovery. When it works, the group provides a substitute for alcohol, a socially valuable form of dependence. It helps alcoholics regain their self-esteem and repair the damage they have done to themselves and others. At one time there was some mistrust between mental health professionals and AA. Many professionals were unsympathetic to AA's quasi-religious features, and AA members often felt that psychotherapists and other professionals had failed them. Mutual trust is much greater now, and most mental health and medical professionals who work with alcoholics recommend AA as part of the treatment.

Despite this universal recognition, it remains uncertain just whom AA helps and how much it helps. Controlled studies are difficult, and the time available for follow ups has usually been insufficient to judge long-term effects. Some skeptics say that recovering alcoholics continue to attend AA meetings only because they have already become socially stable enough to maintain abstinence. Many patients seen in alcoholism clinics may be there partly because they are so seriously ill that AA has been of no use or would be of no use.

One study suggests that AA may be especially helpful for a particular type of alcoholic. One hundred men treated at an urban alcoholism clinic were followed for eight years. By that time 29 had achieved stable abstinence (three years or more), and 15 of them had been to 300 or more AA meetings. Only one of the 71 still active alcoholics in the group had attended AA meetings that often. In general, social stability on admission to the clinic (for example, being married, being employed, having no arrests for drunkenness) made abstinence after eight years more likely, but social instability on admission increased the likelihood of faithful participation in AA. Both higher social stability and AA were important for recovery; alcohol abusers who started with fewer family and community ties were more likely to need AA. A warm early family life and high intelligence also improved the chance of success through AA.

Abstinence

A sometimes intense and angry dispute about the necessity for abstinence began in the 1960s when studies reported that some former alcoholics could continue to drink moderately. Most advocates of controlled drinking are behavioral or cognitive-behavioral therapists who see alcohol abuse as a bad habit or a personal or social problem. Defenders of abstinence, including Alcoholics Anonymous and many medical and mental health professionals, believe that loss of control is inevitable for an alcoholic once drinking starts. They tend to regard alcoholism as a disease whose progress can be arrested only by removing the poison that causes it.

Mark and Linda Sobell conducted the most famous study that reported a successful return to moderate drinking. They offered 20 severely alcoholic patients a program of intensive therapy including practice in controlled drinking. For comparison they treated three other groups of patients; two were given less intensive therapy and one was trained for abstinence. The Sobells found that after two years the patients who learned controlled drinking had significantly fewer alcohol problems than the others. Advocates of abstinence quickly challenged their methods and results. Ten years after treatment, outside researchers found that nine of the patients in the controlled drinking group were still alcoholic, six were abstinent, and four were dead. Only one could be regarded as a moderate drinker. Critics also questioned a study by the Rand Corporation suggesting that alcoholics could become social drinkers; outside researchers again found that many patients described in the study as social drinkers were actually still alcohol abusers. Because alcoholism is an episodic disorder, a short follow-up may give an illusory impression of control in a person who is destined to relapse.

After a quarter of a century, despite some unresolved questions, more and more professionals concerned with alcoholism are coming to a consensus on controlled drinking; it seems to be an option only for alcohol abusers who are not severely dependent and have relatively few drinking problems. They may still have a choice about how and when to drink, although they must observe rigid rules. Once the problems have become serious enough to require admission to an alcoholism clinic, returning to moderate drinking is rarely possible. The habit is too well-entrenched to be modified, and abstinence is the only way to correct it.

In one recent study patients discharged from several alcoholism treatment facilities were followed for three years. At the end of that time two-thirds were still alcoholic, 15 percent had been abstinent the whole time, and 12 percent were heavy drinkers (seven or more drinks a day at least four times a month) who nevertheless apparently had no serious problems. Only 6 percent drank moderately or occasionally. Although these patients had not been trained in controlled drinking, it is doubtful whether that would have changed the result. In fact, some authorities think that even when moderation is possible, aiming at abstinence may be the best way to achieve it, just as a low speed limit causes even the people who exceed it to drive more slowly than they otherwise would.

Benefits of Abstinence

How much does abstinence change the life of an alcoholic? Some studies suggest that serious tension, depression, feelings of inadequacy, and personality disorders often persist. The best evidence now is that abstinence does make a big difference, but only after a long time, as much as two or three years. This is a corollary of the episodic nature of alcoholism. Trying to stop drinking is one of the symptoms, and even succeeding at it for many months is no guarantee of recovery. One long-term study found that although alcoholics who had not had a drink in ten years were hardly distinguishable from people who had never been alcoholic at all, those who had been abstinent for less than three years had most of the same psychological and social problems as active alcoholics. (They were, however, less likely to die of illness caused by alcohol.)

Alcoholics in the first few years of abstinence have been compared with returning prisoners of war. Their world is unfamiliar, because they have been living in an environment created by alcohol. Feelings that have been blunted or suppressed come back to trouble them. They have lost a great deal of time and must start where they left off. Being sober, like being free after imprisonment, entails new responsibilities. Thus alcoholics in the early stages of abstinence often suffer from anxiety and depression and may find it difficult to hold a job or preserve a marriage. The resolution of these problems comes when they establish new personal relationships, rebuild old ones, and begin to develop confidence in their power to control their lives.

Spontaneous Recovery

Most recovery from alcoholism is not the result of treatment. Probably no more than 10 percent of alcohol abusers are ever treated at all, but as many as 40 percent recover spontaneously. Alcoholics with a stable job and family life have the best chance; age, sex, and the duration of alcohol abuse matter less.

It is naturally important to understand how and why alcoholics cure themselves. One way is by changing their social situation through marriage, a new job, a new love, or the self-esteem and sense of community provided by a religious commitment. Moments of crisis and conversion are often important. In one study, 29 alcoholics were interviewed after a year of abstinence sustained entirely on their own. Sixteen said they stopped drinking because they "hit bottom"—fell into despair or lost a job, a husband, or a wife. Six had become physically ill, and three had developed a physical aversion to alcohol (one while taking lithium). Three mentioned an incident (such as a drunk driving accident) that made them realize they had lost control, and four had a religious or spiritual experience. After a year, two still had a physical aversion to alcohol, and eleven, surprisingly, had lost the desire to drink soon after stopping. Sixteen still had to make themselves resist temptation, mainly by associating images of drinking with images of suffering.

Answers of this kind are worth attention, but they leave much to be explained. Crises and confrontations are common in the lives of alcoholics, but rarely lead to recovery. 'Hitting bottom' means different things to different people; some are ready to change their drinking habits after a serious family argument, while others are not moved even by landing on skid row.

Outcome

Recent research has made it clearer than ever that alcoholism is not always a progressive disease. Patterns of abuse are complicated, with remissions and relapses at varying intervals. The average problem drinker is 25 to 35, married, and working, and has never been treated for alcoholism. Fewer alcohol abusers are over 40; 'maturing out' is common, as in heroin addiction. Older alcoholics are more likely to have been treated but less likely to recover than younger ones, even when their symptoms are apparently similar.

The influence of treatment on these patterns is unclear. One of many difficulties in studying the outcome of this cyclical, episodic disorder is that patients usually come into treatment at a low point and therefore almost always improve for a while. Years of follow-up are needed to judge the effects of a treatment, and by that time the issue has often been complicated by intervening therapy and inability to find some of the original patients. Multimodality programs try to assign patients to forms of treatment that seem intuitively appropriate for them, but there is little solid evidence that any approach works better than any other, either for alcoholics in general or for a particular group of alcoholics. Time after time a method that was seemingly effective when applied by its enthusiastic originators has failed when other researchers repeated the experiment.

Clients who faithfully attend an alcoholism clinic are more likely to recover, but then people who already have stable marriages and jobs are more likely to attend consistently. The National Institute for Alcohol Abuse and Alcoholism (NIAAA) has reported that more than half of the patients treated for alcoholism at St. Elizabeth's Hospital in Washington, D.C. are sober after periods of one to five years. A Rand Corporation study found that two-thirds of patients at federally funded alcoholism clinics showed significant improvement after 18 months. But according to the best controlled study, elaborate and extensive treatment, including months-long hospital or sanitorium stays, does not have an unequivocal advantage over brief counseling or no treatment at all. (Some authorities question the increasing involvement of profit-making institutions in residential alcoholism rehabilitation.) In the eight-year follow-up of treated alcoholics discussed earlier, most continued their therapeutic contacts (Alcoholics Anonymous, alcoholism counseling, or group therapy), but most (71 percent) also continued to drink.

Cirrhosis of the liver, heart disease, and other illnesses caused by alcohol account for a very large share of medical costs. An estimated 25 percent to 40 percent of patients in general hospitals are being treated for complications of alcoholism. Alcoholics use health services four times more than non-alcoholics, and the medical expenses of their families are twice as high. Here at least treatment seems to help in the short run. Several studies suggest that outpatient alcoholism clinics pay for themselves by reducing the cost of medical care and the number of work days lost to sickness. But in the long run death rates are just as high in more intensively treated as in less intensively treated alcoholics, maybe because patients in poor physical health get preferential admission to detoxification facilities from which they are referred to counseling and therapy.

Prevention

Obviously, preventing alcohol abuse would be better than having to treat it, but less is known about prevention than about treatment. According to some studies, taxes that raise the price of alcohol and therefore reduce a society's total consumption have a more than proportionate effect on serious alcohol abuse. There are usually fewer alcohol problems in countries where the price of alcohol is high relative to the average income. It is less clear whether merely treating alcohol advertising is effective.

Some authorities believe that alcohol abuse would become rare if people were taught how to drink from an early age. This preventive behavioral therapy emphasizes taking alcohol only with food, only at certain times of day, and only to celebrate rather than to escape. Binge drinking and drunkenness should be subject to strong social disapproval. It should be made very clear when drinking is appropriate and what the informal penalties are for inappropriate drinking; weak, vague, and ambiguous rules and sanctions promote uncontrolled alcohol use. This kind of customary restraint is historically well established in some cultures and ethnic groups, but difficult to impose through public policy. People tend to resist any official demand for more restraint than their entrenched attitudes already endorse. There is also the question of which comes first—ability to drink safely and moderately, or effective customary restraints. It may be the absence of alcohol abuse that explains the survival of these customs, rather than the other way around.

A Debate

Whether alcoholism should be regarded as a disease is so important and controversial an issue that we have asked two experts to debate it. Herbert Fingarette, Ph.D., is Professor of Philosophy at the University of California, Santa Barbara and the author of Heavy Drinking: The Myth of Alcoholism as a Disease *(University of California Press, 1988). He has been a consultant on addiction to the World Health Organization. George E. Vaillant, M.D., is Raymond Sobel Professor of Psychiatry at Dartmouth Medical School and the author of* The Natural History of Alcoholism *(Harvard University Press, 1983).*

We Should Reject the Disease Concept of Alcoholism

by Herbert Fingarette, Ph.D.

Why do heavy drinkers persist in their behavior even when prudence, common sense, and moral duty call for restraint? That is the central question in debates about alcohol abuse. In the United States (but not in other countries such as Great Britain) the standard answer is to call the behavior a disease, 'alcoholism,' whose key symptom is a pattern of uncontrollable drinking. This myth, now widely advertised and widely accepted, is neither helpfully compassionate nor scientifically valid. It promotes false beliefs and inappropriate attitudes, as well as harmful, wasteful, and ineffective social policies.

The myth is embodied in the following four scientifically baseless propositions: (1) Heavy problem drinkers show a single distinctive pattern of ever greater alcohol use leading to ever greater bodily, mental, and social deterioration. (2) The condition, once it appears, persists involuntarily: the craving is irresistible and the drinking is uncontrollable once it has begun. (3) Medical expertise is needed to understand and relieve the condition ("cure the disease") or at least ameliorate its symptoms. (4) Alcoholics are no more responsible legally or morally for their drinking and its consequences than epileptics are responsible for the consequences of their movements during seizures.

The idea that alcoholism is a disease has always been a political and moral notion with no scientific basis. It was first promoted in the United States around 1800 as a speculation based on erroneous physiological theory, and later became a theme of the temperance movement. It was revived in the 1930s by the founders of Alcoholics Anonymous (AA), who derived their views from an amalgam of religious ideas, personal experiences and observations, and the unsubstantiated theories of a contemporary physician.

The AA doctrine won decisive support in the 1940s when a reputable scientist, E. M. Jellinek, published an elaborate statistical study of the "phases of alcoholism." He portrayed an inevitable sequence of ever more uncontrollable drinking that led progressively to such symptoms as blackouts, tolerance, and withdrawal distress, until the drinker "hit bottom" as a derelict, became insane, or died. Jellinek's work seems to put a scientific seal of confirmation on the AA portrait of the alcoholic. That was hardly surprising, since he had taken his data from questionnaires that were prepared and distributed by AA and answered by fewer than 100 self-selected members. Jellinek conscientiously acknowledged the source of his data and his reservations about its scientific adequacy. Nevertheless, his dramatic-tragic portrait of the alcoholic became widely accepted and is now part of American folk beliefs.

Recent scientific literature shows that in reality the typical pattern of heavy drinking fluctuates. Some drinkers with numerous and severe problems deteriorate; others markedly improve, or develop different problems. Some claim loss of control; others do not. Many heavy drinkers report no serious social problems associated with their drinking and are not recognized as alcoholics by friends, colleagues, or even their families.

The idea that alcoholics are constantly drunk is quite false. One leading researcher points out that "in any given month one half of alcoholics will be abstinent, with a mean of four months of being dry in any one-year to two-year period." During any ten-to twenty-year period, about a third of alcoholics "mature out" into various forms of moderate drinking or abstinence. The rate of maturing out is even higher among heavy problem drinkers not diagnosed as alcoholics. Undoubtedly there is a small group who follow a pattern resembling Jellinek's four phases; one objection to the disease concept of alcoholism is that it focuses attention mainly on this marginal group.

It is now widely believed that a biological cause of alcoholism has been discovered; some people are said to have a biochemistry or a genetic predisposition that dooms them to be alcoholics if they drink. The truth is less dramatic. There are certain so-called biological markers associated with heavy drinking, but these have not been shown to cause it. One supposed marker is the metabolism of alcohol into acetaldehyde, a brain toxin, in the bodies of people who are independently identifiable as being at higher risk of becoming alcoholics. Another proposed marker is the high level of morphine-like substances supposedly secreted by alcoholics when they metabolize alcohol. But almost all people with serious drinking problems have intermittent periods of sobriety during which all metabolic products of alcohol have been excreted. It is implausible that any residual effects, whether physical or psychological, could be so powerful as to override a sober person's rational, moral, and prudential inclination to abstain.

Recent studies have also been said to imply that alcoholism is a hereditary disease. But that is not what the genetic research shows. In the first place, these studies provide no evidence of a genetic factor in the largest group of heavy drinkers—those who have significant associated problems but are not diagnosable as alcoholics. Even among the minority who can be so diagnosed, the data suggest that only a minority have the pertinent genetic background. And even in this category, a minority of a minority, studies report that the majority do not become alcoholics.

It is not only misleading but dangerous to regard alcoholism as a genetic disorder. Heavy drinkers without alcoholism in their genetic backgrounds are led to feel immune to serious drinking problems, yet they have the greatest total number of problems. On the other hand, people who do have some hereditary disposition to alcoholism could easily become defeatist. Their risk is higher, and they should be aware of that, but their fate is still very much in their own hands.

The idea of a single disease obscures the scientific consensus that no single cause has ever been established. Heavy drinking has many causes which vary from drinker to drinker, from one drinking pattern to another. Character, motivation, family environment, personal history, ethnic and cultural values, marital, occupational, and educational status all play a role. As these change, so do patterns of drinking, heavy drinking, and "alcoholism." For example, alcohol is used in many so-called "primitive" societies, but their drinking patterns are not ours, and what we call alcoholism does not exist among them before contact with Europeans. That would not be true if alcoholism were a disease caused by chemical and neurological effects of drinking in conjunction with individual genetic vulnerability. The crucial role of psychology in alcoholics' drinking is demonstrated by experiments in which they are deceived about whether the beverage they are drinking contains alcohol. Their drinking patterns then reflect their beliefs; the actual presence or absence of alcohol is irrelevant.

Alcoholics do not "lack control" in the ordinary sense of those words. Studies show that they can limit their drinking in response to appeals and arguments or rules and regulations. In experiments they will reduce or eliminate drinking in return for such rewards as money, social privileges, or exemption from boring tasks. To object that these experiments are invalid because they occur in protected settings is to miss the point, which is precisely that the drinking patterns of alcoholics can vary dramatically in different settings.

True, alcoholics often resist appeals to cease their alcohol abuse, and they ignore obvious prudential and moral considerations. The simplistic explanation that attributes this to an irresistible craving obscures a more complicated reality: they have developed a way of life in which they use drinking as a major strategy for coping with their problems. They have become accustomed to values, friends, settings, and beliefs that protect and encourage drinking. When they encounter drastically changed circumstances in a hospital, clinic, or communal group, they are capable of following different rules. Even some who "cheat" where abstention is expected nevertheless limit their drinking to avoid being found out. They do not automatically lose control because of a few drinks. Our focus of attention must shift from drinking per se to the meaning of drink for certain persons and the way of life in which its role has become central.

Responsible scientists who are familiar with the research but want to preserve the disease concept of alcoholism have had to redefine their terms. What they now mean by "disease" and "loss of control" no longer coincides either with the customary meaning of these words or with what the public is encourage to believe. Thus Mark Keller, one of the early leaders of the alcoholism movement, now reinterprets loss of control to mean that alcoholics who have decided to stop "cannot be sure they will stand by their resolution." This is said to be compatible with anything from constant heavy drinking to remission in the form of permanent moderation or total abstention. Although the medical term "remission" is used, this is not a medical or scientific explanation: we all know that someone who resolves to change a long-standing way of life cannot be sure whether the promise will be kept. Similarly, craving, still popularly understood as an overwhelming and irresistible desire, has now been extended by researchers to include mild inclinations, although this makes nonsense of the supposed compulsion to drink.

The disease concept is sometimes justified on the ground that although scientifically invalid, it is a practical way of encouraging alcoholics to enter treatment. This argument is based on false assumptions and has harmful consequences. The many heavy drinkers who see themselves (often correctly) as not fitting the criteria for alcoholism under some current diagnostic formula are likely to conclude that they have no cause for concern. Their inclination to deny their problems is thus encouraged. As for people who are diagnosable as alcoholics, the vast majority never become permanently abstinent, even after treatment or after they join AA. Yet the disease doctrine may cause them to develop a fatalistic conviction that even one slip is a disaster, since they have been led to believe, falsely, that occasional or moderate drinking is never possible for them.

When behavior is labeled a disease, it becomes excusable because it is regarded as involuntary. This is an important result of the disease concept of alcoholism, and indeed an important reason for its promulgation. Thus special benefits are provided to alcoholics in employment, health, and civil rights law, provided they can prove that their drinking is persistent and very heavy. The effect is to reward people who continue to drink heavily. This policy is insidious precisely because it is well intended, and those who criticize it may seem to lack compassion.

The United States Supreme Court, after reviewing detailed briefs pro and con, has consistently held in favor of those who say that alcoholics are responsible for their behavior, and has concluded that medical evidence does not demonstrate their drinking to be involuntary. Spokesmen for the National Council on Alcoholism (NCA) state publicly that they too believe alcoholics should be held responsible for their misdeeds, but they are being hypocritical. In the less visible forum of the federal courts, the NCA has repeatedly argued that alcoholics should be protected from criminal and civil liability for their acts and excused from the normal regulatory requirements.

But the greatest scandal of the argument for the disease concept as a useful lie is the claim that it helps alcoholics by inducing them to enter treatment. On the contrary, both independent and government research show expensive disease-oriented treatment programs to be largely a waste of money and human resources. Their apparent success proves illusory when they are compared in statistically rigorous studies with other programs, and with the rate of improvement in untreated alcohol abusers (which is a much higher rate than the disease concept has led the public to believe). Very often, perhaps always, brief outpatient counseling works just as well as a long stay in a hospital or other residential clinic costing thousands of dollars. Some studies conclude that professional intervention is slightly better than no treatment, although the treatment method, duration, setting, or cost makes no difference. Other studies find no significant difference in results whether or not there is treatment.

We must refocus our compassion and redefine our policies on alcohol abuse. While continuing biological research, we should loosen the grip of physicians on the chief government agencies and research funding sources, and we should reject their deep bias in favor of the disease concept. Greater resources must be shifted to psychological and sociocultural research. We should consider promising new approaches to treatment that are being used in other countries. The public should be better informed about the scientific facts and above all about our scientific ignorance. Our policies should reflect the fact that heavy drinking is not primarily a biochemical or medical problem but a human and social one.

We Should Retain the Disease Concept of Alcoholism

by George E. Vaillant, M.D.

When I read expert discussions of why alcoholism is not a disease, I am reminded of the equally learned discussions by "the best and the brightest" of why the Viet Nam War was a good idea. These discussants had intelligence, advanced degrees, scholarship, prestige, literacy—every qualification but one. They lacked experience. None had spent much time in Viet Nam. Just so, the philosopher Herbert Fingarette, the psychoanalyst Thomas Szasz, the sociologist and theoretician Robin Room, and provocative, thoughtful psychologists like Stanton Peele and Nicholas Heather have every qualification but one for explaining why alcoholism is not a disease—they have never worked in an alcohol clinic. Why, I wonder, do experienced alcohol workers and recovering alcoholics, the thousands of competent common folk in the trenches, accept the view that alcoholism is a disease? Why is it mainly less competent people, the active alcoholics, who agree with Professor Fingarette that they are just "heavy drinkers"?

I will begin with a summary of evidence provided by the legion of learned academics who have pointed out the folly of the medical model of alcoholism. First, alcohol abuse—unlike coughing from pneumonia, for example—is a habit under considerable volitional control. Second, there is compelling evidence that variations in alcohol consumption are distributed along a smooth continuum, although a medical model would suggest that in any individual, alcoholism is either present or absent. Third, when alcoholism is treated as a disease it can be used both by individuals and by society to explain away major underlying problems—poverty, mental deficiency, crime, and the like—which require our attention if efforts at prevention, treatment and understanding are to succeed. Fourth, to diagnose people as alcoholic is to label them in a way that can damage both self-esteem and public acceptance. Fifth, alcoholism should not be considered a disease if it is regarded as merely a symptom of underlying personality or depression.

Let me try to refute these objections one by one. First, it may be true that there is no known underlying biological defect in alcoholism. Rather, alcohol abuse is a multidetermined continuum of drinking behaviors whose causes are differently weighted for different people and include culture, habits, and genes. But the same can be said of high blood pressure and coronary heart disease. The incidence of hypertension varies with measurement procedures and psychological circumstances. It lies on a physiological continuum which defies precise definition. It has no known specific cause. It is powerfully affected by social factors; for example, it has become epidemic among young urban black males. The point of using the term 'disease' for alcoholism is simply to underscore that once a person has lost the capacity to control consistently how much and how often he or she drinks, continued use of alcohol can be both a necessary and a sufficient cause of a syndrome that produces millions of invalids and causes millions of deaths.

The second objection to the medical model of alcoholism is that only opinion separates the alcoholic from the heavy drinker. Supposedly one either has a disease or does not have it; diagnosis should depend on signs and symptoms, not value judgments. But consider the example of coronary heart disease. We regard it as a medical illness, although its causes are diverse and often poorly understood and there is no fixed point at which we can decide that coronary arteries become abnormal. So it is with alcoholism. Normal drinking merges imperceptibly with pathological drinking. Culture and idiosyncratic viewpoints will always determine where the line is drawn.

The third objection is that alcoholism is affected by so many situational and psychological factors that the drinking must often be viewed as reactive. Some people drink uncontrollably only after a serious loss or in certain specific situations, and some alcoholics return to normal drinking by an act of will. But these observations are equally true of hypertension, which often has an extremely important psychological component. Nevertheless, prospective studies show that alcohol dependence causes depression, anxiety, and poverty far more often than the other way around. In citing psychological problems as a cause of alcoholism, Fingarette reverses the position of cart and horse.

The fourth objection to calling alcoholism a disease is that it involves both labeling and a disparagement of free will. But in this case both labeling and the denial of free will are therapeutic. Some people believe that the label 'alcoholic' transforms a person into an outcast, akin to a leper. Well, should a doctor who knows that a person has leprosy keep the fact secret lest the patient be labeled a leper? Some people believe that if alcoholics are taught to regard alcoholism as a disease they will use this label as an excuse to drink or a reason why they should not be held responsible for their own recovery. It does not work out that way. Like people with high blood pressure, alcoholics who understand that they have a disease become more rather than less willing to take responsibility for self-care. That is why the self-help group, Alcoholics Anonymous, places such single-minded emphasis on the idea that alcoholism is a disease.

Once patients accept the diagnosis, they can be shown how to assume responsibility for their own care. Physicians stress the value of diagnosing hypertension early because it can provide a rational explanation for headaches and other symptoms that were hitherto regarded as neurotic or irrational. For years alcoholics themselves have labeled themselves 'wicked,' 'weak,' and 'reprehensible.' The offer of a medical explanation does not lead to irresponsibility, only to hope and improved morale.

The fifth argument against calling alcoholism a disease is the most compelling; it is said that uncontrolled maladaptive ingestion of alcohol is not a biological disorder but a disorder of behavior. Like compulsive fingernail biting, gambling, or child molesting, this form of deviant behavior can often be better classified by sociologists than by physiologists, and better treated by psychologists skilled in behavior therapy than by physicians with their medical armamentarium.

But unlike giving up gambling or fingernail biting, giving up alcohol abuse often requires skilled medical attention during acute withdrawal. Unlike gamblers and fingernail biters, most alcoholics develop secondary symptoms that do require medical care. Unlike child molesters, but like people with high blood pressure, alcoholics have a mortality rate two to four times as high as the average. In order to receive the medical treatment they require, alcoholics need a label that will allow them unprejudiced access to emergency rooms, detoxification clinics, and medical insurance.

The final argument for regarding alcoholism as a disease rather than a behavior disorder is that it often causes alcoholics to mistreat persons they love. Very few sustained human experiences involve as much abuse as the average close family member of an alcoholic must tolerate. Fingarette's "heavy drinking" model (which conveys a concept of misbehavior) only generates more denial in the already profoundly guilt-ridden alcoholic. Calling alcoholism a disease rather than a behavior disorder is a useful device both to persuade the alcoholic to acknowledge the problem and to provide a ticket for admission to the health care system. In short, in our attempts to understand and study alcoholism, we should employ the models of the social scientist and the learning theorist. But in order to treat alcoholics effectively we need to invoke the medical model.

Let me close with an anecdote. My research associate, reviewing the lives of 100 patients who had been hospitalized eight years previously for detoxification from alcohol, wrote to me that she mistrusted the diagnosis of alcoholism. To illustrate, she described one man who drank heavily for seven years after his initial detoxification. Although the alcohol clinic's staff agreed that his drinking was alcoholic, neither he nor his wife acknowledged that it was a problem. Finally he required a second detoxification, and the clinic staff claimed that they had been right. "How can you call such behavior a disease," my associate wrote, "when you cannot decide if it represents a social problem [i.e. requires a value judgment] or alcohol-dependent drinking?" Then she shifted her attention to the ninety-nine other tortured lives she had been reviewing. Oblivious of the contradiction, she concluded: "I don't think I ever fully realized before I did this follow-up what an absolutely devastating disease alcoholism is." I respectfully submit that if Professor Fingarette were to work in an alcohol clinic for two years, he would agree with the last half of my research associate's letter rather than the first half.

How Does the Law View Alcoholism?

We asked Paul S. Appelbaum, M.D., A.F. Zeleznik Professor of Psychiatry, University of Massachusetts at Worcester.

Is alcoholism a disease, or is it the self-indulgent behavior of people who do not want to stop drinking? In a recent case, *Traynor v. Turnage*, the United States Supreme Court faced that issue, and, if reports in the popular media are to be believed, found that alcoholism is not a disease. In fact, the decision and its aftermath are much more complicated. The controversy is worth examining for the light it sheds on the conflicting ways in which the law deals with alcoholism.

Traynor was a challenge to Veterans Administration (VA) regulations governing eligibility for educational benefits. Ordinarily these benefits must be used within 10 years of discharge from the armed forces, but an extension can be granted if the veteran is unable to use them because of a disability. The VA classified alcoholism as a legitimate disability only when it was secondary to another physical or psychiatric illness. According to the VA, the plaintiff's alcoholism constituted "willful misconduct."

The court was asked to decide whether this policy violated a section of the Rehabilitation Act that forbids discrimination against handicapped persons in federal programs. It ruled that Congress was aware of the VA classification when it amended the Rehabilitation Act to cover federal agencies. Thus the VA policy was not inconsistent with the law. The Court further ruled that Congress could reasonably take this view because there was "a substantial body of medical literature that even contests the proposition that alcoholism is a disease, much less that it is a disease for which the victim bears no responsibility." As the opinion emphasized, the Court was not declaring that alcoholism was not a disease, only saying that Congress and the VA could legitimately come to that conclusion.

Justice Blackmun dissented vigorously, echoing the American Medical Association and American Psychiatric Association, which had argued in amicus briefs that "willfulness" did not distinguish primary from secondary alcoholism. Blackmun said that the presence of willful misconduct should instead be determined individually, case by case.

It is important to understand what the majority opinion did and did not state. The Court found sufficient controversy about the nature of alcoholism to justify a Congressional decision to treat primary alcoholism as willful misconduct for a certain purpose. It did not conclude that alcoholism is not a disease for all legal purposes. Furthermore, the Court did not have the last word even on that limited issue. Several months after its decision, Congress explicitly forbade the VA to classify the effects of chronic alcoholism as a result of willful misconduct.

How is alcoholism viewed elsewhere in the legal system? Many states have laws permitting involuntary treatment of alcoholics. These laws generally apply to people who are said to have lost control over their drinking, which suggests a willingness to embrace the view that alcoholism is an illness. On the other hand, intoxication has never been an excuse for criminal acts, although it may mitigate the legal severity of the offense. The reasoning here is that the offender begins to drink voluntarily and therefore should bear responsibility for whatever illegal acts follow.

Given the uncertainty of medicine and the mental health professions about the nature of alcoholism, it would be surprising if the law was more consistent. Most health professionals regard alcoholism as a disease, but some do not. A prominent critic of the disease theory, Herbert Fingarette, was cited by the majority in *Traynor.* Furthermore, even if alcoholism is acknowledged to be a disease, the legal and medical implications are ambiguous. Although we often say that alcoholics lack control, most treatment programs encourage them to take responsibility for their drinking, and many experts are reluctant to say that willful behavior plays no part in initiating or perpetuating alcoholism. Until the nature of the impairment suffered by alcoholics is better understood, we can expect the law to go on reflecting our own divergent and sometimes inconsistent views.

FRAME the DEBATE

Form at end of book

WiseGuide Wrap-Up

Although few chemical dependency experts argue the existence of alcoholism and addictive behaviors, there is only fractional consensus on the nature of addictions. The disease concept of alcoholism is the most widely accepted theory among health professionals (including the American Medical Association and the American Psychological Association). Reexamination of the early research that formed the basis of the disease concept of alcoholism, however, points out certain methodological flaws.

Clearly, the disease concept has helped many addicts over the years, as evidenced by the success of Alcoholics Anonymous. On the other hand, it may also hamper addicts' efforts and the efforts of concerned others to control abusive and irresponsible drinking or drug use. Reliance on a single causation theory may, in fact, lead to misdiagnosis and ineffective treatment of a drug or alcohol abuser. The disease concept, it is argued, may be too inclusive and thus may misclassify individuals in terms of their drinking habits and the causes of their drinking behaviors.

Should we preserve a theory that seems to work moderately well by conducting supportive research? Or should we expand our paradigm to include a more diverse approach to this health problem?

R.E.A.L. Sites

This list provides a print preview of typical **Coursewise** R.E.A.L. sites. (There are over 100 such sites at the **Courselinks**™ site.) The danger in printing URLs is that web sites can change overnight. As we went to press, these sites were functional using the URLs provided. If you come across one that isn't, please let us know via email to: webmaster@coursewise.com. Use your Passport to access the most current list of R.E.A.L. sites at the **Courselinks** site.

Site name: Alcohol—An Interactive Assessment

URL: http://www.mayohealth.org/mayo/9707/htm/alcohol.htm

Why is it R.E.A.L.? This is an educational tool to help you evaluate either your or other's drinking patterns.

Key topics: alcohol, alcoholism

Try this: Take the self-test at the site. What patterns emerge in your evaluation? Does this site ascribe to the disease concept of alcoholism, or do the authors of the evaluation appear to employ other alternative models of alcohol abuse and addiction?

Site name: Alcohol Runs in Families

URL: http://www.health.org/pubs/alcruns/index.htm

Why is it R.E.A.L.? This site provides links to several alcohol-related informational pages.

Key topics: alcohol, alcoholism

Try this: Read the article "Alcoholism Tends to Run in Families." Does this article tend to bolster support for the disease concept of alcoholism? Does the information presented support a strong social influence on alcohol abuse behavior?

Section 5 Summary

No American college student who has been schooled in America since the 1950s needs to be informed that we have a serious drug and alcohol abuse problem in the United States. The health-care costs of alcohol and drug abuse alone are staggering. The National Institute on Drug Abuse and the National Institute on Alcohol Abuse and Alcoholism state that "The economic cost to society from alcohol and drug abuse was an estimated $246 billion in 1992. Alcohol abuse and alcoholism cost an estimated $148 billion, while drug abuse and dependence cost an estimated $98 billion."*

Conservative estimates for nicotine abuse place the annual death toll at around 420,000, whereas alcohol and illegal drugs account for upward of 133,000 deaths, with the largest proportion of lives lost between 20 and 40 years of age. Tobacco use is related to one in five deaths in America, according to the American Cancer Society. Clearly, the legal drugs—alcohol and nicotine—account for the largest proportion of unnecessary mortality, morbidity, and human suffering in America.

Beyond the extraordinary toll that tobacco, alcohol and illegal drugs take on American health, daily consumption of seemingly harmless substances such as caffeine may also pose a health threat.

In light of these startling statistics and a concern for personal health, the prudent and critical-thinking student is challenged to separate accurate information from the hyperbole and to ask important questions about the relative harm of substance abuse and the viability of proposed methods of control and treatment of abuse disorders.

*Executive Summary, http://www.nida.nih.gov/EconomicCosts/Chapter1.html#1.1.

STAND! **section 6**

Health Care in America

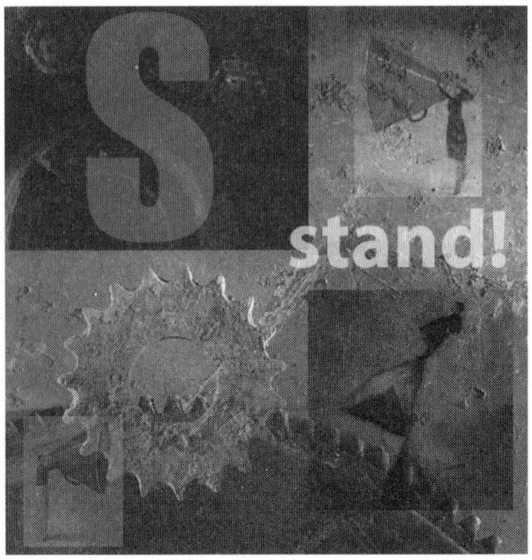

Learning Objectives

- Examine the economic, moral, and ethical issues involved in physician-assisted suicide.
- Debate the relative economic advantages and disadvantages of managed health-care systems and free-market health care.
- Explore the viability of alternative health-care practices in our current health-care delivery system.
- Examine your personal values regarding health care and cost containment.

Introduction

The question of the individual's right to die is a contemporary problem facing the American health-care system. As health care continues to advance, people are living longer and surviving the formerly un-survivable. The question facing the American public and health-care professions is the relative balance between quality and quantity of life. Further, it is a sad but undeniable fact that the majority of the American health-care dollar is spent on people dying of chronic disease in their last 2 years of life. Health and medical ethicists are faced with the issues of physician-assisted suicide and euthanasia.

The health-care industry in America is also facing the challenge of alternative health care in the free marketplace. Many individuals are frustrated with Western medicine and seeking alternative forms of health care. Western science and allopathic medicine have dominated health care in America for a hundred years. Now, the viability of alternatives to allopathic medicine is being considered. According to a study published in the *New England Journal of Medicine,* 25 percent of Americans seek alternative health-care methods. According to studies done by Landmark Health Care Company, nearly half of all Americans use alternative health-care methods regularly. Alternative forms of health care may or may not be effective and safe. However, alternative health care is often cheaper than conventional medicine, which makes it attractive to those wishing to contain health-care costs.

Health care in America is among the best in the world. We have the finest technology and the best medical schools. The availability and accessibility to quality health care is *theoretically* unmatched by any other industrialized nation. However, despite this positive picture, health care in America currently accounts for over 14 percent of the gross national product. From the early 1980s to the late 1990s, the cost of health care in America doubled! The exponential increase in health-care costs has placed quality health care out of the reach of more and more Americans.

As health-care costs continue to rise, cost containment measures are being pursued. One of these is the formation of health maintenance organizations (HMOs). HMOs operate in a similar fashion to other consumer cooperatives. Doctors and health-care practitioners are paid a salary to see patients who are co-op members. Patients and employers (called subscribers), on the other hand, prepay a membership fee and then, in some cases, pay a nominal co-pay fee with each visit. Critics complain that patients are limited in their choice of providers and treatments to only those that the HMO covers.

The readings in Section 6 explore the ethical and economic issues of physician-assisted suicide, the viability of alternative health-care practices, and the pros and cons of managed health-care programs.

Is Physician-Assisted Suicide a Viable Treatment Option for the Terminally Ill?

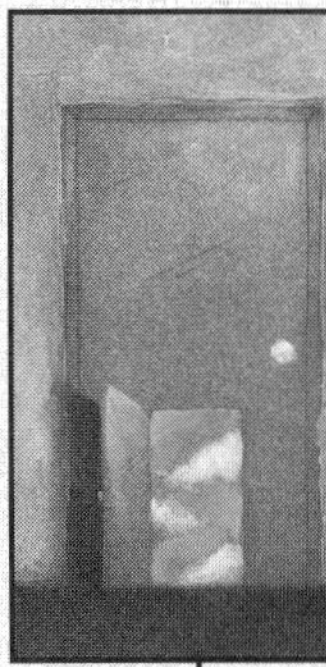

ISSUE 13

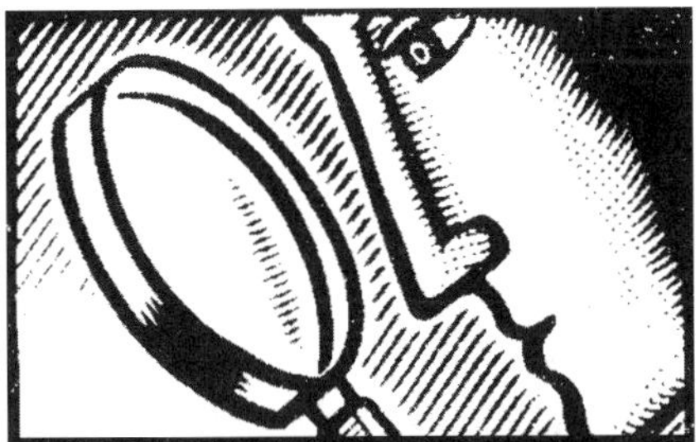

Take a Closer Look

1. In Reading 34, Garrison discusses Holland's physician-assisted suicide laws. About how many people in Holland ask their doctors to help them die each year?
2. Has this number increased as people feared it might when physician-assisted suicide became legal?
3. Garrison uses her mother's story as an example of the need for discussion on physician-assisted suicide. List three important ethical and moral decisions she faced in dealing with her mother's situation.
4. Define physician-assisted suicide.
5. What percentage of physicians support a patient's right to choose to die?
6. Name three organizations mentioned in Reading 35 that are opposed to physician-assisted suicide.
7. According to most medical ethicists and physicians, what are the three conditions that must be met to justify physician-assisted suicide?

WiseGuide Intro

Due to advances in emergency medicine and intensive care in the twentieth century, we are able to prolong life much further than in the past. Despite these advances, however, many trauma and medical patients are still going to die. As they die, the quality of their lives generally decreases, which raises the issue of preserving the quantity of life over the quality of life.

In the past five decades, health-care costs have reached enormous proportions. Continued care for the terminally ill consumes astronomical amounts of health-care dollars and resources, and greatly burdens families, hospitals, and federal and private health-care insurance systems. One answer to the issue of quantity over quality of life and the health-care resource drain is physician-assisted suicide.

There are basically two forms of physician-assisted suicide: (1) active assistance, where a physician actually administers a lethal dose of a drug or substance such as carbon monoxide or provides the patient with the drug or substance, and (2) passive assistance, where health-care professionals withdraw life-support care from the terminally ill and allow "nature to take its course."

Proponents of physician-assisted suicide see it as a responsible way of ending human suffering and of preserving dignity and health-care resources. Opponents argue that it is immoral, unethical, and an irreversible medical decision, and that it may position our society on a slippery slope of deciding who lives and who dies for less than humanitarian reasons.

In Reading 34, "Rushing Heaven's Door: Assisted Suicide—Do We Really Know What We Want?" Jayne Garrison uses firsthand examples to illustrate the slippery moral and ethical slope encountered when considering physician-assisted suicide for a loved one. She also looks at the current state of sanctioned euthanasia in the Netherlands, where physician-assisted suicide is much lower than expected. Garrison uses university study results and expert commentaries to support her opposition to physician-assisted suicide.

In Reading 35, "Legalizing Physician-Assisted Suicide: Some Thoughts and Concerns," Harold Koenig takes an impartial and detached stance regarding physician-assisted suicide by describing related terms and arguments for and against the practice. He presents some statistics regarding the feelings of physicians toward physician-assisted suicide, along with some data on specific California and Washington State laws and initiatives regarding physician-assisted suicide. In the second half of the reading, Koenig explores the ambiguities in terminal illness and suffering, diagnosis, and decision making that physicians, patients, and family members face. He also examines some of the problems facing Dutch physicians and suggests alternatives to physician-assisted suicide as his reading summary.

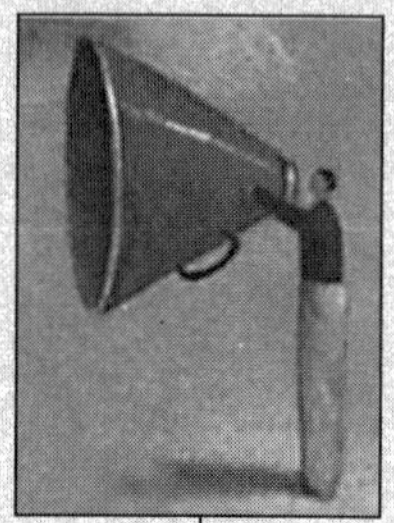

Issue 13: Is physician-assisted suicide a viable treatment option for the terminally ill?

Rushing Heaven's Door:
Assisted Suicide—Do We Really Know What We Want?

Would you help end the life of a parent you were sure wanted to die? I was ready to.

Jayne Garrison

Jayne Garrison is the news editor of Health.

My mother is a woman who didn't go to funerals and who never cried. When her closest friend killed herself after struggling with breast cancer for five years, my mother said only, "This wasn't suicide. It was a reasonable choice." She believed we live once, like every other animal on earth, and when that life is ending there is no reason to hang on or to mourn. And if, through a twist in time, I could show her at age 40 a video of herself today, I can hear what she would say. "Oh Gawd," she'd drawl, exhaling blue smoke from her Virginia Slim. "Not this gal." She never wavered from her unsentimental view of life, and she instilled it in me as well. So when I got the phone call, I knew what we should do. "She's bleeding internally," my younger sister said, crying, a few weeks after she'd taken our ailing mother into her home. "She's got stomach ulcers so bad they can't stop it. They could operate, but Mom might die during the surgery. What do we do?" I took my own shaky breath. "Don't let them do anything," I said. "She wants to go peacefully. Please. We've got to respect her wishes." I was sure I was right. That certainty troubles me now as I listen to the national debate over legalizing assisted suicide. When my elderly and confused mother was dying, no doctor tried to convince us of the need for heroic measures. The hospice nurse even gave us information we could have used to gently speed her death. If my sisters had not hesitated when I insisted our mother wanted no intervention, she probably would have died. And I would never have known that she had changed her mind.

For two years, ever since my father died in his sleep of a heart attack, it had seemed to me my mother was waiting to go. Her greatest fear was that we would take her away from her home in Idaho and force her to live with one of us. When the tenant in the small apartment below our house moved, I put on my best, brightest daughter voice to call her. "It's perfect and just waiting for you!" My mother hung up on me. My sister tried. "The kids want you here so much. They've already figured out which room is yours." My mom laughed and said, "Don't be a pain."

We wanted to save her, but we couldn't give her the younger, healthier self that was gone. So she withdrew, refusing to go to doctors or to allow any help in her home. Finally nature took the stand we could not. Last year the ceiling of my mother's living room collapsed under the weight of freezing snow. She didn't call for help. When the boy next door stopped by, she told him to go away. She slipped into a cold unconsciousness and lay on the floor for three days before neighbors broke in.

The doctors diagnosed vascular dementia: A series of tiny strokes was gradually destroying her brain. My mother, this invulnerable woman who lied about her age and cut short polite ladies in town with, "Oh, darling, that's a load of bull," could never live independently again.

I took her back to San Francisco with me, to live in the apartment downstairs. She blossomed those first few weeks. Despite her frailty, she tapped her foot to the beat at my older son's third-grade sock hop and watched his hockey games in the cold stadium. She petted her grandsons with sarcastic praise—"You know if you got any smarter your head would explode"—just like the old days.

But after a while she began each morning with the same question: "When are you taking me home?" And when her doctor and I sat her down to explain she couldn't return home, ever, she put on her sunglasses in the dim office, hiding her eyes, and quipped in a choked voice, "My, the sun's bright in here." I took her hand and asked, "What can I do to make this easier for you?" She turned away for a minute, then said, "I don't want to live a controlled life."

My mother began to fade then, as if she were willing herself to die. I never thought you could see someone die of old age, like I can't seem to catch my sons growing, though they shoot up inches in months. But I could actually see her let go of life.

One day as we sat on the sofa watching television, she suddenly slumped on my shoulder. "This is it," I thought. I considered calling 911. But the paramedics would crack her ribs to jump-start her heart. The hospital would bruise her with tubes. No. I would let her die in my arms. I sat there for half an hour, feeling frightened but also a little righteous. It was hard, having someone die in your arms, but I could do it, my last gift to her. Then, faintly, just as my arm around her numbed, I heard her snoring. Sheepishly, I put her to bed.

She didn't die that day, of course, but within the next few weeks—a terrible tunnel of time—she would fall on the stairs leading from her apartment to my house and be hospitalized twice. Realizing she could no longer manage the stairs, we decided that she would be better off living in Colorado with my younger sister, Jonna, who had offered to become our mother's full-time caretaker during her final days.

Then came the crisis, and Jonna's call. Sometime in the past couple of years, it seemed, ulcers had begun eating at my mother's stomach. There were three, so big they had perforated the stomach wall, which was hemorrhaging. Surgeons generally operate in such cases; they can cauterize the ulcers to stop the bleeding. But my mother was so fragile that surgery would probably have killed her. So the doctors started giving her blood transfusions, in the hope that the ulcers would stop bleeding on their own.

We were buying time, but our mother was paying the price. Her voice over the long-distance line was thin, raspy. "Get them to take these tubes out," she said. "I want to go home now."

I put down the telephone—and picked it up again to call Jonna. "No more transfusions!" I exploded. "It's cruel. We're just prolonging her pain."

If my sisters hadn't hesitated when I insisted our mother wanted no intervention, she probably would have died.

But Jonna resisted. If we stopped the transfusions, our mother would die in a day or two. My sisters decided that someone would have to ask our mother: Did she want to try to live?

No one wanted to have that conversation. We are a family that leaves things unsaid, especially about death; our mother had never even drawn up a will. We asked a doctor at the hospital to talk to her about her choices: to try the risky surgery, continue the transfusions, or stop treatment entirely. He told us that all she would say was, "Whatever you think is best."

Finally, after nine days and nine transfusions, the doctors said there was nothing more they could do. My older sister and I flew to Colorado. Together, we brought our mother to Jonna's house so she could die under hospice care in peace, surrounded by her daughters.

We fluttered around her, not knowing how to handle ourselves. The hospice nurse instructed us on how to draw the morphine into a syringe. Be careful, she warned. Here's how much you need to ease her pain; twice that amount could kill her. At last, I thought. If she wakes up in the middle of the night bleeding and crying, I'll be able to help her out of this nightmare.

Instead, on the second day at home, my mother grew stronger, more alert than she'd been in a month—and very wary. We'd never told her she was going to die, but she knew what hospice meant. She pushed herself up in bed, pointed out the kids playing, a blue jay on the fence, a cloud that might be bringing rain. She asked for the newspaper and commented on the headlines. It was as if she were saying, "Look, I'm not that sick." And every hour or so she'd ask me for her blood pressure medicine.

My God, I realized, she's afraid we've given up on her. She doesn't want to die.

I wanted to tell her not to worry: We wouldn't withhold her medicine or do anything to hasten her death, not if she didn't want us to. But I didn't, of course. I just held her hand while she got stronger.

On the fifth day of this bizarre reunion, my sisters and I sat around the kitchen table in an awkward silence. My older sister was due to fly home the next morning; my flight would leave the day after that. "So," I said finally, "we came to help her die. Looks like she doesn't want the help. What do we do now?"

Death with dignity. We talk about it a lot these days, and about the way that lifesaving advances often turn out to be mere death-delaying techniques or, worse, death-prolonging. So many of us have come to see the hospital as a place to fear that in two separate cases now being decided, patients have asked the Supreme Court to declare assisted suicide a constitutional right. But over the past year I've begun to believe the very concept of a good death misses a crucial point: Our definition of dignity changes as we grow older.

I'd seen that kind of shift occur even before I faced my mother's illness. My mother-in-law, Toni, was a wily, strong-willed woman who had escaped Hitler's Germany and survived the war in a Shanghai ghetto. She was as fiercely independent as my own mother and just as unsentimental about everything except her children. When she was diagnosed with Alzheimer's disease, my husband feared she would slide into an unrelenting depression because he thought she'd rather die than become a shell of the person she was.

Yet at every point she seemed content. We'd walk into her assisted-living apartment and find her laughing at some sitcom on TV. "What are you watching?" my husband would ask. "Oh, I don't know," she'd reply. And she meant it. In time she could no longer tell a TV comedy from a drama, and she didn't have a clue what she read when she picked up the paper. But she never seemed unhappy.

Age or sickness frequently prompts people to change their minds about what constitutes a tolerable quality of life, says Roger Evans, a sociologist at the Mayo Clinic who studies transplant patients. Early in the course of disease, he says, many people say they'd rather die than become infirm, require dialysis several times a week, or need a respirator to breathe. But when Evans analyzed survey responses of 1,407 transplant patients—including those who were disabled and dying—he found the patients beat out the rest of us in their feelings of contentment and happiness.

Other studies, too, show that insults of age like incontinence or senility, so outrageous when we are 40, can seem acceptable when we're 70. Perhaps that's why surveys have found that while most healthy, young adults support the legalization of assisted suicide, most frail, elderly people oppose it. Perhaps as they grew weaker and sicker they changed their minds about what type of life is worth living. Perhaps they fear that, disdainful of the quality of their lives, we will usher them out too quickly.

Any unease could only be worsened by the fact that we're not being quite honest in our public debate. We politely talk about assisted suicide; the headlines we read are about the desperate few who climb into Dr. Kervorkian's van to claim the right to die as they choose. But is it really the right to commit suicide that most people in the United States want? Or do they want someone else to end their lives for them when they are past all reason and joy?

One afternoon, as my husband and I drove home from visiting his mother at the board-and-care home, he quietly said, "Don't ever let me become like that. Assisted suicide's going to be legal soon. And even if it's not, if I get Alzheimer's, I want you to help me kill myself before I become an empty shell."

While most young adults support assisted suicide, most elderly people oppose it. Perhaps they fear their children will usher them out too quickly.

I twisted in my seat to face him. "At what point?"

He thought. "I don't know. Maybe when I'm not able to recognize anyone." Then, after a minute, "Or maybe, even if I don't recognize you, if I can still enjoy the sun and my food . . . I want you to help me kill myself when I can't enjoy anything anymore."

I grinned, the first wide-open grin I had enjoyed in some time. "That's not *assisted* anything, hon. It's murder. Euthanasia at best. And if I spend five or ten years taking care of you, I'm sure as hell not going to spend the last ten years of my life in prison."

The truth is, few people choose to kill themselves, even if they are in the final days of cancer. Look at the experience in the Netherlands, where assisted suicide and euthanasia have been tacitly allowed for 20 years. Only 400 people in that country of 15 million kill themselves under a physician's supervision each year. Most who want to die ask the doctor to do it for them: Every year 3,300 Dutch people are euthanized. That number has held fairly steady over the past five years (the first official survey on the matter wasn't done until 1990)—an indication that allowing doctors to hasten death doesn't send a nation tumbling helterskelter down a moral slippery slope. But the statistics aren't entirely reassuring. According to a study by the Dutch government, in 1,000 of those cases the doctor simply *assumes* the patient and family would prefer to avoid a slow death. The Dutch call this "termination of the patient without explicit request."

Studies done in the United States indicate that even close family members aren't very good at guessing what their ill or aged relatives want. In the nation's largest study of dying patients, known as the SUPPORT study, researchers asked 1,226 patients at five hospitals whether they wanted aggressive care at the end of life; then the researchers asked the families what they thought the patients would want. The families were wrong a quarter of the time. Often they chose aggressive care when a relative would want no intervention. But in a sizable minority of cases a family's mistake would have let a loved one go quietly when he or she wanted to fight for more time.

A study from Duke University shows that it's the most vulnerable among the elderly—the poor, women, and minorities—who are most likely to resist the notion of legal assisted suicide. Perhaps for good reason, says psychiatrist Herbert Hendin, who has studied the Netherlands's experience with euthanasia. Unlike the Dutch, who have a system of socialized health care, Hendin points out, Americans sometimes must choose between saving for their own old age and paying for a parent's nursing home. That dilemma burdens aged parents as well as their children: Last year data from the SUPPORT Study showed that patients were 30 percent more likely to say they wouldn't want life-prolonging treatment if it would cause economic hardship for their families. Such pressures, Hendin says, might be enough to make assisted suicide seem an obligation.

Hendin, who heads the American Foundation for Suicide Prevention, says most people who ask for assisted suicide really want help, not death. These are the same people who might consider suicide while young and healthy if life took a cruel turn, and professional support can bring them out of their despair. That's the doctor's job, he says: to ease physical pain with medicine and mental pain with talk therapy or drugs.

Internist Timothy Quill at the Genesee Hospital in Rochester, New York, sees the issue quite differently. Quill is among the doctors and patients urging the Supreme Court to declare assisted suicide a constitutional right. He has been identified with the movement since 1991, when he wrote about his experience with a dying patient. Diane had leukemia; Quill prescribed barbiturates, knowing she intended to use them to commit suicide. Doctors have the responsibility to give their patients good health or to make illness bearable, Quill says, and if neither is possible, to help patients find a good death.

Quill has devised a set of criteria for doctors trying to figure out whether a patient is making a clearheaded request for death, feeling pressured to let go of life, or crying out for relief from pain or emotional distress. At least two doctors must determine that the patient is terminally ill and desires to die, he says. The patient must unmistakably and repeatedly ask for help in dying and must be competent to make the decision; a doctor should never assist a senile patient in committing suicide. And because people do change their minds, the request must come at the time of crisis, not in writing years before.

Few people would qualify under these criteria, and only the most determined would succeed. This is Quill's vision. But Hendin is convinced that some doctors would subtly encourage patients to escape those last awful weeks—awful for the patients but also for the people who can't save them. And even if the patient's mind is clouded, making him or her ineligible under Quill's rules, Hendin thinks many doctors may be willing to help death come quickly. Why should a dazed person be denied the easy exit given to a coherent one? Especially if family members are sure, as I was in very different circumstances, that they know what their loved one would want.

Any day now, doctors say, Alzheimer's disease will so paralyze my mother-in-law's brain that it will no longer send the signal to swallow food. At one time we said this would be our signal to sedate her and let her die a natural death; we wouldn't give the order for tube-feeding. We've changed our minds, and not because we think she wants to live longer as a vacant human shell who can't move. We're not sure *what* she wants—or for that matter, if she can think or feel anything. We've changed our minds because we don't want to spend the rest of our lives wondering if we guessed wrong.

My own mother never has told us what she'd want, and after our timid effort in the hospital we've never asked. How can you pose such a question to someone who wakes in the mornings asking how her own mother—dead 40 years—slept the night before? Time and place mean little to her now, though she still knows us and delights in her grandchildren.

I wonder at times what would have happened if assisted suicide or even quiet euthanasia were the norm in this country, if my sisters hadn't resisted when I frantically cried, "No more transfusions! It's cruel." We don't discuss that, of course, being a family that leaves such things unsaid.

There are days when my mother is cranky and days when Jonna is exhausted even with respite help. Most of the time, however, my mother is appreciative. Perhaps she's biting her acerbic tongue, or maybe she no longer remembers that she is, by personality and habit, sarcastic. Whatever the reason, the two of them have fallen into a new relationship: My sister takes gentle but firm care of her, as my mother once cared for us, and my mother compliments Jonna's cooking.

After three months under hospice care, they went to the clinic to check the condition of my mother's ulcers, which the doctor had described as the worst he'd ever seen. They had healed; no one could explain how.

Although I'm only guessing, I think that our independent mother, who once would rather have died than become feeble, simply changed her mind. Somewhere in her primal core, she decided that being sickly, confused, and dependent is better than the alternative.

FRAME the DEBATE

Form at end of book

R E A D I N G 3 5

Issue 13: Is physician-assisted suicide a viable treatment option for the terminally ill?

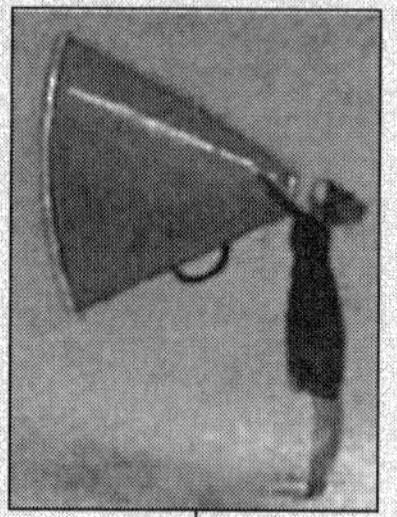

Legalizing Physician-Assisted Suicide: Some Thoughts and Concerns

Harold G. Koenig, M.D., M.H.Sc.
Durham, North Carolina

Surveys show that most Americans favor the decriminalization of physician-assisted suicide in certain circumstances. Several states are now considering legislation to bring this about and make the United States the first place in the civilized world where physician aid in dying is sanctioned. In the Netherlands, where physician-assisted suicide is practiced but officially remains illegal, 85% of assisted suicides occur in the elderly, and most involve the help of general practitioners. In the United States, family physicians provide health care to many older adults with chronic or terminal illness whose numbers will increase as the elderly population expands. The legalization of physician-assisted suicide would affect the way American physicians practice medicine in unpredictable ways, yet physicians are participating relatively little in deliberations concerning this issue. The problem of suffering in persons with chronic and terminal illness cannot be ignored. Compassionate, effective, and ethical solutions must be found. As a former family physician and now geriatric psychiatrist, I review the pros and cons of physician-assisted suicide (emphasizing arguments against legalization) and encourage family physicians to debate this matter.

Most physicians have had patients with advanced cancer, end-stage heart failure, severe chronic obstructive pulmonary disease, or other disabling and painful diseases. Many of these persons experience great physical and emotional suffering during the final few weeks or months of their lives. In such circumstances, it is our professional, ethical and moral duty to do everything possible to relieve such apparently meaningless suffering. Should physicians be allowed to honor requests by terminally or chronically ill patients to assist them in ending their lives? This subject has special relevance for older adults, who are most likely to be affected by terminal or chronic diseases, and for family physicians who care for them. In the Netherlands, more than 85% of euthanasia cases occur in medically ill persons aged 50 years or over, and most are performed by general practitioners.[1]

Clarification of Terms

To discuss this topic intelligently, one must carefully define one's terms, or risk ambiguity and confusion. First, withdrawal of life support, or *passive euthanasia*, involves the removal of tubes, respirators, or any other type of artificial support that may prolong life. The excess use of medical technology to extend apparently meaningless life and prolong suffering, especially in cases of terminal or near-terminal illness, is one of the factors that have stirred a public outcry for physician assistance in dying. *Physician-assisted suicide* occurs when a physician intentionally and willfully takes actions that help a suicidal patient to end his or her life. This may involve providing information on ways of committing suicide, supplying a prescription for a lethal dose of medication, providing a syringe filled with a lethal dose of medication, inserting an intravenous line so that the patient can inject the drug, or providing a suicide device that the patient can operate (such as the "suicide machine" invented by Jack Kevorkian, MD). *Active euthanasia* involves a physician willfully and intentionally performing an action that directly and immediately results in the patient's death. Here, the physician is the actor, but acts at the patient's request.

Watts and Howell[2] argue that there are clear philosophical distinctions between passive forms of assisted suicide (providing information), more aggressive assisted suicide (providing a lethal dose of medication or apparatus to inject it), and active euthanasia (physician injecting a lethal drug), pointing to the differing degrees of physician influence or control over the process leading to death. Others, however, contend that legalizing any form of physician-assisted suicide may open a door that is not easily closed. They refer to the strategy taken by advocates of

Legalizing Physician-Assisted Suicide: Some Thoughts and Concerns, Harold G. Koenig. THE JOURNAL OF FAMILY PRACTICE, Volume 37, Number 2, 1993. Reprinted by permission.

euthanasia in the Netherlands, who gradually won widespread acceptance of active euthanasia by first endorsing more palatable, less offensive categories.[3] Making distinctions between forms of assistance, while easy in theory, is difficult in practice. If one can justify providing support and advice, a lethal dose of medication, or a suicide device to a patient who is both intent on and capable of killing himself or herself, it becomes difficult to ignore the desperate pleas of another severely ill patient who needs assistance to die but cannot complete the act because of problems with swallowing, physical frailness, or a lack of emotional fortitude.

If one can justify that it is ethical and safe for a physician to assist the suicidal patient, then it is difficult to argue against more active interventions in more complex, and perhaps more appropriate, circumstances. Physicians in the Netherlands acknowledged this obvious conclusion almost a decade ago, when the Royal Dutch Medical Association (KNMG) recommended that the distinction between euthanasia and assisted suicide be abolished on grounds that the intent in both cases is to bring about the patient's death.[3] For these reasons, the arguments proposed in this article will apply to all forms of assistance in dying, including active euthanasia.

Proponents of Assisted Suicide

Between one half and two thirds of Americans today favor the legalization of physician-assisted suicide in certain circumstances.[4,5] The public's attitude toward assisted suicide has changed during the past 15 years. In 1975, a Gallup poll showed that 41% of respondents believed that persons in great pain without hope of improvement had a moral right to commit suicide; in 1990, the figure had increased to 66%.[6] Similarly, a survey by the Harvard School of Public Health reported that 61% of all Americans would vote for an initiative legalizing physician-assisted suicide; 52% said they would consider some option to end their life if they had an incurable illness and were in a great deal of pain.[5]

Leading and organizing the effort to legalize physician-assisted suicide is the Hemlock Society, founded in Los Angeles in 1980 and now numbering over 40,000 members. Englishman Derek Humphry, its principal founder, was the organization's leader and spokesman until 1992 when, following adverse publicity surrounding the suicide of his second wife,[7] he stepped down as executive director. Humphry's most recent book, *Final Exit,*[8] marketed as a "how to do it" manual for those wishing to commit suicide, sold over 500,000 copies within 6 months of publication.

The Hemlock Society has led initiatives to legalize assisted suicide in Washington and California that were only narrowly defeated (both by a 54% to 46% margin). The issue, however, remains very much alive, and similar measures are expected to qualify for the 1994 ballot in California, Oregon, and Washington.[9] In a speech to the 1992 annual meeting of the Academy of Psychosomatic Medicine, Humphry emphasized that he hoped that future legislation would be as carefully considered and well reasoned as the California initiative. A number of California psychiatrists, on the other hand, argued that Initiative 161 was "a potential disaster" because of a lack of safeguards to prevent persons with treatable mental illnesses, e.g., depression, from committing suicide.

Proponents' View

Almost two decades ago, philosopher James Rachels[10] argued that there was no ethical distinction between passive and active euthanasia. If one can justify not treating or withdrawing treatment from hopelessly ill patients to quicken death and reduce suffering, then providing them with more active assistance in ending their lives should pose no moral or ethical dilemma. In a more recent article, Weir[11] argues that assisted suicide is morally justifiable. Rather than harm the patient, physician-assisted suicide benefits him or her by relieving intolerable and useless suffering, some of which may not be amenable to even the most expert palliation. Assisted suicide enhances patient autonomy and reduces fear by giving the person control over the dying process. The argument for physician-assisted suicide has also been presented in several recent articles by Timothy Quill and Christine Cassel in *The New England Journal of Medicine.*[12–14] Death with dignity and control is seen as better than an agonizing, prolonged, and unpredictable death. Furthermore, the right to die is guaranteed in the first and fourth amendments to the Constitution, and therefore the right to end one's life is seen as being as important as the right to life.[15] Finally, assisted suicide can benefit society by reducing the use of scarce medical resources on hopeless cases. The latter argument is seldom stressed, since proponents believe that if assisted suicide became available, it would be chosen by relatively few persons, and thus have little impact on resource conservation or on discouraging efforts by society to care for the needs of persons with debilitating illnesses.[2] Dr. Quill has recently published a book entitled *Death with Dignity,*[16] which poses a very serious challenge to all physicians who would oppose physician-assisted suicide across the board.

Proponents believe that guidelines can be developed that would protect the safety of patients and prevent physicians, patients, and society from abusing this privilege.[12] Such guidelines, according to Quill et al.,[14] include the following: (1) the patient must have a condition that is incurable (not necessarily terminal) and associated with severe suffering without hope of relief; (2) all reasonable comfort-oriented measures must have been considered or tried; (3) the patient must express a clear and repeated request to die that is not financially or emotionally coerced; (4) the physician must ensure that the patience's judgment is not distorted; (5) physician-assisted suicide must be carried out only in the context of a meaningful physician-patient relationship; (6) consultation must be obtained from another physician to ensure that the patient's request is voluntary and rational; and (7) there must be clear documentation that the previous six steps have been taken and a system of "reporting, reviewing, and studying such deaths" must be established.[14(p 1382)] A number of these guidelines are already in place in the Netherlands, where proponents believe the system works quite well.[17] As a final safeguard in the United States, ethics committees could be established to remove the responsibility for such decisions from any one physician. The practical aspects of exactly how monitoring would take place to ensure that guidelines were being followed, however, have yet to be worked out to everyone's satisfaction.

Opponents of Assisted Suicide

Those who oppose physician-assisted suicide include many influential and respected groups in America, among which are several professional organizations. The American Medical Association,[18,19] the American Geriatrics Society,[20] and the American Bar Association[21] have all spoken out against the practice and legalization of physician-assisted suicide. A recent article in the *American Journal of Psychiatry* by Herbert Hendrin (director, American Suicide Foundation) and Gerald Klerman (former director of the federal Alcohol, Drug Abuse, and Mental Health Administration) voices considerable concern within the psychiatric community about physician-assisted suicide.[22] I focus here on four major groups that tend to oppose physician-assisted suicide: physicians, bioethicists, the elderly, and religious organizations.

Physicians

Information on physicians' attitudes toward assisted suicide was sparse until recently. Evidence for opposition comes from the state of Washington, where the state medical society in 1990 voted 114 to 22 against Initiative 119, which would have legalized physician-assisted suicide. Similarly, the majority of the members of the California state medical society voted to oppose Initiative 161, which also failed to gain the majority vote from the public in the November 1992 election. A survey of Florida internists in 1991 found that 87% would not administer a lethal dose of a drug under any circumstances.[23] Opposition, however, is not uniform. A survey by the American Board of Family Practice found that 90% of 300 internists, family physicians, and psychiatrists agreed that terminally ill patients had a right to choose to die; however, this opinion primarily reflected support of withdrawal of life-sustaining therapy (passive euthanasia) rather than assisted suicide.[23] However, evidence of increasing support within the medical community for physician-assisted suicide comes from a recent decision by Michigan physicians to reverse their stand against the practice, preferring that it not be considered a felony.

Perhaps the best data are available from a study conducted by Watts and colleagues,[24] who surveyed 727 internist geriatricians on their attitudes toward assisting suicide among dementia patients. Fourteen percent of physicians said Dr. Kevorkian's assistance of Janet Adkins' suicide in 1990 was morally justifiable; 26% favored easing restrictions on assisted suicide for competent, nondepressed dementia patients; and 21% would themselves consider assisting in the suicides of such patients. Again, these findings suggest that only a minority of physicians support physician-assisted suicide. Finally, a recent survey of hospice physicians, nurses, and volunteers found overwhelming opposition to assisted suicide.[25] Hospice physician David Cundiff provides an articulate and well-reasoned case against physician-assisted suicide in his book entitled *Euthanasia Is Not the Answer.*[26]

Medical Ethicists

A number of medical ethicists oppose the legalization of physician-assisted suicide in the United States.[27–33] Leading this group is Daniel Callahan, director of the Hastings Center of Bioethics.[34] In his book *Setting Limits,*[35] Callahan warns against the legalization of physician-assisted suicide, arguing that such an action may send unintended messages to older persons in our society. Callahan fears that elders will come to feel that "old age can have no meaning and significance if accompanied by decline, pain and despair." He is also concerned that younger persons will come to believe "that pain is not to be endured, that community cannot be found for the old, and that a life that is not marked by good health, by hope and vitality, is not a life worth living." [35(pp 193–197)] In a December 1990 international meeting of euthanasia experts at the Institute of Bioethics (Maastricht, the Netherlands), Callahan's strong opposition to physician-assisted suicide became explicit.

> To legitimize active euthanasia is to add a new category of killing. It is to add indeed the worst category of killing, namely private, self-determined killing between people, not for the sake of protecting the nation (as in war), not for the sake of justice (as in capital punishment), and not for the sake of saving a life (as in self-defense), but rather to satisfy private wants and desires.[35(p 29)]

The Elderly

Proponents of physician-assisted suicide argue that older persons should be allowed to end their lives if they choose. Humphry has supported the right of elderly couples to commit double suicide to avoid bereavement after one spouse has become terminally ill.[7(pp 96–99)] Although old age may be a criterion for physician-assisted suicide proposed by some advocates, many elders feel quite differently about this. Age has a strong impact on the percentage of Americans who favor physician-assisted suicide. The Harvard survey mentioned earlier found that whereas 79% of 18- to 34-year-olds favored physician-assisted suicide, only 64% of 35- to 49-year-olds and 53% of those over the age of 50 did so.[5] Although information was not given on the views of persons aged 65 years or older, the downward trend among the above three age groups suggests that the percentage of persons in this age group favoring physician-assisted suicide would probably fall below 50%.

Why does age make a difference? First, older persons tend to have more conservative values. Second, older persons may be less fearful of death and thus less desperate to be in complete control of the process. Finally, there may be concern that if physician-assisted suicide were legalized, elders with chronic or terminal illness might be manipulated, either consciously or unconsciously, into viewing themselves as unnecessary burdens and therefore pressured into committing suicide. Elders who have chosen to live rather than die may be made to feel guilty because they are consuming their family's inheritance or placing a burden on their caregivers. Besides guilt, this is likely to arouse feelings of resentment toward those (family members or others) who would put them in a position of having to choose between life and the more "heroic" or "dignified" option of assisted suicide.[28] The current law provides a buffer against pressures that might prompt elders to end their lives for others' sake. Legalizing physician-assisted suicide could subject the 998 out of 1000 terminally or chronically ill older persons who choose life over death to experience unnecessary psychological turmoil over their decisions to live.[36]

Religious Organizations

Although some religious denominations in the United States have spoken out in favor of legalizing physician-assisted suicide (Unitarian Universalist Church), most oppose it. Traditional doctrines in Christianity, Judaism, and Islam oppose the killing of oneself to avoid personal pain or suffering, and no major world religion condones suicide for self-serving purposes.[37] While this article does not explore the religious arguments for or against the legalization of physician-assisted suicide, a strong religious faith can make even the most intolerable suffering tolerable for some persons.[38] It does so by providing a framework in which suffering can have meaning and purpose.[39]

The Opponents' View

Opponents argue that although there may be cases where physician-assisted suicide could be considered an ethical alternative, it is one thing to justify an act, but quite a different thing to justify a general practice.[36] Undoubtedly, there are circumstances in which even the most stringent opponents would agree that assisted suicide is the best and possibly only ethical solution, particularly in cases where optimal medical care and pain relief are unavailable. Nevertheless, the risks of legalizing physician-assisted suicide on a more general basis are seen as far outweighing the benefits that it might provide to a few, especially given that sensible and safer alternatives exist.[32,36,40–42]

Concerns about Assisted Suicide

I will present here five reasons for displaying caution in legalizing physician-assisted suicide. The focus is primarily on medical and psychiatric considerations; social factors will be touched on only briefly. These concerns, which are hardly exhaustive, include the following: (1) ambiguous indications, (2) physician biases, (3) the "slippery slope," (4) failure to follow guidelines, and (5) the existence of sensible alternatives.

Ambiguous Indications

Most agree that three conditions must exist for physician-assisted suicide to be justifiable: (1) intolerable suffering and intractable pain, (2) terminal illness, and (3) a request by a rational patient. None of these conditions are easily verified.

Intolerable Suffering and Intractable Pain

We all suffer to some extent over losses, failures, unmet expectations. There comes a point, however, when the severity of suffering crosses a threshold from tolerable to intolerable. That threshold varies widely from individual to individual for a given level of physiological pain. There is reason to believe that this "toleration threshold" can be affected without changing the level of physiological pain, since the psychological aspects of suffering often far outweigh the physical aspects. Suffering includes emotions such as fear, hopelessness, discouragement, fatigue, anger, and feelings of entrapment. Even if the level of pain remains unchanged, suffering can still be lessened, at least to the point that it is tolerable, by addressing emotional elements through psychological or psychosocial interventions.

Next, one must establish the intractability of pain or other physical discomforts such as nausea or breathlessness. According to Saunders,[43] approximately 10% to 15% of terminal cancer patients die with pain that cannot be entirely eliminated. Many of these patients, however, *choose* to tolerate pain to maintain mental alertness to take care of "unfinished business" in their final days. "Intractable pain" is actually a misnomer, since pain can always be reduced or even eliminated, if by no other means than by continuous anesthesia. Under such circumstances (when food and fluids are not forced), death quickly follows.

It is hard to say exactly how much suffering might be *made* tolerable, given adequate pain relief, support, and nurturance from others, and maximization of autonomy by providing personal control over health care decisions. Unspoken personal and interpersonal issues are commonly involved in a request for assisted suicide: fear of loneliness or abandonment, fear of dependency on others, frustration over a dismal situation, and anger toward family members or health care providers over unmet expectations. It may also represent a cry for someone to demonstrate that this patient's life is important, valuable to others, and worth the struggle to continue living. If the physician agrees to assist in the suicidal plan, the patient may interpret this as a confirmation of his or her worst fears: that life is indeed without purpose, meaning, or value, and *cannot become otherwise* during the patient's time remaining.[36,44]

Terminal Illness

The accuracy of diagnosis for many diseases is imprecise. Even when the diagnosis is correct, predictions about the timing of death are quite unreliable. This is true for Alzheimer's disease, cancer, and many other disorders. After a complete medical evaluation, including extensive bloodwork and brain scans, physicians correctly diagnose Alzheimer's disease only about 75% to 80% of the time.[45] Cognitive impairment may be reversible with the treatment of various medical or psychiatric conditions, or at least may not progress if appropriate medical measures are taken (control blood pressure, stop excess alcohol use, replace thyroid medication, remove toxic drugs). Thus, it is hard to say when an illness is terminal and prospects for reversal or stabilization are no longer present.

Unimpaired Reasoning

This condition requires that a person is rational, has no significant impairments in judgment, and can freely choose between alternatives. Psychiatrists report that at least 95% of suicide victims have a preexisting mental illness.[46,47] In a study of terminally ill patients, Brown and colleagues[48] found that it was not "normal" for even severely ill patients to either desire death or wish to end their lives. Other studies indicate that a high proportion of elders with chronic or terminal illness experience depression, with rates as high as 40% to 45%.[49,50] When emotional pain reaches a certain level, consciousness becomes constricted to the point where choices other than suicide cannot be appreciated by the patient. In such cases, treatment that lessens the emotional pain will broaden consciousness so that alternatives may be considered. Rather than infringe upon autonomy, the prevention of suicide and treatment of underlying emotional illness act to preserve and restore autonomy. Requests for assistance in committing suicide, then, often mean more than a simple expression of autonomy or individual choice. Although cases probably do exist, "rational" suicidal thinking in the setting of chronic and disabling medical illness is not common.[51]

On the other hand, one study by Lee and Ganzini[52] examined attitudes toward life-sustaining therapy in 50 depressed and 50 nondepressed elderly veterans hospitalized with medical illness. They found that depressed subjects desired fewer interventions (nasogastric tubes, kidney dialysis, ventilator support, etc) than control subjects in hypothetical scenarios with a good prognosis and in their *current* state of health; however, there were no differences between groups in poor prognosis scenarios. Based on the latter finding, one might conclude that depression does not have a major effect on the decision making of chronically or terminally ill patients. Note, however, that failure to document attitudinal differences between depressed and nondepressed patients occurred only for *hypothetical* poor-prognosis scenarios, not real-life situations. Furthermore, attitudes toward acceptance or rejection of painful or cumbersome life-sustaining procedures may be quite different from attitudes toward suicide.

During the Durham Veterans Administration Mental Health Survey,[53] we examined the relationship between psychiatric disorder and suicidal thoughts in 444 consecutively admitted younger and older hospitalized medical patients. Among those under age 40 (n = 115), 19% of 57 patients with depression or other psychiatric disorder had at least fleeting suicidal thoughts at the time of evaluation; none of the 58 patients without mental disorder had such thoughts. Among patients aged 70 years or older (n = 329), 14% of 159 patients with depression or other psychiatric disorder had suicidal thoughts, compared with 1% of 170 patients without mental disorder (author, unpublished data, 1991). This suggests that suicidal thoughts almost always occur in the setting of psychiatric disorder.

Ruling out depressive illness and establishing rationality, particularly in the setting of chronic pain, suffering, or terminal illness, is a challenge for even the most expert clinician. Studies have shown that only 9% to 20% of depressed, medically ill older patients are diagnosed with this disorder by their medical physicians.[54,55] Part of the reason is that depression is very difficult to identify in these patients. Many symptoms of physical disease are identical with those of psychological distress. For example, chronic pain is usually accompanied by insomnia, fatigue, decreased concentration, and other psychological and physiological symptoms that are indistinguishable from depression and can impair judgment and reasoning.

Adding to this problem is that depression in the elderly may present *without sadness or dysphoria.* Approximately 50% of all depressed persons seen by physicians come in complaining about physical symptoms, aches and pains, that either have no organic basis or represent an exaggeration of real but minor physical problems.[56] This syndrome has been called "masked" depression.[56,57] Physical symptoms are often more acceptable to elders than emotional ones, which are seen by many as embarrassing and indicative of weak or unstable character. Thus, deciding whether mental illness is present in a suicidal patient with chronic illness often boils down to subtle perceptions, distinctions, and judgments. Such decisions are almost always made subjectively and with some degree of uncertainty, and are therefore easily swayed by the physician's own biases.

Physician Biases

Quill and colleagues[14] see safety for the patient in the stipulation that the physician involved ought to have an ongoing and, ideally, long-standing personal relationship with the patient. Indeed, it is precisely that relationship that will aid the physician in identifying intolerable suffering and unimpaired reasoning. Nevertheless, as the physician weighs the various factors noted above, his or her personal attitudes, feelings, and other factors invariably come into play. From a young healthy physician's standpoint, the disabled, chronic or terminally ill elder may appear to lack an acceptable "quality of life." If so, the physician may be more likely to agree that it is "reasonable" and "rational" for that patient to choose to end his or her life, while ignoring symptoms suggesting a reversible depressive illness.

Other factors that may influence a physician's decision include experiences within his or her own family, personal ethical and moral values, anxiety over death, feelings about the patient, and burden of treating that patient. The physician's objectivity may be further compromised by pressure from the patient's family (who are often paying the bills) whose motivations may not reflect the patient's best interests. Leaving the physician as the sole person responsible for deciding the patient's competence and rationality, then, can be problematic.

One solution, noted earlier, is to require that all such decisions either be reviewed by a hospital ethics committee or be reassessed by a second physician. Ethics committees, while preventing a single professional from taking full responsibility for such decisions, do not solve the central problem—that is, establishing with some degree of certainty that the conditions necessary to justify physician-assisted suicide are present. It is also unclear who would be chosen to sit on such committees or how these committees would be monitored and regulated. Many final decisions would ultimately rest on judgments made by the personal physician who knew the patient best. If that physician also had an active role in choosing the consultant who would provide a second opinion, consultation would become a farce.

Slippery Slope

The "slippery slope" argument contends that once the legal barrier to physician-assisted suicide is broken, there will be little justification for limiting this practice to the terminally ill. Wennberg[37(p 194)] notes that "once voluntary active euthanasia for the terminally ill is legalized, one can reasonably expect pressure to mount to secure legalized euthanasia for those with illness or physical impairment that is incurable, of a distressing character but not terminal." This would include the nonterminal accident victim who, unlike terminally ill patients, has to face suffering for the rest of his or her lifetime. The same argument could be used to justify physician-assisted suicide for those suffering from chronic, degenerative diseases like Alzheimer's disease and other disabling conditions associated with old age.

In Holland, where physician-assisted suicide has been tolerated since 1973, 3% to 15% of all deaths occur by this method. Physician assistance with dying has now extended from terminal patients with cancer to chronically ill patients with paraplegia, multiple sclerosis, and "gross physical deterioration at advanced age." [58] According to Dr. T. van Berkestijn, secretary general of the KNMG, this Dutch medical organization is now openly preparing guidelines for terminating the lives of incompetent patients: the demented elderly, the mentally handicapped, and defective newborns.[3] The eight cases of assisted suicide by Dr. Kevorkian between 1990 and 1992 involving middle-aged or elderly women suffering from chronic but not terminal illnesses demonstrate that such things can happen in America, too.[59]

Social and Financial Pressures

Powerful social and financial forces exist that could influence the circumstances in which physician-assisted suicide could be carried out in the years ahead if it were legalized.

The cost of health care in this country has been spiraling upward, and the pressure to contain costs has been accelerating. With these trends, we can expect an increasing tendency to limit the provision of health care for those who are less productive or seen as profiting least from such expenditures.[35] Physician-assisted suicide, then, would provide an all too expedient solution to the problem of an expanding, chronically ill elderly population.

Substituted Judgment

How might a society implement physician-assisted suicide for incompetent patients? "Substituted judgments" made by either the physician or family member might be called on to justify such acts. Substituted judgments would have merit if it could be established that physicians and relatives accurately predict how patients might feel in such circumstances. Unfortunately, evidence for this is lacking.[60] Proponents of physician-assisted suicide argue that assisting the death of incompetent patients or of patients against their will would never happen; the situation in Holland, however, speaks loudly to the contrary. A recent survey of Dutch physicians' participation in patient deaths found that about 3% of all deaths in Holland could be attributable to physician-assisted suicide.[1] Physicians admitted, however, that nearly 28% of such deaths (500 to 1000 per year) were performed "without an explicit and persistent request" by the patient. Given this fact, it is difficult to argue that similar abuses could not occur in the United States.

Generation Effect

While the current generation may be reluctant to liberalize conditions necessary to justify physician-assisted suicide, the next generation and the one following that may have other ideas, especially if they have been reared in a society where assisted suicide among the chronic or terminally ill is the norm. Wennberg[37(p 202)] notes that "It is hard to introduce for the first time a practice that conflicts with long-standing moral, social, and legal prohibitions; it is easier the second time."

Failure to Follow Guidelines

If physician-assisted suicide were legalized in America, how likely would it be that physicians would follow (or could follow) established guidelines for this practice? This is not a moot point. Dutch physicians have had many problems in this regard. In Holland, the only safeguard for assisted-suicide is the review of deaths by a coroner (a requirement by law). If physician-assisted suicide accounts for between 2000 and 10,000 deaths per year in that country, then one would expect a similar number of reports to coroners. Dutch coroners, however, say that they receive only about 200 reports of physician-assisted suicide per year.[36] Enforcing laws that standardize physician-assisted suicide has proven difficult in Holland, as it likely would in America. Because of the negative attitudes our society has toward suicide, maintenance of privacy has been a central component of initiatives for physician-assisted suicide in the states of Washington and California. Balancing this need with the need to control the practice and monitor for abuses would be a difficult task.

Sensible Alternatives

Rather than assist and support patients in ending their lives, physicians may choose to seek the underlying causes for suffering and then aggressively implement measures to correct them. This may include arranging for companionship to alleviate loneliness, mobilizing family members to dispel a sense of abandonment, providing assistive devices to help limit disability, or allowing the patient's participation in medical decision making to maximize autonomy and self-care. More research could be directed into improving medical control of distressing symptoms such as pain, nausea, and breathlessness, and conditions such as constipation, incontinence, and other intolerable physical problems associated with dying. Likewise, comprehensive psychological and spiritual care could be offered to help lessen emotional discomfort, relieve anxiety or depression, and convey hope. Each of these actions requires more effort, more money, and more time than simply allowing patients to terminate their lives. Nevertheless, these actions preserve the traditional role of the physician as healer, sustainer of life, and afforder of comfort. Furthermore, such efforts prove to our elderly and young people that disabled and chronically and terminally ill persons are valuable to society, that life is worth fighting for, and that tough problems sometimes require tough answers.

Improving Care for the Dying

With good hospice care, most terminally ill patients can be made comfortable, even if pain cannot be entirely eliminated.[43,61] Adequate analgesia can be maintained with high doses of narcotics that are either self-administered by patient-controlled infusion devices or administered by a continuous intravenous drip monitored by health care providers. The emotional aspects of suffering (feelings of isolation, dysphoria, and anxiety) can be greatly diminished by having a close relationship with another person (family, friend, or hospice staff member), by supportive counseling, or in cases of severe depression, by use of antidepressants, tranquilizers, or sometimes, electroconvulsive therapy.

Allowing to Die

Humane care for the dying includes recognizing when provision of comfort must become the primary goal. This is particularly true for terminally ill patients with only a few weeks or months to live who are suffering to the point that life has lost its meaning. This may also be true for certain patients with severe and irreversible dementia, those with irreversible coma, and those who exist in a persistent vegetative state (alive but with only minimal brain activity). Family members and friends should be encouraged to visit and spend time with their loved one. If suspected, depression or anxiety should be vigorously treated in conscious patients.

After arriving at a consensus by patient (when conscious), family, and health care providers (in that order), an agreement can be made to use whatever means necessary to provide comfort and relieve symptoms, even at the risk of hastening death. This plan should be clearly documented in the chart. Advanced directives may guide family and health care providers in making such decisions for unconscious, or incompetent patients. At this point, all life support measures, including administration of food and water, may be withdrawn and interventions to prolong life avoided in circumstances where death is imminent and suffering is intolerable, or where consciousness has been obliterated by continuous anesthesia.

While the popular press portrays starvation and dehydration as the epitome of neglect, medical experts are aware that when death approaches, discomfort from hunger or thirst becomes minimal or absent. Starvation in this setting may even cause a release into the bloodstream of natural analgesic substances that act to relieve pain.[62,63] Similarly, limiting fluids will minimize secretions, ease respirations, decrease incontinence, and cause little discomfort to the patient.[64–65] Thus, forcing food or fluids into terminally ill patients who have little desire for these substances is not only counterproductive but cruel.

Instead all efforts should be directed at simple comfort measures, such as providing good skin and oral care, maintaining a fresh and clean environment, and allowing the patient as much freedom as possible in deciding how and where to spend his or her final days. A narcotic analgesic such as morphine should be used freely and unrestrictedly to relieve pain, nausea, or shortness of breath. In some cases, an excess dose of such medication may inadvertently hasten or cause the patient's death. This risk should be acknowledged and is unavoidable.

Need for Research and Ongoing Debate

Sensible alternatives to physician-assisted suicide do exist and must be pursued. Nevertheless, the case for legalizing physician-assisted suicide is a strong one that cannot be ignored. Further research is needed on attitudes toward physician-assisted suicide held by the elderly and those with chronic or terminal illness, with and without mental illness. In addition, this topic needs continuing debate among those within medicine so that all sides of the question can be carefully considered. If we decide to legalize physician-assisted suicide, then guidelines should be carefully established, with physicians having an active role in the process. Family physicians must debate and voice their support or concerns, since they are the physicians who would assist patients in committing suicide if the practice were legalized.

References

1. Van der Maas PJ, Van Delden JJ, Pineborg L, et al. Euthanasia and other medical decisions concerning the end of life. *Lancet* 1991; 338:669–74.
2. Watts DT, Howell T. Assisted suicide is not voluntary active euthanasia. *J Am Geriatr Soc* 1992; 40:1043–6.
3. de Wachter MAM. Euthanasia in the Netherlands. *Hastings Cent. Rep* 1992; 22:23–31.
4. Giving death a hand; rending issue. *New York Times* 1990 June 14; Sect A:6
5. Lawton K. The doctor as executioner. *Christianity* Today, 1991; Dec 16:50–2.
6. Ames K, Wilson L, Sawhill R, et al. Last rights. *Newsweek,* 1991; Aug 26:40–1.
7. Marker R. *Deadly compassion.* New York: William Morrow, 1993.
8. Humphry D. *Final Exit.* New York: Dell Publishing, 1991.
9. Newman A. Psychiatry urged to get ready for major debate on assisted suicide. *Clin Psychiatry News* 1992; 20(12):1, 14.
10. Rachels J. Active and passive euthanasia. *N Engl J Med* 1975; 292:78–80.
11. Weir RF. The morality of physician-assisted suicide. *Law Med Health Care* 1992; 20:116–26.
12. Cassel CK, Meier DE. Morals and moralism in the debate over euthanasia and assisted suicide. *N Engl J Med* 1990;323:750–2.
13. Quill TE. Death and dignity: a case of individualized decision making. *N Engl J Med* 1991; 324:691–4.
14. Quill TE, Cassel CK, Meier DE. Care of the hopelessly ill: proposed clinical criteria for physician-assisted suicide. *N Engl J Med* 1992; 327:1380–4.
15. Palmore E. Arguments for assisted suicide. *Gerontologist* 1991; 31:854.
16. Quill TE. *Death with dignity.* New York: WW Norton, 1993.
17. Rigter H, Borst-Eilers E, Leenen HJJJ. Euthanasia across the North Sea. *BMJ* 1988; 297:1593–5.
18. American Medical Association Judicial Council. Opinions of the Judicial Council, 1982. In: *President's Commission for the Study of Ethical Problems in Medicine and Biomedical and Behavioral Research. Deciding to forego life-sustaining treatment.* Washington, DC: Government Printing Office, 1983:299–300.
19. Orentlicher D. Physician participation in assisted suicide. *JAMA* 1989; 262:1844–5.
20. American Geriatrics Society, Policy Statement. Voluntary active euthanasia. *J Am Geriatr Soc* 1991; 39:826.
21. American Bar Association. House of Delegates meeting, voting on report from ABA's Commission on Legal Problems of the Elderly. Dallas, Texas, February 3, 1992.
22. Hendrin H, Klerman G. Physician-assisted suicide: the dangers of legalization. *Am J Psychiatry* 1993; 150:143–5.
23. Charnow J. Most internists support patients' "right to die," surveys find. *ACP Observer* June 8, 1991.

24. Watts DT, Howell T, Priefer BA. Geriatricians' attitudes toward assisting suicide of dementia patients. *J Am Geriatr Soc* 1992; 40:878–85.
25. Miller RJ. Hospice care as an alternative to euthanasia. *Law Med Health Care* 1992; 20:127–32.
26. Cundiff D. *Euthanasia is not the answer: a hospice physician's view.* Totowa, NJ: Humana Press, 1992.
27. Foot P. Euthanasia. *Philosophy Public Affairs* 1977; 6:85–112.
28. Kamisar Y. Euthanasia legislation: some nonreligious objections. In: Beauchamp TL, Perlin S, eds. *Ethical issues in death and dying.* Englewood Cliffs, NJ: Pretince-Hall, 1978:220–32.
29. Gaylin W. Doctors must not kill. *JAMA* 1988; 259:2139–40.
30. Callahan D. Can we return death to disease? *Hastings Cent Rep* 1989; 19(Suppl):4–6.
31. Wolf S. Holding the line on euthanasia. *Hastings Cent Rep* 1989; 19(Suppl):13–5.
32. Singer PA, Siegler M. Euthanasia: a critique. *N Engl J Med* 1990; 322:1881–3.
33. Sprung CL. Changing attitudes and practices in foregoing life-sustaining treatments. *JAMA* 1990; 263:2211–5.
34. Callahan D. When self-determination runs amok. *Hastings Cent Rep* 1992; 22:52–5.
35. Callahan D. *Setting limits.* New York: Simon & Schuster, 1987.
36. Teno J, Lynn J. Voluntary active euthanasia: the individual case and public policy. *J Am Geriatr Soc* 1991; 39:827–30.
37. Wennberg RN. *Terminal choices: euthanasia, suicide, and the right to die.* Grand Rapids, Mich: Eerdmans, 1989.
38. Koenig HG, Cohen HJ, Blazer DG, et al. Religious coping and depression in hospitalized elderly medically ill men. *Am J Psychiatry* 1992; 149:1693–700.
39. Koenig HG. *Aging and God.* Binghamton, NY: Haworth Press, 1993.
40. Parkes CM. Psychological aspects. In: Saunders CM, ed. *The management of terminal disease.* London: Edward Arnold, 1978:56.
41. Lynn J. Euthanasia—not in America. *Washington Post* 1990 April 19; Sect A:26.
42. Gillett G. Euthanasia, letting die and the pause. *J Med Ethics* 1988; 14:61–8.
43. Saunders C. Principles of symptom control in terminal care. In: MM Reidenberg, ed. *The medical clinics of North America: clinical pharmacology of symptom control.* Philadelphia: WB Saundcrs, 1978:1169–83.
44. Montalvo B. The patient chose to die: why? *Gerontologist* 1991; 31:700–3.
45. McKhann G, Drachman D, Folstein M, ct al. Clinical diagnosis of Alzheimer's disease: report of the NINCDS-ADRDA work group under the auspices of Department of Health and Human Services task force on Alzheimer's disease. *Neurology* 1984; 34:939–44.
46. Kaplan HI, Sadock BJ. *Synopsis of psychiatry.* Baltimore: Williams & Wilkins, 1988:453.
47. Conwell Y. Suicide in the elderly. American Association for Geriatric Psychiatry annual meeting. San Francisco, February 1992.
48. Brown JH, Henteleff P, Barakat S, et al. Is it normal for terminally ill patients to desire death? *Am J Psychiatry* 1986; 143:208–11.
49. Kitchell MA, Barnes RF, Veith RC, et al. Screening for depression in hospitalized geriatric patients. *J Am Geriatr Soc* 1982; 30:174–7.
50. Koenig HG, Meador KG, Cohen HJ, et al. Depression in elderly men hospitalized with medical illness. *Arch Intern Med* 1988; 148:1929–36.
51. Conwell Y, Caine ED. Rational suicide and the right to die. *N Engl J Med* 1991; 325:1100–3.
52. Lee MA, Ganzini L. Depression in the elderly: effect on patient attitudes toward life-sustaining therapy. *J Am Geriatr Soc* 1992; 40:983–8.
53. Koenig HG, Meador KG, Shelp F, et al. Depressive disorders in hospitalized medically ill patients: a comparison of young and elderly men. *J Am Geriatr Soc* 1991; 39:881–90.
54. Rapp SR, Walsh DA, Parisi SA, et al. Detecting depression in elderly medical inpatients. *J Consult Clin Psychol* 1988; 56:509–13.
55. Koenig HG, Meador KG, Cohen HJ, et al. Detection and treatment of major depression in older medically ill hospitalized patients. *Int J Psychiatry Med* 1988; 18:17–31.
56. Fisch RZ. Masked depression: its interrelations with somatization, hypochondriasis and conversion. *Int J Psychiatry Med* 1987; 17: 367–79.
57. Lesse S. The multivariant masks of depression. *Am J Psychiatry* 1968; 124(Suppl):41–53.
58. Pence GE. Do not go slowly into that dark night: mercy killing in Holland. *Am J Med* 1988; 84:139–41.
59. Prodis J. Assisted-suicide advocate helps 2 women end lives. *Durham Herald-Sun* 1992 Dec 16; Sect A:6.
60. Seckler AB, Meier DE, Mulvihill M, et. al. Substituted judgment: how accurate are proxy predictions? *Ann Intern Med* 1991; 115: 92–8.
61. Murphy DJ, Lynn J. Care near the end of life. In: Cassel CK, Reisenberg DE, Sorensen LB, Walsh JR, eds. *Geriatric medicine.* 2nd cd. New York: Springer-Verlag, 1990:607–14.
62. Hamm RJ, Lyeth BG. Nociceptive thresholds following food restriction and return to free-feeding. *Physiol Behav* 1984; 33: 499–501.
63. Hamm RJ, Knisely JS, Watson A, et al. Hormonal mediation of the analgesia produced by food deprivation. *Physiol Behav* 1985; 35:879–82.
64. Billings JA. Comfort measures for the terminally ill: is dehydration painful? *J Am Geriatr Soc* 1985; 33:808–10.
65. Terminal dehydration [editorial]. *Lancet* 1986; 1:306.

FRAME the DEBATE

Form at end of book

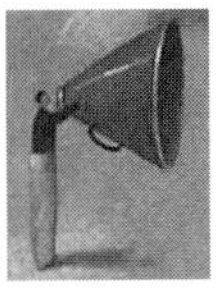

WiseGuide Wrap-Up

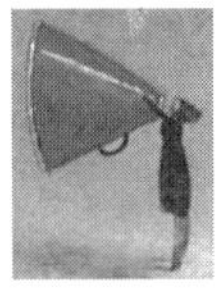

At question is the ethical obligation of the physician to "do no harm" vs. doing what the patient and his or her family desires. As individuals, we are faced with the moral consideration of ending suffering or prolonging our own or a loved one's painful or protracted death. As a society, we are faced with the question of where to draw the line between financial concerns and reverence for human life. Proponents of physician-assisted suicide cite humane and dignified treatment of the dying, while opponents stand firm on the moral conflict of hastening death and the possibility of the practice being misused to dispose of the weak, old, afflicted, or unwanted in our society.

R.E.A.L. Sites

This list provides a print preview of typical **Coursewise** R.E.A.L. sites. (There are over 100 such sites at the **Courselinks**™ site.) The danger in printing URLs is that web sites can change overnight. As we went to press, these sites were functional using the URLs provided. If you come across one that isn't, please let us know via email to: webmaster@coursewise.com. Use your Passport to access the most current list of R.E.A.L. sites at the **Courselinks** site.

Site name: Euthanasia and Physician-Assisted Suicide: All Sides of the Issues
URL: http://www.religioustolerance.org/euthanas.htm
Why is it R.E.A.L.? This site reviews both sides of the euthanasia issue. The authors state, "Ultimately, euthanasia is a question of choice: empowering people to have control over their own bodies."
Key topics: euthanasia, physician-assisted suicide
Try this: Read the article "Euthanasia and Physician-Assisted Suicide: All Sides of the Issue." Focus especially on the subsection titled "Ethical Aspects of Euthanasia." Answer the following questions: Some terminally ill patients are in intractable pain and/or experience an intolerably poor quality of life. They would prefer to end their life rather than continue until their body finally gives up. Does the state have a right to deny them their wish? Should the disabled or terminally ill be given the same access to the suicide option as able-bodied people have? Is denying them physician-assisted suicide a form of discrimination?

Site name: Suicide Watch
URL: http://abcnews.go.com/dispatches/bureaus/euthanasia032298/suicide_profile2.html
Why is it R.E.A.L.? This time line illustrates the controversy, from the original passage of the Death with Dignity Act to the dispute between the state and federal governments.
Key topics: euthanasia, physician-assisted suicide
Try this: Review the time line of news events. Other than the actual right to physician-assisted suicide provided by the law, what additional ethical and legal issues are at hand?

Are Alternative Medicine Practices Viable Health-Care Options or Quackery?

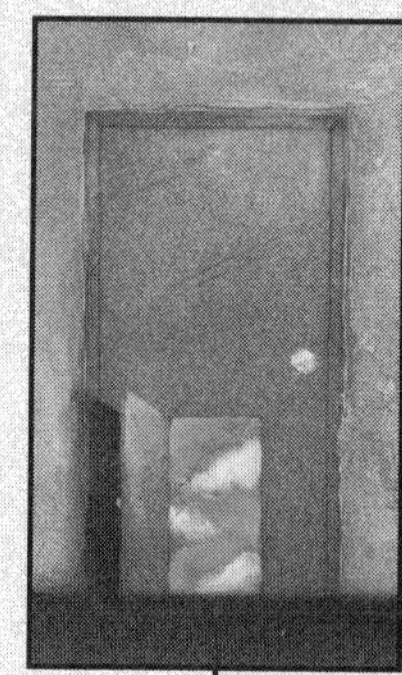

ISSUE 14

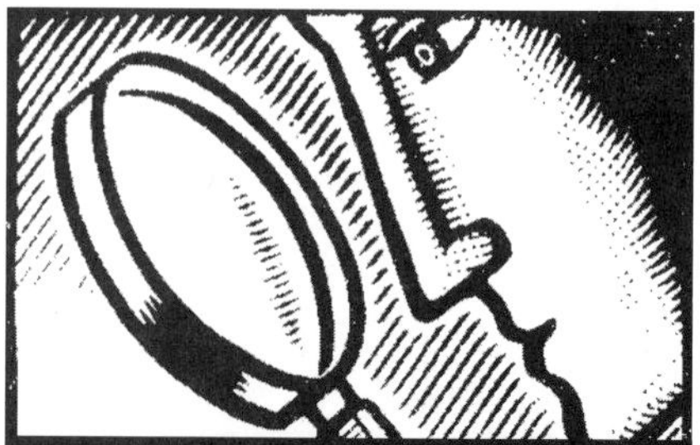

Take a Closer Look

1. List at least three reasons cited in Reading 36 why Americans seek nonmedical practitioners.
2. According to Campion, how should a medical doctor react when a patient brings up nonmedical alternative treatments?
3. Describe Andrew Weil's concept of "Integrative Medicine" fellowships.
4. What is Andrew Weil's opinion of the placebo effect?
5. In Reading 38, how does Barrett define the following three alternative health-care methods: (1) genuine alternative, (2) experimental, and (3) questionable?
6. Barrett is critical of "vitalism." Describe vitalism and why Barrett is opposed to philosophies of health that espouse it. Give an example of "life force."

WiseGuide Intro

A recent study published in the *New England Journal of Medicine* showed that nearly a third of Americans use some sort of alternative medicine in addition to conventional health care. Alternative forms of health care cover a wide selection of practices, ranging from the well-known practices of acupuncture, chiropractic, and podiatry, to the more cryptic and obscure practices of aromatherapy, iridology, reflexology, therapeutic touch, and rolfing. Many of these unconventional alternatives involve more than treatment of the patient's injuries or infirmities. They often include spiritual, meditative, and lifestyle practices.

The so-called "alternative health practices" are generally assumed to be those that have not been proven through the Western scientific method of random selection, double-blind studies, clinical trials, and so on. Nonetheless, we are currently seeing widespread use of relaxation response, hypnosis, visualization, and acupuncture incorporated into dentistry, surgery, and even smoking cessation. The public's disappointment with the shortcomings of conventional medicine has produced a growing demand for alternative approaches, practices, and philosophies to be integrated into the American health-care system.

In Reading 36, " Why Unconventional Medicine?" Edward Campion takes a diplomatic though somewhat antagonistic position toward alternative medicine and health-care practices. He first presents several reasons why Americans seek unconventional medicine, including dissatisfaction with conventional medicine, lower costs, and the power of the placebo effect. Campion acknowledges the widespread attraction patients have to alternatives and advises that allopathic physicians be understanding of their patients' needs and desires. At the same time, however, he stands firm on the efficacy of the modern medical doctor with the closing line: ". . . we must act to guarantee every American something that all deserve: a physician."

In Reading 37, "An Interview with Dr. Andrew Weil: Natural Medicine, Natural Health," "natural medicine" advocate Andrew Weil reviews his initial disenchantment with conventional medicine and the education behind it. He supports education in alternative and integrated practices in medical schools. He defends the concept of natural healing and sees the physician as a proponent of that healing. Weil believes that medicine should be focused on maximizing the body's "healing system" while minimizing the effects on the rest of the body. This "maximizing," he feels, may often come from methods outside of the scope of most allopathic medical practitioners.

In Reading 38, "Be Wary of 'Alternative' Health Methods," health consumer advocate Steven Barrett cautions against accepting alternative methods as being safe and effective. He points out the motivations for and contemporary trend to seek alternatives to conventional medicine. Barrett supports the scientific method of inquiry and encourages readers to regard with a critical eye those questionable practices that lack measurable effects. Interestingly, Barrett views the placebo effect of alternative health practices as "insufficient reason to justify its use," whereas Weil (Reading 37) views it as a positive outcome that completely justifies the use of alternative methods.

Issue 14: Are alternative medicine practices viable health-care options or quackery?

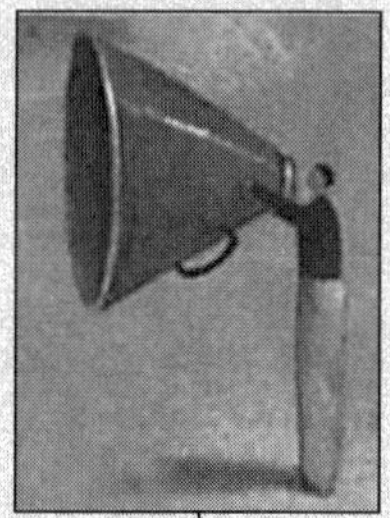

Why Unconventional Medicine?

Edward W. Campion, M.D.

The careful national survey reported by Eisenberg et al. in this issue of the *Journal*[1] tells us that in a given year about a third of all American adults use unconventional medical treatments, such as relaxation techniques, chiropractic, therapeutic massage, special diets, and megavitamins. Unconventional techniques are most often used for back problems, headache, arthritis, musculoskeletal pain, insomnia, depression, and anxiety. The most frequent users are educated, upper-income white Americans in the 25-to-49 year age group, and they are more likely to live in the West than elsewhere in the country. The cost is over $10 billion a year, 30 percent of which is paid for by public or private health insurance.

Has the American public forsaken medicine for herbs and crystal healing? Not exactly. The great majority of those surveyed had seen physicians, as had everyone with major medical problems such as cancer, diabetes, and hypertension. But 12 percent of the respondents visited unconventional practitioners (averaging an astonishing 19 visits in a year), and about a quarter of the respondents used unconventional methods of healing on their own without seeking help from nonphysicians. Of those who saw a physician for their principal medical condition, about a quarter (28 percent) also used some unconventional treatment for the same problem, but most (72 percent) did not tell their physicians about it.

The survey defined unconventional therapies broadly, but the analysis excluded prayer and exercise (which, sadly, are less popular). Some of these treatments are probably quackery; some of them are just the American version of the health spa. Many of the relaxation techniques, massage therapies, special diets, and self-help groups could be considered to be lifestyle choices more than therapeutic interventions. "Lifestyle diets" include everything from simply not eating meat to diet fads that claim to boost virility or cure cancer. Self-help groups include both invaluable organizations such as Alcoholics Anonymous and bizarre ones that preach mysterious chemical sensitivities. Roughly a third of unconventional practices entail theories that are patently unscientific and in direct competition with conventional medicine: for example, chiropractic, spiritual healing, herbal medicine, "energy healing" (with crystals or machines), homeopathy, and acupuncture. Even here, judgments are blurred because some of these treatments are dispensed or recommended by physicians.[2] Unfortunately, this survey does not define the extent of physicians' involvement in prescribing unconventional therapies.

The reason people go to nonmedical practitioners is simple: they want to feel better. Access is easy. Invitations to be healed are everywhere.[3] It's cheaper than seeing a physician. The presenting symptoms are chronic irritations that are difficult for anyone to treat successfully. Many begin unconventional treatments empirically or out of curiosity to see whether they will feel better. Anecdotes and testimonials from friends are powerful persuaders. For such subjective responses as pain and fatigue, about a third of the affected people will respond to any placebo.[4] In addition, many are dissatisfied with the medical establishment. Though Americans want all that modern medicine can deliver, they also fear it. They may resent the way visits to physicians quickly lead to pills, tests, and technology. Most now know of iatrogenic disasters from medicine gone wrong. Consumers also may seek out unconventional healers because they think their problems will be taken more seriously. They receive the benefit of time and attention, with invitations to return often.

Some may think of unconventional therapies as a type of risk-free supplementary insurance that buys a higher state of wellness, a symptom-free, stress-free existence. Hollywood and Madison Avenue tell us we should be energy-packed, physically perfect, and pain-free. The media barrage us with news of medical mishaps, misdiagnosed diseases, and dangers that lurk in food, air, and water, not to mention hospitals. Scientific research seems only to make matters worse, as it identifies risk factors beyond number and hazards in everything from milk to sunshine. We want to feel securely healthy with firm control over our bodies and over disease.[5] There is an unspoken belief that if we think right, feel right, eat right, and breathe right, we will never be afflicted by a terrible disease.[6] We also seek escape from the turbulence, worry, and malaise that plague this rich but troubled society.

Unconventional therapies are not a new or temporary fad.[3] They have been a growth industry even in European countries with universal access to medical care.[7] Some years ago Lewis Thomas wrote about how we were becoming obsessed with health, feeling in "constant jeopardy of disease and death."[8] The irony is that while our poor are too often unwell and undertreated, most Americans are healthier than ever before. The average 40-year-old man can expect to live until he is 75, and the average 40-year-old woman until she is 81.[9] But the statistics don't lessen our worry when we hear and read so much about such fearful diseases as cancer, coronary disease, and dementia.[10] Unconventional treatments often seem to make people feel more comfortable, even when their accompanying theories are silly.

For physicians the first step is to understand what our patients are up to. An adequate medical history should include nonjudgmental inquiries about the use of unconventional therapies. Physicians should resist the immediate temptation to condemn, since that simply cuts off further communication. As Ingelfinger observed, "An establishment indictment of a popular remedy is one of the best advertisements."[11] If the patient feels humiliated by the physician, he or she may conclude correctly that the alternative practitioner is less judgmental and more understanding. The physician should be honest about any possible risks, but it is unwise and unethical to scare the patient with fearful predictions of nasty but unlikely toxicity. A practical approach can actually strengthen the doctor-patient relationship and avert fruitless debate about the theories that underlie most unorthodox therapies. The physician should try to understand the patient's motivation. If it is the hope for better control of hypertension or dyspepsia with less medication, then there can be agreement on the goals. If the purpose is stress reduction, the physician should discuss the problem and offer support. Often the patient's goal is simply to feel healthier and prevent disease. The physician can concur with the goal while being honest about the lack of scientific evidence supporting most unorthodox therapies. Above all, the physician should retain the patient's trust and try not to feel threatened because an intelligent patient is taking garlic pills or meditating to influence his lymphocytes. Almost invariably, the patient continues to rely on the physician to diagnose, treat, and explain major disease and to deliver effective primary and preventive care.

The public's expensive romance with unconventional medicine is cause for our profession to worry. We need to demonstrate more effectively our dedication to caring for the whole patient—worries, quirks, and all. This can be done partly by helping to reform our health care system so that it proves our commitment to primary care for all, commercial deception for none, and simple acceptance of most human foibles. As a profession we must act to guarantee every American something that all deserve: a physician.

References

1. Eisenberg DM, Kessler RC, Foster C, Norlock FE, Calkins DR, Delbanco TL. Unconventional medicine in the United States—prevalence, costs, and patterns of use. *N Engl J Med* 1993; 328:246–52.
2. Cassileth BR, Lusk EJ, Strouse TB, Bodenheimer BJ. Contemporary unorthodox treatments in cancer medicine: a study of patients, treatments, and practitioners. *Ann Intern Med* 1984; 101:105–12.
3. Murray RH, Rubel AJ. Physicians and healers—unwitting partners in health care. *N Engl J Med* 1992; 326:61–4.
4. Beecher HK. The powerful placebo. *JAMA* 1955; 159:1602–6.
5. Gillick MR. Common-sense models of health and disease. *N Engl J Med* 1985; 313:700–3.
6. Angell M. Disease as a reflection of the psyche. *N Engl J Med* 1985; 312:1570–2.
7. Smith T. Alternative medicine. *BMJ* 1983; 287:307–8.
8. Thomas L. *The medusa and the snail: more notes of a biology watcher.* New York: Viking Press, 1979: 49.
9. National Center for Health Statistics. *Vital statistics of the United States, 1988.* Vol. 2. Mortality. Part A. Washington, D.C.: Government Printing Office, 1991. (DHHS publication no. (DHS) 90–1102.)
10. Barsky AJ. *Worried sick: our troubled quest for wellness.* Boston: Little, Brown, 1988.
11. Ingelfinger FJ. Laetrilomania. *N Engl J Med* 1977; 296:1167–8.

FRAME the DEBATE

Form at end of book

Issue 14: Are alternative medicine practices viable health-care options or quackery?

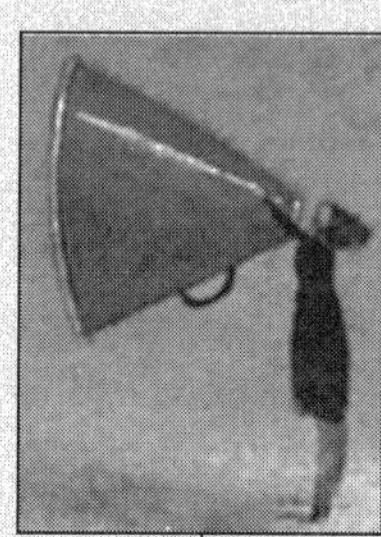

An Interview with Dr. Andrew Weil: Natural Medicine, Natural Health

Daniel Redwood

Dr. Daniel Redwood is a chiropractor and writer who lives in Virginia Beach, Virginia. He is the author of A Time to Heal *and* Contemporary Chiropractic, *and is Associate Editor of* The Journal of Alternative and Complementary Medicine. *A collection of his writings can be found at www.wholeliving.com/redwood.*

Andrew Weil, M.D. has for the past two decades made a unique contribution to the mainstreaming of natural medicine. He has set a high standard in a field that needs high standards, presenting a well reasoned, impeccably documented and intriguingly creative body of work. He is one of a small number of holistic physicians to hold a faculty position at a major medical school, and is an internationally recognized expert on medicinal plants, drugs and drug abuse, altered states of consciousness, and alternative and natural medicine.

Born in Philadelphia in 1942, Dr. Weil received an A.B. degree in biology (botany) from Harvard in 1964, and an M.D. from Harvard Medical School in 1968. After completing a medical internship at Mt. Zion Hospital in San Francisco, he worked for a year at the National Institute of Mental Health, and then wrote his first book, *The Natural Mind.*

From 1971–75, as a Fellow of the Institute of Current World Affairs, Dr. Weil traveled widely in North and South America and Africa collecting information on drug use in other cultures, medicinal plants, and alternative methods of treating disease. From 1971–84, he was on the research staff of Harvard Botanical Museum and conducted investigations of medicinal and psychoactive plants.

At present, Dr. Weil is Associate Director of the Division of Social Perspectives in Medicine of the College of Medicine at the University of Arizona, where he teaches alternative medicine, mind-body interactions, and medical botany. He has a general practice in Tucson, focusing exclusively on natural and preventive medicine and diagnosis of difficult health problems. He is the President of the Center for Integrative Medicine and the Beneficial Plant Institute.

Dr. Weil writes a regular column for *Natural Health* magazine, and is the author of many scientific and popular articles and five books: *The Natural Mind, The Marriage of the Sun and Moon, Chocolate to Morphine* (with Winifred Rosen), *Health and Healing,* and *Natural Health, Natural Medicine.*

Dr. Redwood (DR): What led you into the Healing Arts in the first place?

Dr. Weil (AW): I was always interested in things biological. I went to medical school with the idea of getting a medical education, not of becoming a doctor. I had an intuition that a medical degree would be very useful to me, and I wanted that education. It also put off making a decision about what I wanted to do. So I really didn't see myself as practicing the healing arts for a long time. I became very disillusioned with the kind of medicine that I was being taught, so when I finished my basic clinical training, I really dropped out of that world, and found ways to travel around. I was mostly living as a writer, and observing other kinds of healing practices. It was only after some time that very gradually I was drawn into practicing.

DR: If you were to briefly summarize the principles of natural health, what would you say they are?

AW: The first is that the body has a healing system, an innate healing potential that can be accessed in many different ways. That is the foremost principle of natural health and natural medicine. Secondly, that the optimal treatment is that which minimally impacts the physical body and maximally accesses the healing system.

DR: To what degree has our knowledge of body-mind interactions grown in recent years, and how much of this knowledge is being well-utilized by physicians and other health practitioners on a daily basis?

AW: There has been a tremendous increase in public consciousness of mind-body interactions, but I'm not sure we know any more about it than we ever did. You can look back to the last century and people obviously had a lot of observations about mind-body interactions. The problem is building these into our conceptual framework of health and healing. My sense is that in conventional medicine today, although there is lip service given to the mind and mind-body interactions, despite all of these books and television programs, there is very little use being made on a practical level of that theoretical knowledge.

DR: What kind of changes in medical education and practice do you think could improve that?

AW: I think they would have to be sweeping. And sometimes, at my most cynical, I think the only way we'll see that is if alternative kinds of medical schools start. I really am deeply pessimistic about the prospect of curriculum reform. They are constantly talking about reforming the medical curriculum, and all it is is reshuffling the deck and dealing it out in a different order. I don't see fundamental change happening.

I am working on a project now which I'll give my best shot. We have a unique chance at the University of Arizona College of Medicine to make some change. We're going to start a fellowship program in "Integrative Medicine." We'll start by offering one year fellowships to people who have completed family practice and internal medicine residencies. This will be a one-year fellowship in training on how to combine the best ideas and practices of conventional and alternative medicine, with a strong emphasis on healing, natural healing, mind-body interactions, and so forth. Our hope is that this will grow into a residency program, and eventually into a track that will begin in the first year of medical school. So we're going to try.

DR: Are there other such pilot projects taking place elsewhere in the medical education world?

AW: There are individuals like me at various schools, mostly teaching elective courses. Columbia University was just given a large grant to start a center in alternative medicine. I don't know of any place that has the full institutional support of a medical school, with good prospects for financial backing, that we have at the University of Arizona. We really have a very large vision of trying to start a residency training program in a new kind of medicine.

DR: What were the circumstances at Arizona that brought this about?

AW: Well, an odd combination of things. I am here by pure chance—my car broke down here 21 years ago. It took six weeks to get fixed, and I never left.

DR: What a great story.

AW: I would never have thought I would be living in Arizona. I always had a vision of Arizona being very politically conservative . . .

DR: Which in some ways it is.

AW: Yes, although Tucson is a liberal pole of it. But the regulatory laws in Arizona, including the medical licensing laws, have a kind of Wild West *laissez faire* flavor which is unique, except for Nevada. Nevada and Arizona are the only two states that have a Homeopathic Board of Medical Examiners under which people doing unusual practices can get licensure, that rivals the regular Board of Medical Examiners. So Arizona has been a kind of haven for people practicing alternative medicine. The third naturopathic college in the United States just opened here in Phoenix. Canyon Ranch is here, which is the spa that has the greatest commitment to preventive and alternative medicine. And I'm here, and have been teaching courses in alternative medicine. It's just a continuing set of favorable circumstances that have made this possible.

DR: Some holistic medical physicians are pressured by their state boards to discontinue some or all of their unconventional practices. Some have lost their licenses. What do you think is a fair way for boards to both protect the public and allow for something other than lowest common denominator care?

AW: I think that boards should have consultants who are experts in alternative medicine, that they should inform themselves about what is legitimate and what might not be legitimate in alternative medicine. I think the first criterion always has to be whether there is a potential for harm. In general, boards are unlikely to take action against physicians unless there are complaints by patients. A lot of this comes down to the relationship that doctors form with patients, rather than what they're doing. But I think there is great need for education of medical boards.

DR: I want to ask your opinion of the Clinton Administration's health reform proposals, and the other health reform plans in congress.

AW: I am delighted that at long last the federal government is looking at this issue, which should have been addressed a long time ago. It seems unconscionable to me that the richest nation in the world can't provide basic access to health care for all its citizens. At the same time, having seen a little bit of Medicare, I am not very enthusiastic about the prospect of having the federal government run this. And also, I think that the Clinton proposals don't go to the level at which change needs to happen.

DR: What is that level?

AW: I think there really has to be complete rethinking of the nature of medicine, and people's expectations of it. Not simply worrying about who pays for it, as it's now set up.

DR: Tell me more about the deeper level at which public policy should address this.

AW: I think we have an economic crisis in health care because this is an outward sign that the paradigm from which medicine operates has really reached the end of the line. The philosophy of medicine that's in place now is one that says diseases mostly have external causes, that you deal with diseases by developing weapons against agents of diseases, that there's extensive reliance on technology, and that we don't look at the natural healing mechanisms of the body. All of that has led us in a direction that has us on the edge of bankruptcy. And we're not going to change that just by figuring out different ways of reimbursing.

DR: Do you believe that modern Western medicine is a sustainable system for the long run? And if not, why not?

AW: No just because it's too expensive. For that simple fact it just cannot be delivered to the people who need it. And it has become so wedded to technology and so ignoring of natural healing potentials of other methods of intervention which are much more cost-effective.

DR: When there's an emergency situation that requires high-tech care, I don't think anyone I know would be in favor of withholding it. But how do we break out of this cycle where we lurch from crisis to crisis?

AW: First of all, I think a lot of hospitals are going to go bankrupt, and we're going to be left with regional centers at which all the high-tech stuff is done. The main problem is to teach both doctors and patients to sort out those conditions which should go to conventional medicine. You know, of the total number of sick people going to doctors, maybe 20 percent of them have conditions for which conventional allopathic medicine is appropriate. If we restricted that kind of medicine to that percent, we would not be in the kind of economic trouble we're in now. But we're trying to use this for every thing, and it doesn't work for the vast majority of problems.

DR: What do you think are the pros and cons of managed care and HMOs with regard to these questions?

AW: A major con is that doctors who work in them lose all autonomy. They are essentially told how to practice, how much time to spend with patients, what to do in certain conditions. It really has taken away all of the individual autonomy that has made the practice of medicine very interesting and very rewarding. I guess on the pro side, as a stopgap measure it has made the delivery of care economically viable, at least for a time.

DR: Do you see any way in which HMOs could become true wellness centers?

AW: That would be nice. I don't know. One idea that I have that I'd like to see happen, something that I'm going to work at, is that I would like to see a new kind of institution that's somewhere between a spa and a hospital coming into existence. I think a lot of people now go as inpatients to hospitals who could much more profitably be treated in centers of that sort, where they would learn about what healthy lifestyles is, how to do it, and come out knowing more than they went in with about how to keep themselves healthy.

DR: Is there any country whose health care system provides a good model both for holism and social justice?

AW: I would look at Germany and maybe Switzerland. There are definite areas in which they're ahead of us. There is much greater interest in natural medicine. There are more doctors who practice it, there are natural pharmaceutical companies, there is a system of reimbursement for stays in spas and healing centers. So there are certainly things there that we can learn. But with that possible exception, I don't know that there are any other models to look at.

DR: I know that you travel to Japan periodically. What is their health care system like and what lessons can we learn from the Japanese experience?

AW: A lot. We can see many of the faults of our own system blown up to even greater proportions. Japan has national health insurance—there are no competitors. National health insurance in Japan pays 100 percent for procedures and zero percent for consultations, so there is no incentive for a doctor to talk to a patient, and there's a great deal of incentive for doctors to do expensive tests. The average doctor may see 30 patients an hour. Two minutes with a patient—they're called "two-minute doctors." Patients never ask doctors questions. That's just not done. It's very authoritarian. There are enormously lengthy hospital stays.

DR: Why?

AW: Because everybody makes money from it. It's fully paid for by insurance. It's very common to put patients in hospitals for four months, or six months for things where we'd put them in for a few days. But this is fully reimbursable under Japanese health insurance.

DR: Is there no co-payment? Is it 100 percent reimbursement?

AW: Yes. There is also a very unhealthy relationship between doctors and pharmaceutical companies in Japan. A pharmaceutical company will often supply a new doctor in practice with a year's worth of free drugs, which the doctor then sells to patients.

DR: In our country we have historically had a division between the prescribing physician and the dispensing pharmacist, specifically to avoid this sort of conflict of interest.

AW: Exactly. You can see how that's a real area of abuse in Japan. The Japanese build a lot of the machines that we use in our medical centers, CAT scanners and MRI scanners. Every local Japanese hospital has one. The same problem exists here, but it's worse in Japan, because there are more of the machines around. And in order to recover the costs, there is enormous incentive to use them, and this is also payable through insurance. So there is a tremendous amount of [diagnostic] testing.

The rate of coronary heart disease in Japan is much lower than in the United States, probably because of diet primarily. But the rate of doing coronary angiograms is the same. So that means that if you have the misfortune to have chest pain anywhere in the vicinity of a Japanese hospital, they're going to do an angiogram on you, whether you need it or not. These are just some of the ways where you can see the kind of problems we have, blown up even bigger.

DR: Which traditional healing systems from other cultures do you have the most familiarity with, and how compatible are they with contemporary medical practice?

AW: I have a fair amount of familiarity with Chinese medicine, which I think at root is not very compatible with Western medicine. It's based on totally different conceptions of health, illness and energy. And yet it's odd that it has become one of the most established in this country. Acupuncture is practiced by many physicians in medical centers. There is increasing use of Chinese herbal medicine. It's become very accepted.

I'm a great fan of manipulative medicine [manual manipulation of the spine and other joints], and I see that beginning to be incorporated into more mainstream medicine. I think that's potentially very compatible with conventional medicine, as is naturopathic medicine.

I'm really interested in all the mind-body interventions, which I think are all potentially very compatible with standard medicine. It's just that most standard doctors don't know how they are used or don't think to use them.

DR: If you were to attempt to project a generation or two into the future, what kinds of changes would you anticipate in terms of the boundaries between the health professions.

AW: I certainly think we're going to see the appearance of wellness centers and healing centers. Some will be these inpatient facilities that I mentioned and others may be clinics where many kinds of practitioners work under the same roof. I think that's definitely going to happen. And we'll see about this effort that I'm making to create a field of integrative medicine. There's high potential there to turn out medical doctors who are familiar with these other techniques and willing to work with other practitioners.

DR: I've found your writings on the placebo effect to be both original and fascinating. What is your current thinking on placebos and on spontaneous remission from disease?

AW: I still think that placebos are really the meat of healing interactions. They are examples of pure healing responses from within that are triggered through the mind by belief. The mind is only one avenue to the healing system, but it's a very interesting one and the advantage of it is that it requires little external paraphernalia, and there's no [side effect of] toxicity involved. So I think the placebo response is the greatest ally that a practitioner has, and that the best kind of medicine is that which elicits the maximum placebo response with a minimum direct impact on the physical body. So I'm a big fan of placebo response, and I really try to get people to think differently about them.

DR: And remissions?

AW: I'm working on a new book called *Spontaneous Healing,* which should be published next year by Knopf. I'm not using the term "remission" in the title, for two reasons. First of all calling it remission implies that it's temporary, that it's going to come back. And in genuine healing, the problem is dealt with. Secondly, remission has a strong connotation of cancer, and I am interested in all healing responses, not just cancer. One of the problems I see made in the field (such as it is, it's a very tiny field) has been to look entirely at cancer. I think that's a mistake, because if you look only at cancer, you get very little sense of how powerful the body's healing system is, and how widespread are the kinds of conditions in which it operates.

I'm very much interested in the complete disappearance of back pain, autoimmunity, allergies, all sorts of conditions, including serious conditions. I'm looking at all of these examples of healing, I think that in general this is a field that has been just totally ignored by medical research. When doctors come across cases of it, they tend to wonder at it, maybe they ignore it, maybe they look at it, but they tend not to let these kinds of cases influence their general thinking about health and illness. And I think this should be a major focus, or the major focus, of medical research and practice as well.

FRAME the DEBATE

Form at end of book

Be Wary of "Alternative" Health Methods

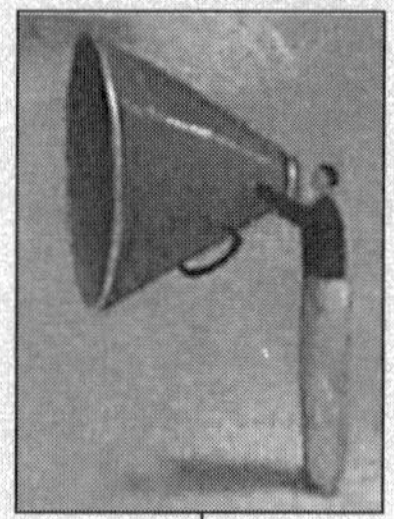

Stephen Barrett, M.D.

"Alternative medicine" has become the politically correct term for questionable practices formerly labeled quack and fraudulent. During the past few years, most media reports have contained no critical evaluation and have featured the views of proponents and their satisfied clients.

To avoid confusion "alternative" methods should be classified as genuine, experimental, or questionable. *Genuine* alternatives are comparable methods that have met science-based criteria for safety and effectiveness. *Experimental* alternatives are unproven but have a plausible rationale and are undergoing responsible investigation. The most noteworthy is use of a 10%-fat diet for treating coronary heart disease. *Questionable* alternatives are groundless and lack a scientifically plausible rationale. The archetype is homeopathy, which claims that "remedies" so dilute that they contain no active ingredient can exert powerful therapeutic effects. Some methods fit into more than one category, depending on the claims made for them. Blurring these distinctions enables promoters of quackery to argue that because some practices labeled "alternative" have merit, the rest deserve equal consideration and respect. Enough is known, however, to conclude that most questionable "alternatives" are worthless.

An even better way to avoid confusion is sort methods into three groups: (1) those that work, (2) those that don't work, and (3) those we are not sure about. Most methods described as "alternative" fall into the second group. A recent editorial in the *Journal of the American Medical Association* made the same point in another way:

> There is no alternative medicine. There is only scientifically proven, evidence-based medicine supported by solid data or unproven medicine, for which scientific evidence is lacking. Whether a therapeutic practice is "Eastern" or "Western," is unconventional or mainstream, or involves mind-body techniques or molecular genetics is largely irrelevant except for historical purposes and cultural interest. We recognize that there are vastly different types of practitioners and proponents of the various forms of alternative medicine and conventional medicine, and that there are vast differences in the skills, capabilities, and beliefs of individuals within them and the nature of their actual practices. Moreover, the economic and political forces in these fields are large and increasingly complex and have the capability for being highly contentious. Nonetheless, as believers in science and evidence, we must focus on fundamental issues—namely, the patient, the target disease or condition, the proposed or practiced treatment, and the need for convincing data on safety and therapeutic efficacy.[1]

Yet Another Editorial in the AMA Archives

The "alternative movement" is part of a general societal trend toward rejection of science as a method of determining truths. This movement embraces the postmodernist doctrine that science is not necessarily more valid than pseudoscience.[2] In line with this philosophy, "alternative" proponents assert that scientific medicine (which they mislabel as allopathic, conventional, or traditional medicine) is but one of a vast array of health-care options. "Alternative" promoters often gain public sympathy by portraying themselves as a beleaguered minority fighting a self-serving, monolithic "Establishment."

Under the rules of science, people who make the claims bear the burden of proof. It is their responsibility to conduct suitable studies and report them in sufficient detail to permit evaluation and confirmation by others. Instead of subjecting their work to scientific standards, promoters of questionable "alternatives" would like to change the rules by which they are judged and regulated. "Alternative" promoters may give lip service to these standards. However, they regard personal experience, subjective judgment, and emotional satisfaction as preferable to objectivity and hard evidence. Instead of conducting scientific studies, they use anecdotes and testimonials to promote their practices and political maneuvering to keep regulatory agencies at bay. As noted in a recent *New England Journal of Medicine* editorial:

> What most sets alternative medicine apart . . . is that it has not been scientifically tested and its advocates largely deny the need for such testing. By testing, we mean the marshaling of rigorous

evidence of safety and efficacy, as required by the Food and Drug Administration (FDA) for the approval of drugs and by the best peer-reviewed medical journals for the publication of research reports. Of course, many treatments used in conventional medicine have not been rigorously tested, either, but the scientific community generally acknowledges that this is a failing that needs to be remedied. Many advocates of alternative medicine, in contrast, believe the scientific method is simply not applicable to their remedies. . . .

Alternative medicine also distinguishes itself by an ideology that largely ignores biologic mechanisms, often disparage modern science, and relies on what are purported to be ancient practices and natural remedies (which are seen as somehow being simultaneously more potent and less toxic than conventional medicine). Accordingly, herbs or mixtures of herbs are considered superior to the active compounds isolated in the laboratory. And healing methods such as homeopathy and therapeutic touch are fervently promoted despite not only the lack of good clinical evidence of effectiveness, but the presence of a rationale that violates fundamental scientific laws—surely a circumstance that requires more, rather than less, evidence.[3]

The AMA *Archives of Dermatology* recently published the parallel views of a German physician:

When deliberating on the essence of alternative medicine we should simultaneously reflect on the intellectual and moral basis of regular medicine. . . . (1) alternative and regular medicine are speaking different languages; (2) alternative medicine is not unconventional medicine; (3) the paradigm of regular medicine is rational thinking; (4) the paradigm of alternative medicine is irrational thinking; (5) the present popularity of alternative medicine can be explained by romanticism; (6) some concepts of alternative medicine are falsifiable and others are not; (7) alternative medicine and evidence-based medicine are mutually exclusive; (8) the placebo effect is an important factor in regular medicine and the exclusive therapeutic principle of alternative medicine; (9) regular and alternative medicine have different aims: coming of age vs faithfulness; (10) alternative medicine is not always safe; (11) alternative medicine is not economic; and (12) alternative medicine will always exist. The fact that alternative methods are presently an integral part of medicine as taught at German universities, as well as of the physician's fee schedule, represents a collective aberration of mind that hopefully will last for only a short time.[4]

When someone feels better after having used a product or procedure, it is natural to credit whatever was done. This is unwise, however, because most ailments resolve by themselves and those that persist can have variable symptoms. Even serious conditions can have sufficient day-to-day variation to enable useless methods to gain large followings. In addition, taking action often produces temporary relief of symptoms due to a placebo effect. This effect is a beneficial change in a person's condition that occurs in response to a treatment but is not due to the pharmacologic or physical aspects of the treatment. Belief in the treatment is not essential, but the placebo effect may be enhanced by such factors as faith, sympathetic attention, sensational claims, testimonials, and the use of scientific-looking charts, devices, and terminology. Another drawback of individual success stories is that they don't indicate how many failures might occur for each success. People who are not aware of these facts tend to give undeserved credit to "alternative" methods.

The fact that an "alternative" method may exert a placebo effect that relieves symptoms is not sufficient reason to justify its use. Therapy should be based on the ability to alter abnormal physiology and not on the ability to elicit a less predictable placebo effect. Placebo therapy is inherently misleading and can make patients believe something is effective when it is not. Without controlled clinical trials, any treatment that is used could receive credit for the body's natural recuperative ability.

Medical "facts" are determined through a process in which hundreds of thousands of scientists share their observations and beliefs. Editors and editorial boards of scientific journals play an important role by screening out invalid findings and enabling significant ones to be published. Expert panels convened by government agencies, professional groups, voluntary health agencies, and other organizations also contribute to this effort. When controversies arise, further research can be devised to settle them. Gradually, a shared set of beliefs is developed that is considered scientifically accurate.

Many "alternative" approaches are rooted in vitalism, the concept that bodily functions are due to a vital principle or "life force" distinct from the physical forces explainable by the laws of physics and chemistry and detectable by scientific instrumentation. Practitioners whose methods are based on vitalistic philosophy maintain that diseases should be treated by "stimulating the body's ability to heal itself" rather than by "treating symptoms." Homeopaths, for example, claim that illness is due to a disturbance of the body's "vital force," which they can correct with special remedies, while many acupuncturists claim that disease is due to imbalance in the flow of "life energy" (*chi* or *Qi*), which they can balance by twirling needles in the skin. Many chiropractors claim to assist the body's "Innate Intelligence" by adjusting the patient's spine. Naturopaths speak of "Vis Medicatrix Naturae." Ayurvedic physicians refer to "prana." And so on. The "energies" postulated by vitalists cannot be measured by scientific methods.

Although vitalists often pretend to be scientific, they really reject the scientific method with its basic assumptions of material reality, mechanisms of cause and effect, and testability of hypotheses. They regard personal experience, subjective judgment, and emotional satisfaction as preferable to objectivity and hard evidence.

Some "alternative" proponents are physicians who have strayed from scientific thought. The factors that motivate them can include delusional thinking, misinterpretation of personal experience, financial considerations, and pleasure derived from notoriety and/or patient adulation.

"Alternative" promoters often claim that their approach promotes general health and is cost effective against chronic health problems. In a recent article, for example, the American Holistic Association's president claimed that various "basic healthy habits" would "tap a well-spring of physical energy experienced as a state of relaxed vitality."[5] In addition to exercising, eating a nutritious diet, and getting sufficient sleep, the list includes abdominal breathing; taking "a full complement of antioxidants and supplements; and "enhancing the body's ability to receive and generate bioenergy" through regular acupuncture treatments, acupressure, healing touch, craniosacral therapy, qigong, and several other nonstandard modalities. As far as I know, there is no published evidence that "alternative" practitioners are more effective than mainstream physicians in persuading their patients to improve their lifestyle. Nor have any vitalistic approaches been proven effective or cost-effective against any disease.

National Council Against Health Fraud president William T. Jarvis, Ph.D., has noted:

> Some techniques referred to as "alternative" may be appropriately used as part of the art of patient care. Relaxation techniques and massage are examples. But procedures linked to belief systems that reject science itself have no place in responsible medicine. Useless procedures don't add to the outcome, just to the overhead.

Many news reports have exaggerated the significance of the National Institutes of Health (NIH)'s Office of Alternative Medicine (OAM). Creation of this office was spearheaded by promoters of questionable cancer therapies who wanted more attention paid to their methods. Most of OAM's advisory panel members have been promoters of "alternative" methods, and none of its publications have criticized any method. In 1994, the OAM's first director resigned, charging that political interference had hampered his ability to carry out OAM's mission in a scientific manner.[6] The OAM has funded many studies related to "alternative" methods. However, it remains to be seen whether such studies will yield useful results. Even if some do, their benefit is unlikely to outweigh the publicity bonanza given to questionable methods. In 1998, Congress upgraded OAM into an NIH center with an annual budget of $50 million. The agency is now called the National Center for Complementary and Alternative Medicine (NCCAM).

References

1. Fontanarosa PB, Lundberg GD. Alternative medicine meets science. *JAMA* 280:1618–1619, 1998.
2. Sampson W. Antiscience trends in the rise of the "alternative medicine" movement. In Gross PR, Levitt N, Lewis MW (editors.). *The Flight from Science and Reason.* New York: New York Academy of Sciences, 1996, pp. 188–197.
3. Angell M, Kassirer J. Alternative Medicine—The Risks of Untested and Unregulated Remedies. *New England Journal of Medicine,* Sept 17, 1998.
4. Happle E. The essence of alternative medicine. A dermatologist's view from Germany. *Archives of Dermatology* 134:1455–1460, 1998.
5. Inker R. Basic training for holistic medical practice: Nurturing your body. *Holistic Medicine,* Winter 1997, pp. 4–5.
6. Marshall E. The politics of alternative medicine. *Science* 265, 2000–2002, 1994.

FRAME the DEBATE

Form at end of book

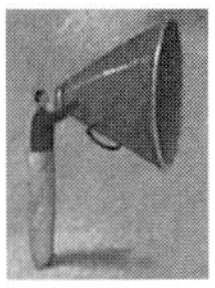

WiseGuide Wrap-Up

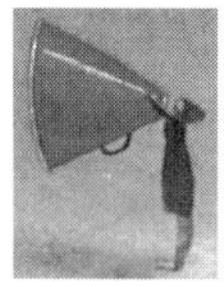

Proponents of alternative health care cite the need for an expanded approach to health, healing, and health care and denounce the American Medical Association as being myopic and exclusive. Opponents' arguments to alternative health care center around the lack of measurable proof behind alternative health theories and the possibilities of persons being harmed or their conditions worsened by ineffective and unfounded treatments.

R.E.A.L. Sites

This list provides a print preview of typical **Coursewise** R.E.A.L. sites. (There are over 100 such sites at the **Courselinks**™ site.) The danger in printing URLs is that web sites can change overnight. As we went to press, these sites were functional using the URLs provided. If you come across one that isn't, please let us know via email to: webmaster@coursewise.com. Use your Passport to access the most current list of R.E.A.L. sites at the **Courselinks** site.

Site name: Alternative Health News Online

URL: http://www.altmedicine.com/

Why is it R.E.A.L.? If you want to keep current with alternative medicine, this site, developed by a journalist, is a great resource.

Key topics: alternative/complementary medicine

Try this: Click on the "Alternative Medical Systems" link. Select one of the seven systems displayed. Read about the theory behind the practice. Become familiar with at least four basic principles of the practice. Do you feel your selected practice should be used as a primary form of health care, or is it more suitable as a complimentary form of care to be given along with Western medicine? What concerns do you have about the alternative health-care practice you selected? What would you like to know before trying it out?

Site name: Quackwatch

URL: http://www.quackwatch.com/

Why is it R.E.A.L.? This site has a variety of articles and essays related to consumer health issues. Particular attention is given to critical thinking and the use of the scientific method of inquiry to expose common health scams.

Key topics: quackery, questionable services and products, alternative health care

Try this: Select an article on a common form of quackery. Identify five questions that an informed, critical thinker might want to ask a practitioner of this form of quackery.

Site name: Alternative Health

URL: http://www.bewell.com/healthy/alternative/index.asp

Why is it R.E.A.L.? This site offers a wide variety of information on alternative health care and herbal remedies.

Key topics: alternative medicine, herbal medicine

Try this: Visit the site and select a featured ailment or alternative treatment. Print a copy to share with your classmates. Is the article well supported? What methods of persuasion (for example, documented facts, proper/improper use of statistics, emotional appeals, superlatives, science or pseudo-science, provable statements, etc.) does the article's author employ?

Site name: Ask Dr. Stoll

URL: http://bcn.net/~stoll/index.html

Why is it R.E.A.L.? This site is a collection of brief essays written by a medical doctor who was trained in allopathic (Western) medicine but now espouses the benefits of alternative medical practices. The site includes an interactive bulletin board that promises that "Dr. Stoll personally reads and responds to all posts directed to him within three days (unless he is ill or travelling)."

Key topics: alternative medicine, aromatherapy, American Medical Association conspiracy, health coaching

Try this: Read the articles "How to Be Healthy," "Modern Medical Interpretation of Stress," and "Why My License Was Revoked." Does Dr. Stoll offer sufficient valid evidence to support his contentions? Discuss the relative strengths or weaknesses of his arguments.

ISSUE 15

Who Benefits from Managed Health Care?

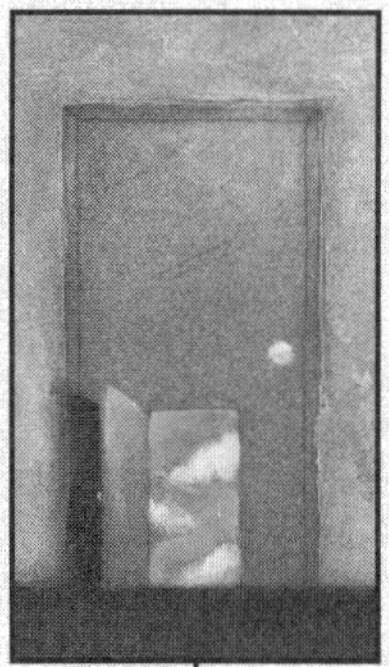

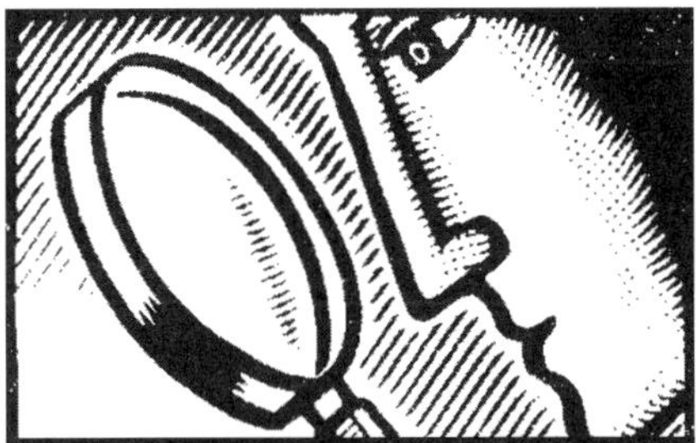

Take a Closer Look

1. What did a researcher at the American Heart Association find concerning surgical procedures and heart attack patients at HMOs?
2. According to the *New York Times,* about how many people were enrolled in HMOs in 1996?
3. What did the Commonwealth Fund survey of HMO physicians find regarding physicians' ability to make decisions regarding patient care and the amount of time physicians are able to spend with their patients?
4. About how often do managed-care facilities deny coverage for physician-recommended care?
5. Some people are concerned that HMOs disallow physicians from telling patients about certain medical procedures or therapies that might help but are expensive. What did the General Accounting Office find regarding so-called gag orders in physician contracts at HMOs?
6. In Reading 41, how does Ehrmann suggest that patients actively protect themselves from becoming involved in a conflict of interest regarding patient care and their HMO's bottom line?

WiseGuide Intro

The philosophy of managed health care centers around the concept of a single company or group coordinating the services of medical service providers. Managed-care programs are generally made up of groups of health-care providers, such as physicians, nurses, and medical technicians, who may work for a single company, as in the case of health maintenance organizations (HMOs), or they may be individual contractors who provide services for companies or groups. The managed-care system can be a privately owned corporation, or it can be controlled by the government, as in the case of socialized medicine.

Proponents of managed care feel that it provides quality health care at minimum cost due to cost-containing systems of care standards, referrals, and reviews. Opponents to managed care state that it limits access to providers, health-care choice, and competition, and affects the concept of a free market system. They fear that concerns for cost containment may result in managed-care systems discouraging doctors from ordering tests or making referrals necessary for proper patient diagnosis and care.

Reading 39, "Problems with Managed Care," is a composite of articles from periodicals and news sources that highlight specific problems and incidents where managed care has failed to meet the needs of consumers. The brief articles are organized under subheadings that focus on common criticisms of HMOs and managed-care systems. The articles that review political bills and new types of programs are likely included in this collection as "solutions" to the perceived problems of HMOs and managed health-care programs.

Reading 40, "Dispelling Managed Care Myths," addresses the common criticisms and concerns raised about managed health care. The authors discuss twelve issues and make counterarguments for each of the criticisms, including the popular concerns regarding limiting physicians' scope of practice and time with patients, and limiting consumers' free choice and access to health care. Much of the discussion is centered on customer satisfaction and cost containment issues.

In Reading 41, "Preserving the Best Health Care Possible," Paul Ehrmann, the president of the Community Coalition for Concerned Providers and Patients, opposes prepaid managed care and HMOs. He describes several key pitfalls to the system, which he perceives will lessen the quality of care that consumers receive. He accuses physicians and HMOs of making financial decisions that create a conflict of interest and compromise the quality of patient care. Ehrmann encourages concerned patients to question their health-care providers and personnel services at their workplace as to their relationship with third parties, such as insurance companies and HMOs.

Issue 15: Who benefits from managed health care?

Problems with Managed Care

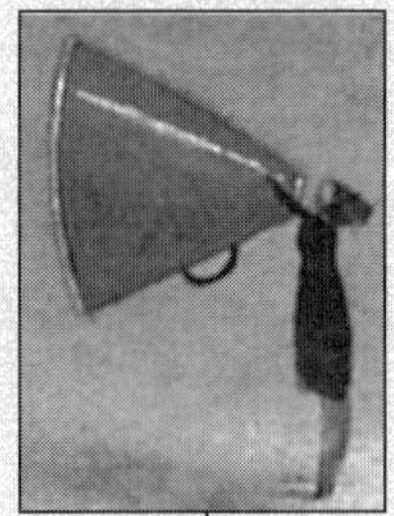

Companies Rebel against Managed Care*

A little more than a year ago, Minneapolis businesses launched a program to overhaul local health delivery systems. Their objective was to bypass the region's three large health maintenance organizations (HMOs), contract directly with doctors and inject a dose of free-market economics into medicine.

No fewer than 26 of the region's largest corporations—including 3M, Honeywell, Dayton Hudson, Pillsbury and Carlson Companies—entered into the arrangement, which has been described as a rebellion.

- In the new scheme, doctors are free to charge, organize and operate as they choose.
- But employees get booklets which rank doctor groups on what they charge and how they fare in terms of customer satisfaction—and employees who choose expensive doctors must pay the extra out-of-pocket.
- Payments to doctor groups are raised if they wind up attracting sicker-than-average patients—who cost more to treat.
- Physician groups which find ways to treat patients more efficiently get to keep the savings—while inefficient or wasteful doctors who go over budget are penalized.

Proponents of the new arrangement say it avoids the most vexing pitfalls of HMOs—such as lack of information among patients, the incentive for doctors to avoid treating sicker patients and the tendency for HMOs to cut the fees of doctors who find ways to reduce costs and treat patients more efficiently.

About 100,000 employees are participating in the experiment, which is being closely monitored by health care specialists throughout the country.

*Source: Brian O'Reilly, "Taking on the HMOs," *Fortune,* February 16, 1998.

Heart Attack Death Rate Higher in HMOs†

Health Maintenance Organization (HMO) enrollees with cardiac disease are twice as likely to die after a heart attack as those with traditional fee-for-service coverage, says cardiologist Paul Casale in a report to the American Heart Association.

- Casale studied 4,000 heart attack patients admitted to Pennsylvania hospitals in 1993.
- He found HMO patients are less likely to receive two surgical procedures common after heart attacks—heart catheterization and angioplasty.
- However, Casale's study did not have data on how long patients waited to get care—considered the best predictor of heart attack survival rates.

But Casale notes that HMO policies discouraging emergency room use could have delayed patients seeking treatment.

Dangers of HMOs‡

A number of studies and press reports indicate that the financial arrangements Health Maintenance Organizations (HMOs) make with doctors reward physicians and hospitals for deferring or withholding care that is deemed too expensive, pitting the financial interest of the doctor against the medical needs of the patient. For example:

- The brain tumor of a 5-year old Florida girl was repeatedly misdiagnosed as the flu until her mother took her to a facility outside the HMO—which refused to pay for the surgery resulting from the correct diagnosis.

†Source: News & Trends, "Are HMOs Trouble for Cardiac Patients?" *Business & Health,* December 1997.

‡Source: "More Trouble with Managed Care," *Consumers' Research,* September 1995.

- Long Island Jewish Hospital in Queens replaced private doctors in its anesthesia department with lower-paid and less-experienced salaried physicians, and in one 10-week period four patients died from anesthesia-related complications after successful surgery.
- A California HMO was fined $500,000 by the state for refusing to refer a young girl to a specialist for her Wilm's tumor and instead assigning a physician who had never operated on children or on a Wilm's tumor.

A Department of Health and Human Services survey of more than 4,000 enrollees and disenrollees from 45 Medicare HMOs across the country found an "alarmingly high level of dissatisfaction" among chronically ill and disabled patients.

- It found that 20% to 25% of disenrollees said they failed to receive primary care, referrals to specialists and HMO coverage of emergency care they needed.
- Of those who received care, 16% of enrollees and 18% of disenrollees reported waiting more than 12 days to see their primary care doctor.
- And, 24% of enrollees and 26% of disenrollees reported having to wait more than 12 days to see a specialist.

HMOs often reimburse doctors a fixed amount of money per covered patient, together with "withholds" and bonuses for delivering frugal care. Thus, incentives discourage doctors from referring patients to a specialist, authorizing high-tech procedures or approving costly operations. There is usually a review board the doctor can appeal to if HMO management refuses to cover a treatment or procedure, but it also has the power to deny care.

Clamp-Down Coming on HMOs?[§]

Politicians in both parties say public frustration with health maintenance organizations is causing them to introduce bills to set treatment standards. The HMOs and employers are fighting the proposed new rules and regulations. Employers fear the regulations would hamper their ability to control costs through use of HMOs.

- The number of people in HMOs has doubled in the past eight years—to 64 million in 1996.
- Nearly three-fourths of American workers with health insurance receive that coverage in HMOs or other managed-care plans.
- New federal laws and regulations covering HMOs would mark a departure from past practice—whereby states historically regulated insurance.

[§]Source: Robert Pear, "Congress Weighs More Regulation on Managed Care," *New York Times,* March 10, 1997.

- Managed-care companies charge that the drive for federal regulation rests mostly on "anecdotal evidence" based on isolated complaints, and that there is no solid proof of abuses.

They also warn that the effect of federal regulation would be to drive up costs, and mandating new benefits could potentially jeopardize consumers' access to coverage.

HMO Misunderstanding[||]

Most Americans don't understand what managed health care is, how it works, or how it differs from traditional health insurance, according to a current poll.

In a survey last year of 1,081 persons, conducted by Louis Harris and Associates for the consulting firm Towers Perrin, it was found that:

- Some 55 percent said they have either never heard the term "managed care" or didn't have a good understanding of what it means.
- Nearly one-third said they have never heard the term "health maintenance organization"—or had heard it but didn't know its meaning.
- Only 52 percent knew that HMOs put emphasis on preventive care.
- One in three who knew what HMOs were didn't know that they provide coverage for set monthly fees.
- Moreover, one in four in an HMO didn't know that their choice of physicians was limited.

About 60 percent of the U.S. workforce and their dependents—about 140 million Americans—are currently covered by some form of managed care plan.

New Flexibility in Managed Care?[#]

With the threat of new federal and state mandates and regulations hanging over them, managed health-care plans are stepping up efforts to allow greater flexibility in their systems and operations, according to reports.

- An estimated 160 million Americans are now enrolled in some form of managed care—usually HMOs.
- A prime example of the trend toward more consumer-friendly services are so-called Point of Service plans, in which enrollees pay a 10 percent to 15 percent higher premium, and 30 percent of a physician's or hospital's

[||]Source: Steven Findlay, "Survey on HMOs Finds Widespread Ignorance," *USA Today,* November 11, 1996.

[#]Source: Steven Findlay, "Trend in Managed Care is Flexibility," *USA Today,* April 16, 1997.

bill, for the privilege of going to any doctor, hospital or health facility they wish.

- About half of the nation's 630 HMOs now offer this option—up from 20 percent in 1990.
- More plans are reported to be allowing enrollees to see specialists without getting permission from primary care doctors.
- While enrollments in old-style "closed" HMOs has been stalled at about 24 million in the last two years, about 18 million Americans insured through their employers are now enrolled in the new POS plans—up from about 4.5 million as recently as 1992.

Physicians Dissatisfied with Managed Care**

Managed care is expanding to cover an ever broader share of the population, and more and more physicians are allying themselves with managed care organizations in order to keep patients or attract new insured patients.

However, a survey of 1,710 physicians by Louis Harris and Associates found that many of them believe managed care—such as provided by health maintenance organizations (HMOs), preferred provider organizations (PPOs) and point-of-service (POS) plans—has had a negative impact on their ability to care for patients and on their own satisfaction with medical practice.

The 1995 survey was designed by the Commonwealth Fund, which recently released its analysis of the data. Among the findings:

- Nearly two in five physicians (38 percent) report that their ability to make decisions they think are right for their patients has declined in the past three years.
- Forty-one percent report a decrease in the amount of time spent with their patients over the previous three years.
- Almost half of those in discounted fee-for-service or capitated plans rate their ability to get necessary treatment for their patients as fair or poor, and almost two-thirds (62 percent) give low ratings to their ability to get approval for care without delay.
- Sixty percent report very or somewhat serious problems with external review and with limitations on their clinical decisions.

**Source: Karen Scott Collins et al., "The Commonwealth Fund Survey of Physician Experiences with Managed Care," March 1997, Commonwealth Fund, One E. 75th Street, New York, NY 10021, (212) 535-0400. For full text: http://www.cmwf.org/physrvy.html

By contrast, among physicians in traditional fee-for-service plans, nearly two-thirds say they have encountered no serious problems in referring patients to specialists of their own choice, and 57 percent have had no serious problems with reviews of clinical decisions prior to a patient's receiving care.

Wide Variations in HMO Care††

In the most comprehensive national survey ever done among health maintenance organizations and their members, the managed care industry's leading accreditation organization discovered that the quality of health care varies widely among HMOs.

The survey, conducted by the National Committee for Quality Assurance (NCQA), used information gathered by 329 HMOs serving 37 million people, or 64 percent of the nation's 58 million HMO members.

Among the survey results:

- Some 56 percent of about 130,000 HMO enrollees said they were completely or very satisfied with their HMOs, 25 percent were somewhat satisfied and 19 percent reported being dissatisfied.
- Only 39 percent rated their HMOs as excellent or very good at telling them how the plan operates and what services are covered.
- And only 40 percent were satisfied with the number of doctors they could choose from and the length of time it took to get an appointment for routine care.

On the other hand, 85 percent of HMO enrollees said they did not have problems getting medical care recommended by their doctors.

According to Margaret E. O'Kane, president of the NCQA, patients in the average health plan appeared to get as good or better care than patients covered by traditional fee-for-service insurers.

For instance, a broader industry report released by the NCQA, "The State of Managed Care Quality," measured the extent to which heart-attack patients were receiving beta-blockers—which can reduce chances of a subsequent heart attack by 25 percent and chances of death by 10 percent.

- It found that the average health plan was providing beta-blockers to 61.9 percent of patients who could benefit from them.

††Source: Steven Findlay, "Survey Finds HMO Care Varies Widely," *USA Today,* and Ron Winslow, "Quality of HMOs in U.S. Varies Widely, Report by Accreditation Group Finds," *Wall Street Journal,* both October 2, 1997.

- But plans differed in the extent to which they supplied beta-blockers—from a low of 15 percent to a high of 100 percent.
- If all health plans made sure that at least 85 percent of heart patients who would benefit received them, about 1,600 heart-related deaths would be avoided annually.

In contrast, the NCQA says just 25 percent of traditional fee-for-service heart patients who need them receive beta-blockers—although they cautioned that the data doesn't allow saying whether HMOs actually perform better than traditional care.

The Woes of HMOs[‡‡]

Some of the biggest health maintenance organizations are racking up huge losses, grappling with unexpected rises in medical bills and feeling the heat from patients who want more services while paying less.

Here are some of the headaches:

- Subscriber growth could be curtailed as health plans raise premiums as much as 10 percent next year.
- Consumers and doctors are complaining that managed care has compromised quality or at least disrupted the way they want the medical system to work.
- At least 40 states have passed pro-consumer, anti-managed-care regulations, and Congress is considering a wide-ranging bill to do the same.
- Some leading health plans have had to take back charges against earnings because they lost track of how much they owed to doctors and hospitals.

Point-of-service plans—under which an HMO member can go outside the network to see a favorite specialist, subject to higher copayments—have more than tripled in popularity this decade, and now cover 26 million with employer-funded health care.

Until recently, federal payments for Medicare HMO patients were rising as much as 10.5 percent a year. But last summer, Congress enacted tougher limits that will boost premiums by just 2 percent a year.

The HMO industry is adding members at a rate of more than 10 percent a year, with some companies growing as rapidly as 50 percent a year. Observers point out that record-keeping work in medicine is already extraordinarily complex. They question whether the added burden of so many new enrollees might not completely bog down computer systems.

[‡‡]Source: George Anders and Ron Winslow, "HMOs' Woes Reflect Conflicting Demands of American Public," Wall Street Journal, December 22, 1997.

FRAME the DEBATE

Form at end of book

Issue 15: Who benefits from managed health care?

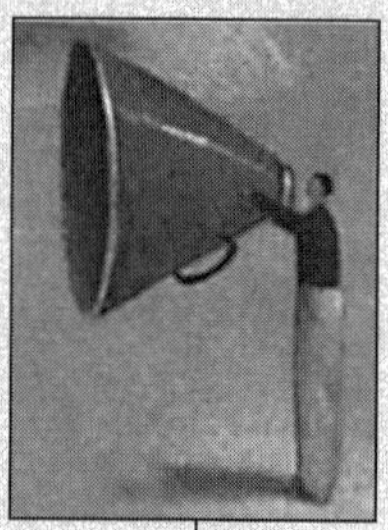

Dispelling Managed Care Myths

Policymakers are increasingly confronted with legislation that would impose a new level of prescriptive federal regulation on managed care plans. Opponents of managed care often promote this legislation by developing caricatures of managed care plans based on anecdotes and myths. Time and again the evidence does not support these claims, and the facts regarding the quality and affordability of the medical care offered by managed care plans are rarely offered or considered. Proceeding without the facts serves only to harm patients by misleading them and undermining their trust in the health care system.

To illustrate the wide gap between the claims and the facts about managed care plans, this Issue Brief presents a few examples of the myths about managed care plans and offers facts that dispel them. By highlighting these examples of health plan myths and correcting the record, AAHP is promoting a more informed debate about the changes occurring in the nation's health care system.

Myth: Managed care plans force physicians to see too many patients, requiring physicians to spend too little time with each patient.

- **Fact: Physicians are spending more time with patients.**

According to calculations based on data reported in the American Medical Association's *Socioeconomic Characteristics of Medical Practice 1997,* physicians spend more time on direct patient care activities per patient visit in 1996 (26.9 minutes) than in 1985 (24.3 minutes). This time encompasses patient visits in all settings, including office and hospital visits, interpreting tests, and consultations.[1]

Myth: Managed care plans are not regulated.

- **Fact: Managed care plans are regulated at both the state and federal level.**[2]

In the areas of quality and access, for example, many states require that HMOs and PPOs monitor the quality of care delivered by plan providers, make all covered services available, have a sufficient number of providers in the network who are accessible, provide information to members on plan policies, and have appeals and grievance procedures in place. Specific regulation of HMOs and PPOs varies by state.

State regulatory requirements for HMOs and PPOs are supplemented by (1) extensive federal program requirements for plans participating in Medicare, Medicaid, and the Federal Employees Health Benefits Program, (2) the Federal HMO Act, for federally qualified HMOs, and (3) the Health Insurance Portability and Accountability Act, among other laws.

In addition, many HMOs are voluntarily accredited by the nationally recognized National Committee for Quality Assurance, Joint Commission on Accreditation of Healthcare Organizations (JCAHO), or American Accreditation HealthCare Commission (AAHCC/URAC). PPOs are voluntarily accredited by AAHCC/URAC and JCAHO.

Myth: Many employees are forced into managed care plans that limit choice of providers.

- **Fact: Plans offer a broad choice of providers. Moreover, nearly all employees are given a choice of joining a plan that covers care by out-of-network physicians.**

Nearly 92 percent of American workers who receive health coverage by their employer are offered at least one plan that covers care provided by out-of-network physicians and hospitals, i.e., PPO, point-of-service (POS) or fee-for-service (FFS) plans, according to KPMG Peat Marwick LLP data analyzed for AAHP by the Barents Group. Of the remaining eight percent of workers, one-third are offered a choice of two or more HMOs. The majority of workers who are offered only one HMO are employed by small businesses.

Myth: Employers are making FFS premiums unaffordable to force employees into managed care plans.

- **Fact: Employers provide larger premium subsidies for FFS plans than for managed care plans.**

A study by KPMG Peat Marwick found that in 1996, on average, in dollar and percentage terms, employers required employees to pay *more* in premiums for network-based plans than for FFS plans. Far from being forced into managed care plans, employees are voluntarily choosing to enroll in managed care plans when they have the option to enroll in FFS.

Even though employers charge employees higher premiums when they choose managed care plans, the percentage of employees choosing an HMO far exceeds the percentage whose employers offer HMOs but no other types of plans. For example, according to KPMG's *Health Benefits in 1996* report and a report prepared by the Barents Group, slightly less than two percent of employees in firms with 5,000 or more employees were offered only one or more HMO, but 38 percent of employees in firms with more than 5,000 employees enrolled in HMOs.

Myth: Managed care plans force patients out of the hospital before it is medically appropriate.

- **Fact: Length of stay patterns for managed care plan enrollees are very similar to those for FFS enrollees.**

AAHP analysis of data prepared by The MEDSTAT Group found that 95 percent of both HMO and FFS hospital admissions had a length of stay that fell within or exceeded the high end of the length of stay range recommended by surgeons surveyed by the American College of Surgeons (ACS) regarding ACS-identified procedures. The other five percent of admissions fell below the recommended length of stay range *for both HMO and FFS enrollees.*

Myth: Managed care plans frequently deny coverage of care recommended by physicians.

- **Fact: Managed care plans rarely deny coverage of care recommended by physicians.**

A recent study of over 2,000 physicians caring for patients in plans that utilize managed care techniques found that the denial rate for all types of care was at most 3.0 percent, and much less for most types of care. For example, coverage for hospitalization was denied only 1.0 percent of the time, surgical procedures 1.2 percent, and specialist referrals 2.6 percent. Initial denial rates were somewhat higher, but between one-half and two-thirds of initial denials were reversed by the health plan, resulting in the lower ultimate denial rates (*Inquiry,* Volume 34, Fall 1997).

Myth: Managed care plans require physicians to practice "cookbook medicine."

According to a *Wall Street Journal* article, "guidelines, which come in thick bound notebooks, have become a standard among managed care plans for deciding length of stay." (November 6, 1996).

- **Fact: Managed care plans support medical care based on the individual needs of each patient.**

An AAHP analysis of The MEDSTAT Group data compared a set of Milliman & Robertson (M&R) guidelines (that represent utilization targets reflective of an ideal delivery system for patients without complications) to plan patients' actual length of stay for procedures identified in a survey by the ACS. The study showed that the length of stay for health plan patients varied widely around the guideline length of stay for specific Diagnostic Related Groups (DRGs). In fact, 61.7 percent of HMO admissions and 67.0 percent of FFS admissions had lengths of stay that exceeded the M&R guidelines.

As expected, within each DRG, length of stay for HMO patients varied. For example, within DRG 105 (Cardiac Valve Procedures Without Cardiac Catheterization), the shortest admission was for one day and the longest admission was for 26 days. Overall, two-thirds of the 52 admissions had a length of stay ranging from three to 10 days (the range reported as appropriate in the ACS survey), and 29 percent had a length of stay exceeding 10 days.

AAHP analysis revealed that in 1995, the severity-adjusted average lengths of stay for capitated plans was greater than the lengths of stay published in the M&R guidelines for all but five of the 28 DRGs that include at least one of the procedures used in ACS's comparison. Of the five DRGs where the severity-adjusted average length of stay was less than the published M&R guideline, one DRG had only four admissions from HMO members. For the four remaining DRGs, the average lengths of stay for both HMO and FFS patients was less than the length of stay published by M&R.

Myth: Managed care plans reduce access to needed care.

- **Fact: Managed care plans have equal, or better, access to physicians and health care facilities as FFS enrollees.**

A recent study using 1992 National Health Interview Survey data found that HMO members were more likely to have visited a physician during the previous year than their FFS counterparts. There was also no difference in the mean number of days spent in the hospital by HMO and FFS patients who had at least one hospital admission.

HMO members with chronic illnesses were more likely to have visited their physician during the previous year and had the same probability of a hospital stay as FFS patients with chronic illnesses. (Fama and Bernstein, *MCR&R,* June 1997). In addition, a number of studies published in peer reviewed journals report that enrollees in health plans have equal or greater access to specialty care than enrollees with FFS coverage.[3–6]

Myth: Managed care plans frequently do not contract with teaching hospitals, and when they do, these plans do not recognize the higher costs associated with a teaching facility.

According to a recent statement by the Association of American Medical colleges, "Teaching hospitals know from long and painful experience that managed care plans are unwilling to pay costs associated with educating doctors or with providing care to the poor." (*Academic Medicine Events and News,* May 2, 1997)

- **Fact: Managed care plans admit a slightly greater percentage of patients to major teaching hospitals than FFS plans.**

A recent AAHP-commissioned study by The MEDSTAT Group found that the percentage of hospital admissions to teaching hospitals for patients in both FFS plans and managed care plans was comparable for all types of hospitals (major teaching, minor teaching, non-teaching), with managed care plans having a slightly higher admission rate (27 percent) to major teaching hospitals than FFS plans (22 percent).

The analysis also showed that managed care plans' payment rates to major teaching hospitals were, on average, about 14 percent higher than their payment rates to non-academic medical centers for a given admission on a geographic- and severity-adjusted basis. The analysis also found that payment rates of managed care plans were lower than those of FFS plans for *all* types of facilities, reflecting successful cost containment. This study examined 1995 data, the most recent available.

Myth: Managed care plans force women to undergo outpatient mastectomy procedures against the advice of their physicians.

- **Fact: A woman's likelihood of having a mastectomy performed on an outpatient basis does not vary by her type of health plan, indicating that the decision is made by physicians in consultation with their patients.**

An AAHP-commissioned study of 1993 and 1994 data by The MEDSTAT Group found that, overall, there was not a statistically significant difference in outpatient mastectomy rates among HMO, PPO/POS, and FFS plans. During these years, 22 percent of mastectomies performed on patients in FFS plans were performed on an outpatient basis, compared to 21 percent in HMOs, and 13 percent in PPOs/POS plans. The study used a subset of the 1993 and 1994 MarketScan database representing the health care experience of about 2.5 million individuals annually.

Data from the New York State Department of Health found that of the 124 outpatient mastectomies performed in New York State in 1995, 72 mastectomies, or 58 percent, were performed on women *in Medicare FFS.* Two mastectomies, or 1.6 percent, were performed on women in Medicare HMOs. Fifteen mastectomies, or 13 percent, were performed in HMOs serving the commercial portion of the market.

Myth: Surveys that reflect high satisfaction are not reliable because most health plan enrollees are healthy and therefore likely to be satisfied with any plan. Enrollees in managed care plans who are sick, and therefore access the health care system the most, are not satisfied with the care they receive.

- **Fact: Health plan members in poor-to-fair health report satisfaction ratings for HMOs and PPOs that are comparable to satisfaction ratings for their counterparts enrolled in FFS plans, and several studies show higher satisfaction rates for health plan members.**

Surveys conducted by the National Research Corporation (NRC) in 1996 and 1997 showed comparable overall satisfaction rates for consumers both over and under the age of 65 in poor-to-fair health. In 1996, overall satisfaction rates for those in poor-to-fair health *under* the age of 65 were 78 percent for HMOs, 75 percent for PPOs, and 77 percent for FFS; 1997 rates changed little, with respective overall satisfaction rates of 77 percent, 76 percent, and 78 percent.

In 1996, overall satisfaction rates for those in poor-to-fair health *over* the age of 65 were 90 percent for HMOs, 92 percent for PPOs, and 86 percent for FFS. In 1997, these respective rates were 85 percent, 91 percent, and 89 percent. Other independent surveys, such as a 1996 Sachs/Scarborough national survey, report significantly higher satisfaction rates for health plan enrollees in poor-to-fair health versus fee-for-service enrollees.

Myth: Managed care plans incorporate "gag clauses" into physician contracts, adversely affecting their ability to communicate with patients.

- **Fact: A recent survey by the General Accounting Office (GAO) found no gag clauses.**

Among the 1,150 physician contracts with 529 HMOs that GAO examined, none used contract clauses that specifically restricted physicians from discussing all appropriate medical options with their patients.

Sixty-seven percent of contracts that have "business clauses," such as nondisparagement, nonsolicitation, or confidentiality clauses, contain specific "anti-gag" provisions, encouraging discussion of all appropriate medical options between physician and patient. The GAO survey concluded that these business clauses "are not likely to have a significant impact on physician practice." Notably, physician-owned plans had the same patterns of using business clauses as other plans.

References

1. The time spent per patient was calculated by dividing the mean number of hours spent in direct patient care activities per week by the mean number of total patient visits per week. This data is not specific to time spent with patients enrolled in managed care plans. However, AAHP analysis estimates that approximately 77 percent of all Americans with group health coverage are enrolled in managed care plans, and approximately 50 percent of all Americans are enrolled in managed care plans (these figures do not include those Americans enrolled in FFS plans that utilize managed care techniques). It is therefore reasonable to assume that a large percentage of physicians' patient visits are with patients enrolled in managed care plans.
2. AAHP, *The Regulation of Health Plans: A Report from the American Association of Health Plans,* Washington, DC, February 1998.
3. Yelin, E. H., "Health Care Utilization and Outcomes Among Persons with Rheumatoid Arthritis in Fee-for-Service and Prepaid Group Health Practice Settings," *Journal of the American Medical Association,* October 2, 1996.
4. Sisk, J., et al., "Evaluation of Medicaid Managed Care: Satisfaction, Access, and Use," *Journal of the American Medical Association,* July 3, 1996.
5. Vernon, Sally W., et al., "Quality of Care for Colorectal Cancer in a Fee-for-Service and Health Maintenance Organization Practice," *Cancer,* May 15, 1992.
6. Preston, J., "The Management of Geriatric Hypertension in Health Maintenance Organizations," *Journal of the American Geriatrics Society,* July 1991.

FRAME the DEBATE

Form at end of book

R E A D I N G 4 1

Issue 15: Who benefits from managed health care?

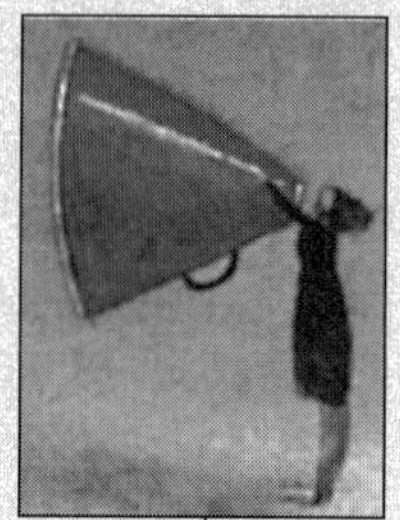

Preserving the Best Health Care Possible

Paul R. Ehrmann, D.O.

President, Community Coalition for Concerned Providers and Patients, Royal Oak

Prepaid (capitated HMO) Managed Care is a subtle form of assisted suicide.

In this setting, if you are sick, you are a financial liability to your doctor.

The formula that your doctor is looking for to thrive financially is as follows: Large volumes of healthy patients come to the office needing a minimum of financial outlay and the other group of patients who feel well stay home. In this prepaid scenario, the doctor receives a monthly pre-payment premium without incurring any overhead or direct medical expense in the management of your care. Therefore, those doctors who sign up with these plans have, in all likelihood, made a conscious decision to sell you out in favor of a self-serving, perceived, advantageous, personal business decision. One would wonder about your doctor's potential conflict of interest in delivering to you the best health care that is available. If your doctor is "stuck" with a bunch of sick and chronically ill patients (and he will be if you believe the axiom that the best doctors are sought out by the sickest patients), he/she is going to be a financial loser. There is more financial outlay for these types of patients. This could discourage and make it more likely that this type of doctor will not be able to survive financially, and therefore be less accessible to serve these types of chronically ill patients.

In the best-case scenario, your doctor may still be accessible because of economic factors but will be forced to restrict or prohibit your medical care to maximize financial return by minimizing expenses and increase revenue by increasing volume in their practices. This increase in volume would, however, make it more difficult for you to get in to see your doctor and longer waits will probably occur.

In the worst case scenario, if your doctor is not available, someone else will deliver your medical care when you are chronically ill. Who that person might be is anybody's guess.

As this present paradigm shift continues toward restricting medical services in favor of the financial bottom line, it is up to those who truly care about their health and the way it is being delivered to step up and support legislation that promotes consumer protection ideas both on a federal and state level.

Become active in joining the many grass-roots groups around the country that promote these issues and bring them to the public light. Ask your present physician if there are any financial relationships they have with your insurance company that has a potential to create a conflict of interest and thereby compromise your care. Discourage your primary care physician in participating with these plans in that as they go, so goes your access to a specialist.

And, finally, talk to your employer benefits managers and let them know the shortcomings that you have experienced. There are other insurance products out there that they may be able to obtain if there is an employee-employer shared-cost arrangements.

The future of the integrity of the profession of medicine and the care of patients therein are in our collective hands. Unless you want to call Dr. K., we better get going today!

FRAME the DEBATE

Form at end of book

Preserving the Best Health Care Possible, Paul R. Ehrmann. THE HMO PAGE. Reprinted by permission of Paul Ehrmann, D.O., P.C.

WiseGuide Wrap-Up

Proponents of managed care state that consumers receive the best treatment for their health-care dollar based on tight federal regulations, medically sound guidelines, and salaried physicians who are not motivated by the profit of expensive tests or procedures. Opponents to managed-care plans accuse the owners of placing profit over the care needs of subscribers. They believe that patient care and patient access to free choice of health-care providers are limited and that physicians are overworked and restricted in their practice.

R.E.A.L. Sites

This list provides a print preview of typical **Coursewise** R.E.A.L. sites. (There are over 100 such sites at the **Courselinks**™ site.) The danger in printing URLs is that web sites can change overnight. As we went to press, these sites were functional using the URLs provided. If you come across one that isn't, please let us know via email to: webmaster@coursewise.com. Use your Passport to access the most current list of R.E.A.L. sites at the **Courselinks** site.

Site name: Managed Care Magazine

URL: http://www.managedcaremag.com/

Why is it R.E.A.L.? This site showcases *Managed Care Magazine.* It contains a variety of articles and monthly postings on the business of running a successful managed-care organization.

Key topics: managed care, health care

Try this: Visit the site and peruse the articles on managed care.

Site name: About.Com Guide to Health Care Industry

URL: http://healthcare.miningco.com/msub13.htm?pid=2770&cob=home

Why is it R.E.A.L.? This site has articles regarding a variety of human interest areas. This page features several articles for and against managed health care.

Key topics: managed care, health care

Try this: Visit the site and peruse the articles on managed care.

Site name: Blue Cross and Blue Shield

URL: http://www.bluecares.com/

Why is it R.E.A.L.? This site provides information about the health insurance and health care industries, along with a virtual tour of the human body.

Key topics: health insurance, managed care

Try this: Enter your zip code to find out about health insurance coverage where you live. Then go to "What's New" and "From Capitol Hill to the State House" to find answers to frequently asked questions about what health-care reform will mean for you.

Site name: MS JAMA Online: Going Hollywood with Patient Rights in Managed Care

URL: http://www.ama-assn.org/sci-pubs/msjama/articles/vol_281/no_9/ms086101.htm

Why is it R.E.A.L.? This site is part of the *Journal of the American Medical Association's* online library of articles. This particular article addresses the effects of patients' rights on managed health care. "As a business that sells health insurance and finances care, managed care should be subject to reasonable consumer protection laws." It also addresses the problems caused by negative images of managed-care companies in movies.

Key topics: managed care, patient's bill of rights

Try this: Consider how recent patient's bill of rights legislation efforts may affect managed care. Explore at least two of the links found in this article. How would this information affect your vote if you were in Congress?

Section 6 Summary

Surveys show that Americans favor the decriminalization of physician-assisted suicide. Despite this prevalent attitude, the issue of physician-assisted suicide is multifaceted and not easily resolved. Several moral and ethical conflicts and financial considerations must first be resolved.

As frustration and disillusionment with modern medicine has increased in the past decade, so has the interest in alternative forms of health care. The American concepts of health, disease, diagnosis, and treatment are centered around empirical science. Little, if any, attention is paid to that which cannot be explained by Western scientific method or that is not supported by rigorous and replicable research. Alternative health-care practitioners and proponents cite the need for expansion of our concept of health to include that which Western science may not be able to explain. Providing consumers with a variety of choices is the cornerstone of the alternative health-care movement.

With ever-rising health-care costs, managed-care health insurance plans are growing in numbers in America, but so are the criticisms of these plans. In the managed-care concept of health insurance, individual subscribers belong to an insurance group, much like members of a retail cooperative. Physicians and health-care providers are paid a salary instead of a fee for individual service. Proponents view it as a way of containing health-care costs, while opponents see it as a way of limiting choices and level of care to improve the profit margin of the owners. Both seek to provide the best care for the least cost to the consumer.

STAND!

section 7 Spiritual Health

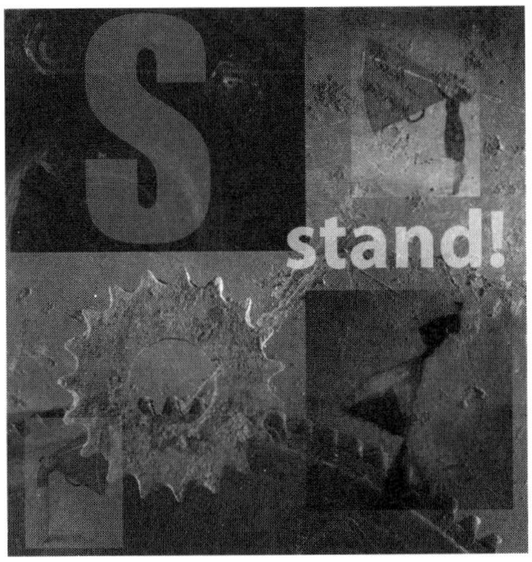

Learning Objectives

- Consider the power of prayer on healing.
- Question your personal beliefs concerning spirituality and its role in health and wellness.
- Establish to what extent prayer and spirituality should be considered part of health and wellness.
- Review current research findings on the effectiveness of prayer on healing.
- Discuss the limitations of prayer research and generalizability of the research findings.

Introduction

In the field of health promotion, considerable efforts have been made since the late 1980s to achieve widespread agreement on the inclusion of a spiritual component in whole-person models of health and wellness. It is now fairly well accepted that, within the spiritual component, lie our values, morals, and sense of right and wrong, as well as our beliefs that we are part of something larger than ourselves. This "larger than ourselves" component may or may not entail belief in a Supreme Being or a spirit or supernatural world. Likewise, one's spiritual sense may or may not be part of a formal religion. Regardless, most health promoters believe that, to be truly healthy, we need to recognize spiritual health as a fundamental and ineffaceable component of wellness.

The concept of body and spirit being linked is not particularly new in America, although it was not popular for most of the twentieth century. Up until the nineteenth century, health in America was largely a spiritual matter. Colonists and pioneers turned to their clergy for guidance in matters of disease prevention and sought divine intervention for healing. In the nineteenth century, many theories of health, such as homeopathy, naturopathy, and Christian Science, developed on the backbones of religious doctrine and the "Rules of God and Nature." It was an easy and logical transition for men of the cloth, such as Reverend Sylvester Graham, the original health-food advocate, to become men of medicine. With the turn of the twentieth century, however, medicine based on the laws of Western scientific thought emerged and has prevailed. Only that which can be explained and measured by science is considered medicinal.

Presently, however, more and more allopathic health practitioners are recognizing the power of spiritual beliefs in the healing of patients. The problem has always been measuring and verifying the power of prayer and spiritual belief in healing. Recently, however, several studies have indicated that spiritual belief and prayer may actually speed healing and perhaps prevent some types of diseases and disorders.

Health educators have long espoused the critical need for the inclusion of spirituality in personal wellness, but have we always had the evidence to support that contention? The readings in Section 7 challenge you to examine your personal beliefs concerning faith, health, and healing.

Can Spirituality Affect Your Physical Health?

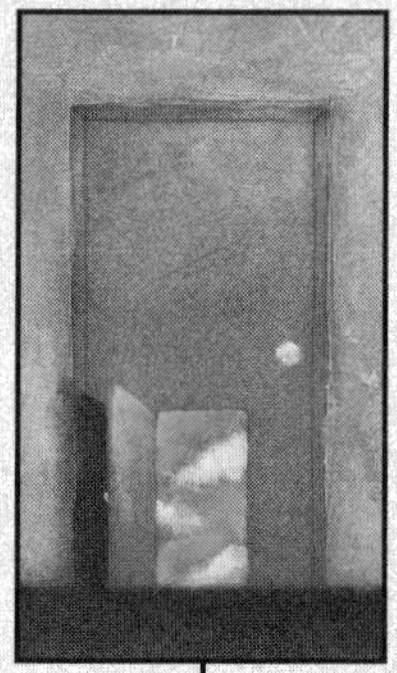

ISSUE 16

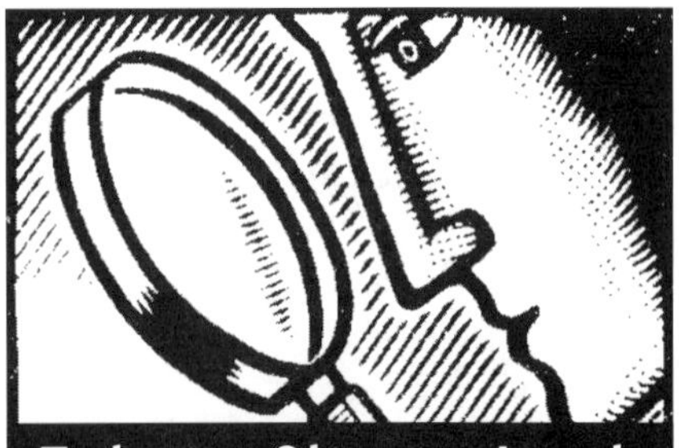

Take a Closer Look

1. What did Dartmouth Medical School discover about heart surgery patients who lacked social support and religious involvement?
2. What have researchers discovered about interleukin-6 levels and religious practice?
3. What has Dr. Herbert Benson found with people who meditate?
4. In Reading 43, the authors provide four plausible medical but nondivine explanations as to why prayer seems to positively affect health. Select one explanation and design a study to test that particular hypothesis. Consider how you will measure your dependent variable, regulate or meter the "dose" of your independent variable, and control for extraneous and interfering variables.
5. Name three positive effects of prayer that research studies have upheld.
6. Give at least two plausible alternative explanations, other than divine intervention, as to why prayer and health studies might have positive findings.
7. According to the *Nature* journal study, what proportion of scientists believe in a God who answers prayers?
8. According to Jaret, what are three problems in researching the power of prayer?
9. What did Walker find regarding recovery rates for substance abusers whose families prayed for their recovery?

WiseGuide Intro

If you were to visit a friend in the hospital today, you'd likely pass a room designated as the "Chapel." The hospital might bear the name of a religious affiliation, such as the Sisters of Providence or Mount Sinai. Most hospitals have priests, ministers, rabbis, and other clergy on staff to assist patients and loved ones in coping spiritually with illnesses, surgeries, births, and deaths. These services are available to all patients and their loved ones but rarely are considered a direct and crucial part of the actual medical treatment at large-scale allopathic hospitals. Religion, prayer, and spirituality are generally seen as supplemental emotional care but not as critical care that has a substantial role in patient outcomes. Regardless, 74 percent of Americans in a recent CBS poll reported that they felt that personal prayer and other spiritual and religious practices can speed or help the medical treatment of people who are ill.*

Recently, the involvement of spiritual services in medicine has begun to go beyond that of mere comfort. Some compelling research indicates that prayer and spirituality may have a direct and profound effect on patients' healing, recovery, and rehabilitation. However, a myriad of uncontrolled extraneous variables can affect measurement of designated dependent variables related to patient care and healing. These uncontrolled variables make measurement of the effects of spirituality on health difficult if not inconclusive. The greatest problems appear to be defining what constitutes prayer and what constitutes success. Further, if prayer and spirituality prove to have a direct effect on healing, physicians are still left with no clear prescriptive guidelines. It has not yet been established how much prayer or spirituality is appropriate for different individuals and conditions. It does not seem likely that prayer, as a healing art, will ever lend itself to druglike dispensation. The key to utilizing spirituality in health and medicine may require the creation of an alternative or new view of health.

Reading 42, "Faith and Healing: Making a Place for Spirituality," begins by pointing out that 75 percent of the physicians polled at a recent meeting of the American Academy of Family Physicians favored the use of prayer as part of the healing process. The authors of the scientifically conservative newsletter *(Harvard Health Letter)* in which this reading appears present data from several research projects that may indicate positive health effects related to prayer and spirituality. They highlight the works of Herbert Benson on the positive calming effects of meditation. They conclude by noting that several medical schools and foundations are currently helping physicians to deal with integrating spirituality into their practices.

*Source: CBS News Poll, "Should Doctors Pray with Their Patients?" April 20–21, 1998, posted at http://www.nihr.org/media/polls.html

Reading 43, "Can Spirituality Uplift Your Health?," presents research on the positive effects of spirituality on health. The reading explores the increases in community support that religious people experience, the fact that regular churchgoers may have different health habits from their non-church-going contemporaries, the stress reduction benefits of prayer, and the relaxation benefits that come from many forms of meditation.

Reading 44, "Health and Spirituality: Medicine Ponders How the Two May Interact," begins by announcing that 90 percent of Americans believe in some sort of God or higher power and that 50 percent of them pray or attend services regularly. The reading then turns to a brief historical review of the role of spirituality in medicine and healing. It itemizes three positive research findings on prayer and health. The major points of debate, such as lack of conclusive evidence, methodological problems, actual measurable effects, and the link between health practices of religious and nonreligious individuals, are explored. In the final paragraphs, the authors warn that spirituality is not a replacement for contemporary and accepted medical care.

In Reading 45, "Can Prayer Heal?," Peter Jaret reviews contemporary research at several leading institutions, including Temple University, the California Pacific Medical Center, the National Institutes for Healthcare Research, and the University of California, that indicates the positive effects of prayer on healing. The work of Herbert Benson with heart patients and prayer is presented as pivotal to the issue. Benson is quoted in the article as saying, "These data suggest that intercessory prayer to a Judeo-Christian God has a beneficial effect in patients admitted to a coronary care unit." Jaret thoroughly explores the scientific limitations and shortcomings of research in this area. He points out alternative explanations that may account for the positive effects of prayer and spirituality, such as lowered stress levels, self-selection of sample subjects, and behavioral similarities between test subjects.

Issue 16: Can spirituality affect your physical health?

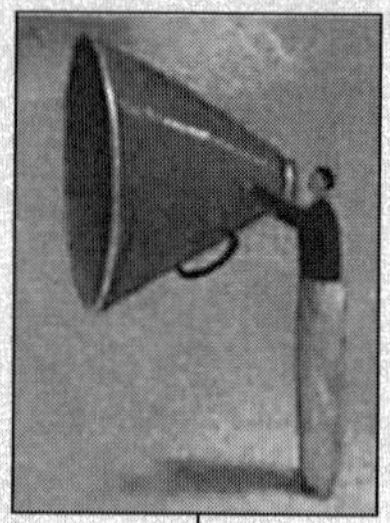

Faith and Healing: Making a Place for Spirituality

In ancient societies, the "medicine man" not only helped relieve physical suffering, he provided spiritual guidance. Indeed, medicine and religion have been linked for centuries. The first hospitals, for example, were opened by monks, and religious orders have historically cared for the sick and infirm.

But as scientific discoveries advanced, religion and medicine were firmly divided into two camps. Armed with antibiotics and other modern medicines, physicians no longer needed to call on a god or spirit to heal people.

Today, the long-standing wall between medicine and religion is crumbling, due in part to the disillusionment of many Americans with what they see as high-tech, impersonal health care. Indeed, there is a growing interest among patients in simpler, "holistic" approaches to healing—through the use of such remedies as herbs and meditation—which, say proponents, aim to treat a host of ills, not just specific symptoms. For an increasing number of Americans and their physicians, this whole-body approach includes spirituality.

Doctors As Believers

Although many physicians are skeptical of alternative remedies, mainly because most remain untested or unproven, some evidence suggests that doctors are surprisingly open to the possibility that religious beliefs can heal. At the October 1996 meeting of the American Academy of Family Physicians, a survey of 296 doctors indicated that nearly all of them felt a person's faith could help the physical healing process. And 75% said they thought the prayers of others might help as well.

Because it is scientifically impossible to prove that belief can heal, the next best way to understand the role of belief in health is to conduct studies that look for an association between the two. Such studies cannot prove a cause-and-effect relationship, but they can uncover apparent connections.

In one small investigation, published in *Psychosomatic Medicine* in 1995, Dartmouth Medical School researchers reported that older people who underwent open-heart surgery for either coronary artery or aortic valve disease—and who lacked either social support from an organized group or said they received no comfort from religion—were three times more likely to die within six months of the operation than those who said they got solace from community groups or religion.

In another study, Duke University researchers found an association between increased immune function and regular attendance at religious services. The investigation, reported in the October 1997 issue of the *International Journal of Psychiatry in Medicine,* involved 1,718 men and women over 65 who were being tracked as part of a larger study on aging and health.

Those who attended services at least once a week were about half as likely as non-attenders to have high blood levels of *interleukin-6,* a protein that regulates immune and inflammatory responses in the body. Elevated levels of interleukin-6 have been associated with some cancers, autoimmune disorders, and heart disease.

One caveat of this study is that healthy people are more likely to attend religious services than those who are sick. The researchers, however, noted that many of the study participants reported that they regularly attended services despite severe illness or disability. The investigators suspect that attending services somehow counteracts stress, which is believed to play a role in immune function. Religious participation not only involves worship of a higher power, but probably also promotes feelings of belonging, both of which may reduce stress and enhance well-being, said the researchers.

A group of Israeli investigators came to a similar conclusion. In a report published in the March 1996 issue of the *American Journal of Public Health,* researchers compared mortality rates in religious and secular communities known as kibbutzim. After accounting for age, sex, and socioeconomic differences, the religious Jewish community had consistently lower mortality rates than the secular group throughout a 16-year period. Living in a supportive religious environment, a belief in God, and frequent prayer may reduce stress and bolster health, the authors noted.

A State of Calm

Herbert Benson, the Mind/Body Medical Institute associate professor of medicine at Harvard, has long believed that prayer elicits the "relaxation response," a form of meditation and the title of his pioneering book on the subject. Dr. Benson found that people who induce this state of calm by focusing on a word, phrase, or prayer for 10–20 minutes a day can decrease blood pressure, heart rate, and breathing and metabolic rates.

In his latest book, *Timeless Healing,* Dr. Benson proposes that the beneficial effects of the relaxation response are enhanced when combined with belief. He calls this union the "faith factor."

Dr. Benson, who believes that humans are "wired for God," is embarking on his most unusual study yet: he will try to measure the effects of praying for others. His team will follow three sets of patients in different parts of the United States who will undergo heart bypass surgery.

One will be prayed for by religious groups and will know that prayers are being said for them. Those who say the prayers, from various faiths, will be told the first names and last initials of the patients for whom they pray. Two other groups won't know if they're the targets of prayer, but one of them will be. Neither the patients nor the physicians will know which group is which. The study will begin shortly and is expected to last for two years.

Confronting the Issue

Doctors typically don't broach matters of religion with patients. Mainly, they worry that raising such issues would violate an individual's privacy or feel that religious discussion does not belong in the doctor-patient relationship.

But this is beginning to change. Eight U.S. medical schools have recently received small grants from the National Institute for Healthcare Research and the John Templeton Foundation to implement courses that explore the relationship between spirituality and health and teach students how to address religious issues in patient care.

At Loyola University Chicago Stritch School of Medicine, for example, students will observe and assist hospital chaplains as they visit patients, and an internal medicine course will focus on how the human spirit confronts chronic pain, long-term illness, and death.

Meanwhile, Harvard Medical School recently held its fourth conference on spirituality and healing for health professionals. Participants learned about the potential physiological and psychological effects of faith on health.

Kenneth B. Schwartz, a health care lawyer in Boston who succumbed to cancer in 1995, believed that physicians and nurses should pay more attention to the nonmedical needs of patients and that broaching personal or emotional issues could be a major source of comfort for patients as well as for the health care workers themselves.

After his death, Mr. Schwartz's friends and family set up a center at Massachusetts General Hospital that sponsors, among other programs, four-month fellowships that enable health care professionals to participate in a pastoral care program, focusing on the spiritual needs of patients and their families.

Although researchers continue to investigate the links among faith, health, and longevity, people who already accept that belief can console and heal don't need scientific studies to convince them. Those who are skeptical may find the results intriguing, but science will never be able to fully assuage their doubts.

In reality, most people probably don't look to religion or spirituality to extend their lives but to provide day-to-day meaning and comfort.

The best part about medicine's growing interest in faith is that some patients may finally get what they have been yearning for: doctors who recognize the needs of the soul as well as those of the body.

FRAME the DEBATE

Form at end of book

Issue 16: Can spirituality affect your physical health?

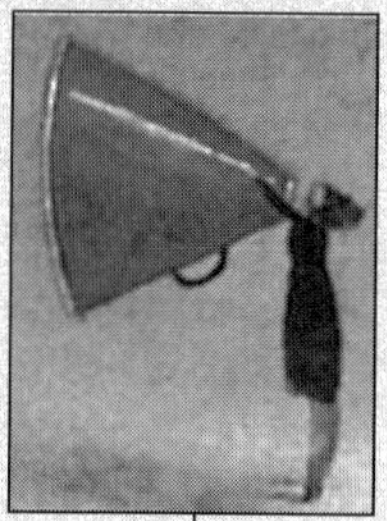

Can Spirituality Uplift Your Health?

Research on the benefits of faith is yielding some intriguing results.

Few people would call a visit to the doctor a spiritual experience. Indeed, modern medicine, with its high-tech wizardry, can do wonders for the body but little for the soul. And until recently, medical research avoided spirituality altogether.

In the past decade or so, a growing number of researchers have put spirituality and religion under the microscope. The number of American medical schools offering courses on spiritual issues has risen from 3 to more than 40 in the past three years. And the research so far does suggest that having a spiritual dimension in your life may help you get healthy when you're sick and stay healthy when you're well.

Religious Results

The research on spirituality consists almost entirely of observational studies. While such evidence can't prove a causal connection, it can suggest possible links. Of the more than 300 studies done so far, over three-fourths have found seemingly positive effects. Certain studies have shown that people with a religious commitment may have fewer symptoms of mental and physical disorders and make fewer doctor visits than other people. Other studies have found that they tend to have a reduced risk of various diseases—including cancer and coronary heart disease.

A 28-year California study published last summer indicated the overall value of those apparent benefits: People who went to weekly religious services had a one-third lower death rate than those who attended less often. After controlling for lifestyle factors, such as smoking, drinking, and social contact, the researchers still found a one-fourth lower death rate.

A recent Duke University study of some 1,700 older people provided one possible biochemical mechanism for those reductions: People who attended weekly services were half as likely as nonattenders to have high levels of interleukin-6, a protein linked to various age-related diseases, such as Alzheimer's disease, cancer, coronary disease, and osteoporosis.

Other studies have examined religion's possible impact on patients' recovery. Researchers from Northwestern University found that women with strong religious beliefs recovered faster after hip replacement than less religious women did. And a study led by Dartmouth researchers, involving 232 open-heart-surgery patients, found that none of the 37 "deeply religious" patients died during the six months after the operation, while 21 of the other patients did.

Spiritual Influences

Researchers aren't sure why religion—and possibly spirituality without organized religion—seems to improve health. Here are the four main possibilities.

Community Support

Just attending weekly services and performing familiar rituals with others can help people feel they're part of a community with similar values. Prayer groups, potluck suppers, bingo nights, and other activities provide additional opportunities to socialize and form lasting friendships.

Numerous studies have linked social support—whether from a church, a synagogue, or a bowling league—with reduced rates of disease and death. In theory, that's because such support may buffer the stress of everyday life and of major crises. And stress may help cause or worsen a wide range of ailments, ranging from infection to cancer.

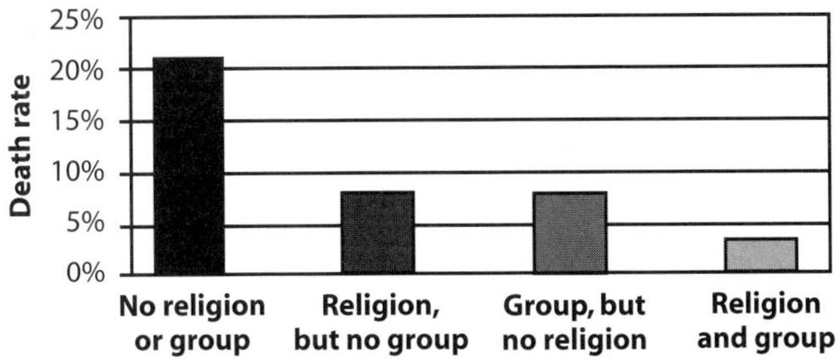

Spirituality and Surgery. The chart shows how the death rate among 232 heart patients varied during the six months after surgery depending on the strength of their religious faith and the degree of their participation in any group activity.

Source: Thomas E. Oxman, M.D., et al., "Lack of social participation or religious strength and comfort as risk factors for death after cardiac surgery in the elderly," *Psychosomatic Medicine*, 1995, Vol. 57, pp. 5–15.

Belonging to a community seems to account for much of the benefit of religious affiliation—but not all of it. In the Dartmouth heart-surgery study, for example, the six-month survival rate was 14 times higher in those who derived "strength and comfort" from religion *and* participated in social groups than in those who lacked both sources of support. After researchers screened out the social factor, religious people were still about three times as likely to survive (see chart).

In another study, Israeli researchers compared death rates of people who lived in secular and religious kibbutz communities. Both types provided similarly high levels of social support. But the death rate was almost twice as high in the nonreligious settlements as in the religious ones.

Healthy Habits

A Dutch study found that the life span of Seventh Day Adventists is nine years longer than average in men, four years in women. One likely reason: Adventists are encouraged to exercise, eat vegetarian diets, and not smoke or drink.

But even people who practice religions with fewer restrictions seem to lead healthier lives than nonreligious people. In one study of some 3,000 people, mainly Protestants, the weekly churchgoers had about half the alcohol-abuse risk of those who attended less regularly. Other studies have shown that religious teen-agers are much less likely to drink or use drugs than less religious teens.

But again, healthy habits aren't the whole story: When researchers control for the effects of lifestyle, spirituality still seems to confer a substantial benefit.

Positive Beliefs

Having an inner spiritual life may promote health by creating a sense of meaning and purpose that helps reduce stress. Studies have shown that religious people tend to be more satisfied with their lives than nonreligious people and to have less anxiety, depression, and mental illness. Other research has linked positive attitudes with better physical health, including less illness, longer survival when serious illness strikes, and a lower overall death rate. Those benefits may occur partly because an upbeat attitude may help patients cooperate with their doctor and participate actively in their own care.

Moments of Relaxation

Prayer, like many forms of meditation, may promote health through a special form of stress relief, according to Harvard researcher Herbert Benson, M.D., who pioneered the "relaxation response." That response involves relaxed muscles and slowed breathing, heartbeat, brain waves, and metabolism. Eliciting the relaxation response regularly can reduce blood pressure in people with hypertension and blood sugar in people with diabetes; it may also ease anxiety, depression, insomnia, headaches, and psychosomatic complaints. And it may have benefits in sick people, such as easing chronic pain and controlling nausea from chemotherapy.

Calmly repeating any emotionally neutral word or phrase, silently or aloud, tends to evoke the relaxation response. But picking a word, phrase, or passage that has special positive meaning for you will generally work better. That could be a prayer—or it could be an inspirational poem or even the name of someone or something you love. Sit quietly in a comfortable position, close your eyes, clear your mind, relax your muscles, and breathe slowly and naturally while repeating the word, phrase, or prayer to yourself for 10 to 20 minutes.

Summing Up

Observational studies have linked religion and spirituality with a reduced risk of disease, faster recovery from surgery, and a lower overall death rate. Such studies can only suggest a connection—they don't *prove* that faith bolsters health. However, there are several plausible explanations for a faith-health link: Religion and spirituality may encourage healthy habits and may help reduce stress, perhaps by promoting social support, an optimistic outlook, and deep relaxation during prayer. Whether or not religion helps, note that it's possible to accomplish all those things without holding any spiritual beliefs at all.

FRAME the DEBATE

Form at end of book

R E A D I N G 4 4

Issue 16: Can spirituality affect your physical health?

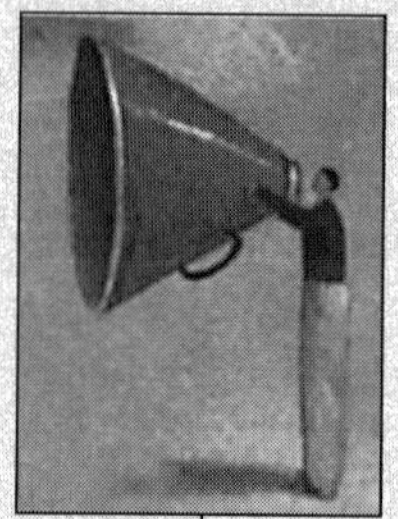

Health and Spirituality: Medicine Ponders How the Two May Interact

Prayer. Worship. Belief in a divine being.

For many people, these are important parts of life. Polls consistently show that more than 90 percent of people in the United States believe in a god or higher power. About half of Americans regularly attend religious services or pray.

Incorporating prayer, faith and worship into your life may give you a sense of community, tradition and spiritual satisfaction. But some studies suggest there may be other benefits. Could spiritual beliefs and practices enhance your health and well-being as well?

More and more, the medical profession is considering that possibility. As a result, spirituality's role in today's high-tech medical world is being increasingly explored.

Medicine's Spiritual Roots

In the 20th century, modern medicine has largely kept health and spirituality separate. But for centuries, the two were linked.

In some early societies, religious leaders were also healers. In the Middle Ages, priests administered medicinal herbs and prayer to the sick, while monasteries recorded medical knowledge. Many modern religions are based on holy men or women whose followers believe they had the ability to heal.

However, during the 20th century, especially in Europe and North America, health and spirituality grew apart as scientific methods and discoveries revolutionized medicine. Medicine focused on the body's physical mechanisms. Physicians who developed long-standing relationships with patients often dealt with spiritual issues as part of the case, but in a world of MRI scans, advanced surgical procedures and electron microscopes, spirituality often became a topic left to theologians and religious leaders.

Patients Spur Interest

Yet spirituality's importance in medicine has remained unchanged for at least one group—patients.

According to polls, about the same proportion of Americans today believe in a god as did 50 years ago. In the meantime, books devoted to spirituality and medicine regularly appear on best-seller lists.

It's this patient interest that's prompted medicine to begin a serious discussion of spirituality, according to doctors at Mayo Clinic and elsewhere. Since the late 1980s, several doctors have written books advocating spirituality's health benefits. Top medical journals have also published articles advocating exploration of the topic.

In addition, studies have been conducted. They've suggested that:

- Prayer may have improved recoveries of patients who underwent heart-bypass surgery at a San Francisco hospital.
- Regular church attendance may have helped reduce hypertension in elderly men.
- Religious faith helped ease the emotional anguish of those facing a cancer diagnosis.

Debate Continues

Still, spirituality's role in medicine remains controversial.

One reason is that other studies haven't shown any significant health benefits. There's also been criticism of the design and methods used in studies that did show benefits.

For example, critics have charged that in the study of heart-bypass patients in a San Francisco hospital, there were no safeguards to prove that prayer groups really prayed for patients. Other studies have drawn similar criticism.

Realistic Expectations

Do you know the difference between curing and healing?

To cure means to completely eradicate a disease or disability. In contrast, healing applies to your state of mind and acceptance of life's circumstances. For example, someone who is terminally ill and who is at peace with his or her situation might be healed but not cured.

Much of medicine's discussion of spirituality has focused on how it might help you "heal," or cope with life's difficulties.

If you're ill, it's unrealistic to expect an instant cure or return to vitality. But when accompanied by traditional medical practices and treatments, your spirituality may help you find the strength and comfort you need to deal with your illness.

If you're healthy, the sense of well-being and satisfaction you get from spiritual beliefs may provide perspective and help keep your stress level in check. In turn, that may help you stay healthier in the long run.

In addition, there's been much debate about the mechanism—the actual way—in which spirituality might affect your body.

Some believe that religious lifestyle practices, such as not drinking or smoking, provide certain health benefits. Others theorize that physical changes may occur in your body from the sense of well-being and community that spirituality can provide.

For example, meditation and relaxation may slow your heart and breathing rate. In addition, your body may produce chemicals, called endorphins, that contribute to a sense of well-being—much like the "runner's high" experienced by long-distance runners.

Changes Taking Place

Although the debate is far from over, you may see changes in medicine because of this discussion.

While it's not likely your doctor will write "prayer" on the prescription pad, he or she may be comfortable discussing how you might benefit from spirituality. Chaplains may be more likely to be on your medical team during hospital stays. And, clinics specializing in cancer and other chronic diseases may also include emotional and spiritual health in patient care.

In addition, a growing number of medical schools are beginning to include courses on spirituality's role in health.

Not a Cure-All

Medicine remains firmly anchored in science, technology and the objective, fact-based methods that have conquered many diseases.

Spirituality is not a replacement for these methods or the medical advances they've spawned. Nor is it a cure-all or guarantee you won't become ill.

Still, a growing number of physicians are considering the idea that spiritual practices and beliefs might strengthen traditional medicine when accompanied by realistic expectations.

FRAME the DEBATE

Form at end of book

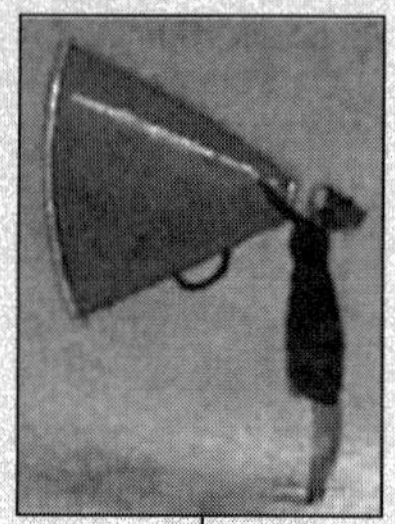

Issue 16: Can spirituality affect your physical health?

Can Prayer Heal?

Researchers with their feet on the ground say it can—but not in the way you might think.

Peter Jaret

Ask Herbert Benson to talk about his latest experiment and the distinguished Harvard researcher clams up. "Don't even ask," he says. "The more we say in public about the study we're doing, the more risk we run of compromising the results."

Neither Benson's silent treatment, however, nor the fact that the study is still in the planning stages has prevented word of his investigation from sparking a heated debate in the journal *Science.*

Small wonder. Benson, who directs the Mind/Body Medical Institute in Boston, has decided to rush in where most scientists fear to tread. In an experiment rumored to include more than 500 heart patients, he hopes to prove what has long been considered a matter of faith alone: the healing power of prayer.

Across the country, in fact, a growing number of scientists are putting prayer to the test. At Temple University in Philadelphia, researchers plan to examine whether the prayers of volunteers can speed the development of premature babies. At California Pacific Medical Center in San Francisco, psychiatrist Elisabeth Targ is studying whether prayer helps AIDS patients. "There are many of us who believe that prayer has enormous power to heal," says psychiatrist David Larson, who heads the National Institute for Health-care Research, a Maryland-based organization devoted to the study of religion and health. "Now, as scientists, we're looking for proof."

Many Americans, it seems, don't need convincing. According to one recent study, 87 percent of adults believe their prayers are sometimes answered. In a survey conducted by the journal *Nature,* two out of five scientists said they believe in a God who answers prayers.

Is science itself beginning to show that they're right? The answer, it turns out, is not so simple. Prayer *can* heal, the latest findings suggest. But not the way most people suppose.

Scientists have been scrutinizing prayer for more than a century, but the first study to make skeptics sit up and take note was published in 1988 by cardiologist Randolph Byrd of the University of California at San Francisco. Byrd had divided 393 heart attack patients randomly into two groups. One group got standard medical care only. The others also received the daily prayers of volunteers who described themselves as born-again Christians. Neither the patients, nor the hospital staff, nor Byrd himself knew who was prayed for and who wasn't.

Reviewing hospital records, Byrd found that patients singled out for prayer required fewer antibiotics, suffered less congestive heart failure, and were less likely to develop pneumonia. His conclusion fairly leaped off the pages of the medical journal in which it was published. "These data," Byrd wrote, "suggest that intercessory prayer to a Judeo-Christian God has a beneficial effect in patients admitted to a coronary care unit."

Since Byrd's study came out, several researchers have ventured into the same territory, seeking to show that so-called remote prayers by one person can help heal another. So far the evidence is iffy.

Last year, for instance, when University of New Mexico psychiatrist Scott Walker tested whether remote prayer could speed the recovery of substance abusers, the results turned out to be a bust. For one thing, the patients who were prayed for by volunteers were no more likely to kick the habit than those who weren't. Walker also asked patients if any friends or relatives might be supplicating on their behalf. Those who said loved ones were praying for them were actually less likely to give up drinking.

Perhaps the prayed-for patients in Benson's proposed study, which is modeled on Byrd's, will fare better. Still, critics ask, what would even the most dramatic results really mean? "Frankly, it's hard to see how studies like this can tell us anything," says Dan Blazer, a professor of psychiatry and the dean of medical education at Duke University.

The problem, he says, is that prayer can't be tracked or measured. No matter how carefully controlled the

Can Prayer Heal? Peter Jaret. HEALTH, March 1998. Reprinted by permission.

experiment, there's no way to know which subjects are being prayed for and which aren't. True, volunteers may be recruited to intercede for only one group. But at least a few family members or friends are probably praying for the others. (Herbert Benson won't talk about his study for fear that people who hear about it might send unsolicited prayers toward his patients, potentially skewing the results.) One could argue that a legitimate scientific study has to measure the "dose" of prayer each subject receives—impossible without some kind of prayer meter.

As it is, critics say, you can interpret any kind of result any which way. "If a study finds no benefits, you can say there weren't enough prayers, or they weren't done right, or by the right people," says Hector Avalos, a former faith healer who is now an assistant professor of religious studies at Iowa State University.

Even negative results can become proof of prayer's power. Consider the study Walker did. You'd think the fact that patients fared worse when they knew family and friends were praying for them would argue against the notion that prayer works. But Walker offers a different interpretation: "Suppose I'm an alcoholic and you're my brother. I've called you up drunk in the night, you've had to bail me out, I've caused scene after scene. Chances are when you sit down to pray for me you're feeling a lot of anger and frustration. What we may be seeing here is the possibility that certain kinds of prayer have the power to do harm."

If Walker is right—and let's hope he isn't—trusting in someone else's prayers may not be such a great idea, especially if you're not on the best of terms with Aunt Martha or Uncle Ed. But that doesn't mean prayer can't help anyone. The surest way to tap its potency, studies suggest, may be by practicing religion yourself.

Indeed, there's growing evidence of the power of belief. In 1990 researchers at Northwestern University Medical School found that among elderly women who'd had hip surgery, those with a strong religious faith got back on their feet faster than did nonbelievers.

Other studies have shown that believers live longer: At Dartmouth-Hitchcock Medical Center in New Hampshire, heart patients who said they drew comfort from their religious beliefs were three times more likely to survive bypass surgery than those of little faith. In one of the latest and largest studies of its kind, epidemiologist William Strawbridge and his colleagues at the California Public Health Foundation tracked more than 5,000 people for 28 years. Death rates of men and women who said they attended religious services regularly were only 65 percent of those for people who rarely entered a church or synagogue.

Well, sure, skeptics say. Churchgoers are less likely to drink, smoke, or carouse. But when researchers figured in such obvious lifestyle differences, worshipers still lived longer and healthier lives.

Why? One explanation may be that a religious community provides strong social support. And the evidence suggests a network of friends and family is crucial to health. According to Strawbridge, social connections explained some of the advantages worshipers enjoyed, but not all. People who went to church were still healthier than those who went to play bridge.

In the Dartmouth study, heart patients with extensive social networks fared as well as those who found solace in their faith. But those with deep religious convictions *and* a strong community of friends and family were almost 14 times more likely to recover than those with few friends and little faith.

Psychiatrist Harold Koenig, director of Duke University's Center for the Study of Religion/Spirituality and Health, thinks belief in God may help people cope with stress and uncertainty. "People who believe in a compassionate, caring God take enormous comfort from that," he says. "They have a hopeful worldview that gives them a sense of control when things go wrong. And the more in control people feel, the healthier they are both physically and mentally."

Prayer itself may reduce stress much the way meditation does—by quieting the mind, slowing heart and respiration rates, reducing blood pressure, and lowering levels of stress hormones like cortisol. Dozens of studies have shown that such hormones can rob immune cells of their disease-fighting abilities.

As intriguing as these findings are, Dan Blazer, for one, doubts that scientists will ever find what Benson and Walker are searching for: irrefutable evidence that the prayers sent by one person can improve the health of another. It's not that Blazer, a former missionary who describes himself as a devout Christian, doubts prayer's power. "I pray for my patients every day," he says. "But that's not a matter of medical science for me. It's a matter of faith."

FRAME the DEBATE

Form at end of book

WiseGuide Wrap-Up

Most Americans believe in some sort of divine being, and the majority of physicians believe that prayer can help their patients, although they do not know precisely how. Research studies seem to indicate that prayer may help speed healing and facilitate recovery. Problems with prayer research are centered on the difficulty in measuring independent variables and controlling extraneous variables. Alternative hypotheses for the apparent effectiveness of prayer in healing suggest the positive effects of social support rather than divine intervention.

R.E.A.L. Sites

This list provides a print preview of typical **Coursewise** R.E.A.L. sites. (There are over 100 such sites at the **Courselinks**™ site.) The danger in printing URLs is that web sites can change overnight. As we went to press, these sites were functional using the URLs provided. If you come across one that isn't, please let us know via email to: webmaster@coursewise.com. Use your Passport to access the most current list of R.E.A.L. sites at the **Courselinks** site.

Site name: Spirituality and Health: Pathfinders

URL: http://www.spiritualityhealth.com/path/xpat.html

Why is it R.E.A.L.? This site offers a variety of articles about spiritual health and links to associated sites.

Key topics: alternative medicine, spiritual health, spirituality, religion

Try this: Visit the site and select two articles to read. Based on your chosen articles as well as your personal experiences, create a definition of spiritual health. Confine your definition to one paragraph.

Site name: Yahoo! Health—Alternative Therapies

URL: http://health.yahoo.com/health/Alternative_Medicine/Alternative_Therapies/Meditation/

Why is it R.E.A.L.? This site offers a variety of articles on alternative health care. This particular page features an article on meditation.

Key topics: alternative medicine, spiritual health, spirituality, religion

Try this: Visit the site and read the article "Meditation." In what ways do you see similarities between meditation and prayer? Are they the same or different? In what ways do you see the healing power of prayer similar or different from the healing power of meditation?

Section 7 Summary

The concept of health being the aggregate of one's mind, body, and spirit is certainly not new. It has, however, been only marginally accepted by modern medicine. The past century has seen extraordinary advances in the fields of physical health and medicine, and psychology and mental health. Spiritual health, however, remains an estranged component in the whole-person concept of health.

The problems with the acceptance of spiritual health and the power of prayer in healing have been the inconsistency of research results, stemming mostly from the myriad of difficulties in measuring prayer or the construct of spirituality. Some positive research findings may indicate change and new acceptance of the role of spirituality and the power of prayer in the healing process.

Index

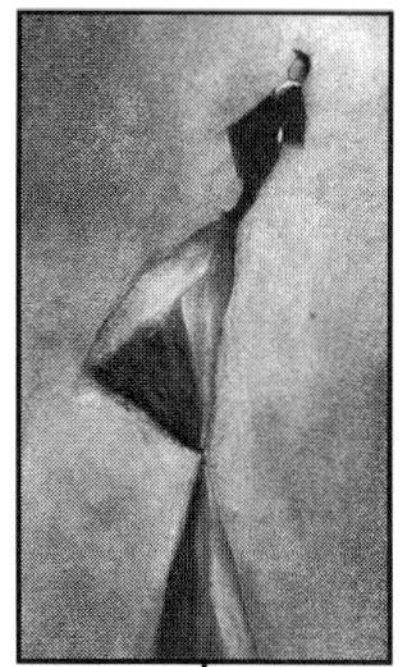

Note: Names and page numbers in **bold** type indicate authors and their articles; page numbers in *italics* indicate illustrations; page numbers followed by *t* indicate tables.

A

B

C

I

J

K

L

M

N

O

P

Q

R

S

STAND!

Frame the Debate

Review Form

Name ______________________ **Date** ______________

Issue ______________________

1. Prior to reading about and discussing this issue, my personal beliefs were:

2. Describe the credentials and/or credibility of experts cited in each of the readings for this issue.

3. Summarize the main idea presented in each of the readings for this issue.

4. Summarize the facts that support each main idea.

5. Identify any opinions expressed.

6. List any examples of bias or faulty reasoning.

7. How does this issue correlate with material presented in class and/or in your textbook?

8. Based on further consideration of this issue, my personal beliefs are now/still:

COPY ME! Copy this form as needed. This form is also available at http://www.coursewise.com
Click on STAND!